MANUAL OF VENOUS AND LYMPHATIC DISEASES

THE AUSTRALASIAN COLLEGE OF PHLEBOLOGY

MANUAL OF VENOUS AND LYMPHATIC DISEASES

THE AUSTRALASIAN COLLEGE OF PHLEBOLOGY

Edited by

KEN MYERS and PAUL HANNAH

with illustrations by Marcus Cremonese

Editorial Committee

Lourens Bester, Phil Bekhor, Attilio Cavezzi, Marianne de Maeseneer,
Greg Goodman, David Jenkins, Herman Lee, Adrian Lim, David Mitchell,
Nick Morrison, Andrew Nicolaides, Hugo Partsch, Tony Penington,
Neil Piller, Stefania Roberts, Greg Seeley, Paul Thibault, Steve Yelland

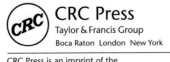

CRC Press
Taylor & Francis Group
Boca Raton London New York

CRC Press is an imprint of the
Taylor & Francis Group, an **informa** business

This manual is an initiative of the Australasian College of Phlebology and Phlebology Foundation of Australia, and is the official text of the Australasian College of Phlebology Training Program.

CRC Press
Taylor & Francis Group
6000 Broken Sound Parkway NW, Suite 300
Boca Raton, FL 33487-2742

© 2018 by Taylor & Francis Group, LLC
CRC Press is an imprint of Taylor & Francis Group, an Informa business

No claim to original U.S. Government works

Printed and bound in India by Replika Press Pvt. Ltd.

Printed on acid-free paper

International Standard Book Number-13: 978-1-1380-3676-5 (Paperback); 978-1-138-03686-4 (Hardback)

Contents

Preface

This book has grown out of a need for a comprehensive syllabus directed to trainees in phlebology, but from there has hopefully developed into a reference book for all practitioners. It started as an effort to bridge a gap between traditional phlebology textbooks and a study guide for prospective examination candidates. It now attempts to provide a summary of venous and lymphatic diseases that will be of value to a broader audience of undergraduates and graduates who have a general interest in the subject or are specialists in diagnostic or interventional aspects of these conditions.

The text is a product of input from members of the Australasian College of Phlebology based on their expertise and experience rather than a range of specific scientific works. The chapters were subsequently submitted to other local and international colleagues to help provide a broader perspective. We recognise the need for evidence to support these views by referral to the recent scientific literature and international consensus documents, and hope that this has helped reduce personal bias. There are likely to be regional attitudes for management that may not be common to all countries, but we hope that allowance can be made for these variations.

There is now a great depth of knowledge about venous and lymphatic diseases and no single group is likely to be experienced in all aspects. With this in mind, major international organizations have commissioned groups of interested experts to produce consensus documents and conduct working parties to study specific aspects of the disease in detail. Our project has leaned heavily on these documents as a source of information, and our summaries of the extensive material are acknowledged in the individual chapters. We thank these working groups for providing the ground work for us to incorporate into our work a synthesis of their deliberations. Any errors or generalizations in interpreting these documents are entirely our responsibility.

References to these consensus documents and to major reviews are listed with internet links to all, generally directing the reader to the full text. Other selected references to contemporary or historical reports have been included if considered to be of special importance. No attempt has been made to provide an extensive reference base for all aspects of the many conditions, as these are listed within the references that we have provided.

The presentation is deliberately didactic but hopefully balanced and comprehensive. Included are many boxed summaries of highlights, tips and warnings. Many of the agents used for treatment carry their Australasian names and will need to be cross-referenced by international readers. Illustrations have been kept simple and may need to be supplemented by reference to more specialized texts for further study. Several procedures in common use have been described in detail, however, it is important to note that the descriptors relating to them are not sufficient for performing any of the indicated processes. Proper training under supervision must be sought.

It is hoped that this manual will help when you next encounter the problem patient or are faced with making a difficult management decision.

Ken Myers and Paul Hannah

Foreword

Dear Readers,

I take this opportunity as President of the International Union of Phlebology (UIP) to introduce this *Manual of Venous and Lymphatic Diseases* on behalf of the Australasian College of Phlebology (ACP), one of the most important member societies in the UIP.

The leadership of the ACP, in conjunction with members of the Editorial Committee has organized, directed, and created this text which will come to be an indispensable tool for all those practicing in the field of venous and lymphatic medicine. This work of the ACP is welcomed and deeply appreciated by the UIP.

The UIP is currently developing several initiatives that will enhance education and research of venous and lymphatic disorders. One initiative may be a certificate of knowledge of phlebology. Also, it is expected there will soon be an independent funding entity available to the UIP that should be able to facilitate and accelerate education and research worldwide. Through such initiatives, it is anticipated that the level of understanding of venous and lymphatic disorders will improve the health of patients suffering from these disorders more uniformly across the globe.

It is a great honour to recognize the work involved in the production of this text, and my congratulations to the editors for their tremendous efforts to elevate knowledge in the field of venous and lymphatic medicine.

With great respect,

Nick Morrison, MD, FACS, FACPh, RPhS
President, International Union of Phlebology

Embryology of veins and lymphatics

The venous system

> Knowing how veins and lymphatics develop provides a basis for understanding their anatomy and helps explain congenital vascular malformations and developmental abnormalities.[1,2]

- The embryo has three systems of paired veins – vitelline veins taking nutrients from the yolk sac, umbilical veins carrying oxygenated blood from the placenta and a systemic system of cardinal veins (Figure 1.1).
- The embryonic vascular system appears as cords of cells in the mesoderm by 15–16 days, and these differentiate into blood cells and vessels. **Veins develop from an irregular capillary network within the first five to six weeks and the architecture is complete by eight weeks.** Lymphatics bud off veins and appear at the end of week five, about two weeks later than blood vessels. **Venous valves appear by 12 weeks as** thickened ridges filled

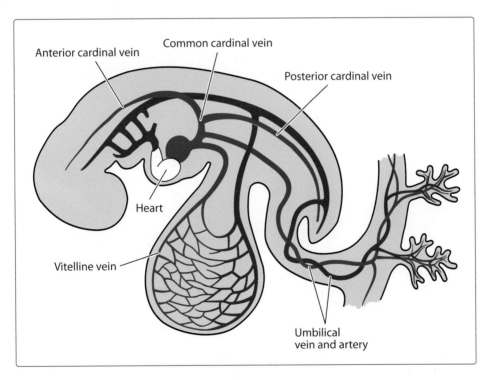

Figure 1.1 Lateral view of the embryo at eight weeks showing components of the foetal venous circulation – the cardinal, vitelline and umbilical veins.

in with mesenchyme, which then widen and thin down to their final shape.[3]

Vitelline veins

- Vitelline veins take blood from the yolk sac to the embryo and are later modified to become the superior mesenteric and portal veins, liver sinusoids and hepatic veins, and the final segment becomes the supra-hepatic section of the inferior vena cava.
- The yolk sac provides a blood supply and a source of nutrients during early development, but the vitelline circulation ceases by the fourth week as the yolk sac atrophies to be incorporated into the primordial gut.

Umbilical veins

- The umbilical circulation is then responsible for provision of all nutrients and oxygenation. The two umbilical veins fuse to form a single trunk in the body stalk but remain separate within the embryo as they pass to the heart. The right umbilical vein gradually disappears and the left umbilical vein becomes dominant, only to be obliterated at birth to form the ligamentum teres.

Cardinal veins

- Anterior cardinal (precardinal) veins return blood from the cephalic part of the body; posterior cardinal (postcardinal) veins drain the rest of the body caudal to the heart, and they join to form common cardinal veins passing into the heart through the sinus venosus.
- Left-sided veins largely disappear or form lesser permanent veins, whereas right-sided and anastomotic veins between the two sides form the final major veins.

Cardiac circulation

- The sinus venosus is the final pathway for flow from the vitelline, umbilical, and common cardinal veins before entering the heart. It is initially paired, but the left side shrinks to form the coronary sinus of the right atrium and oblique vein of the left atrium, while the right side becomes the last part of the superior vena cava as it connects to the right atrium (Figure 1.2).

- In the embryo, blood flows to bypass the pulmonary circulation, either from the right to the left atrium through the foramen ovale or from the right ventricle and pulmonary artery to the aorta through the ductus arteriosus. The septum primum is a flap valve on the left atrial side of the interatrial septum. It allows right-to left flow as the fluid-filled lungs cause high back pressure to the right atrium in utero, but should close when the neonate breathes and the left atrial pressure then exceeds the right atrial pressure.

1.1 Developmental abnormalities

- Vascular malformations result from defective development (see Chapter 26). In the early stages, the reticular network of primitive vessels has not yet evolved into vascular trunks, so malformations arising before the fourth week are termed extratruncular. Those developing later, between weeks four and eight, are classified as truncular. Abnormalities that develop after week eight cause simple anatomical variations.
- A patent foramen ovale results from failure of the septum primum to seal the foramen after birth, and it persists to varying degrees in about 30% of subjects. This can later allow paradoxical right-to-left embolism (see Chapter 22) or passage of foam sclerosant into the arterial circulation with foam sclerotherapy (see Chapter 12).

Veins in the neck and upper limbs

- Veins in the neck develop from the anterior and common cardinal veins (Figure 1.3). The internal jugular veins develop from the anterior cardinal veins, the left brachiocephalic trunk develops from an anastomotic vein between the anterior cardinal veins, and the right brachiocephalic trunk is the more proximal segment of the right anterior cardinal

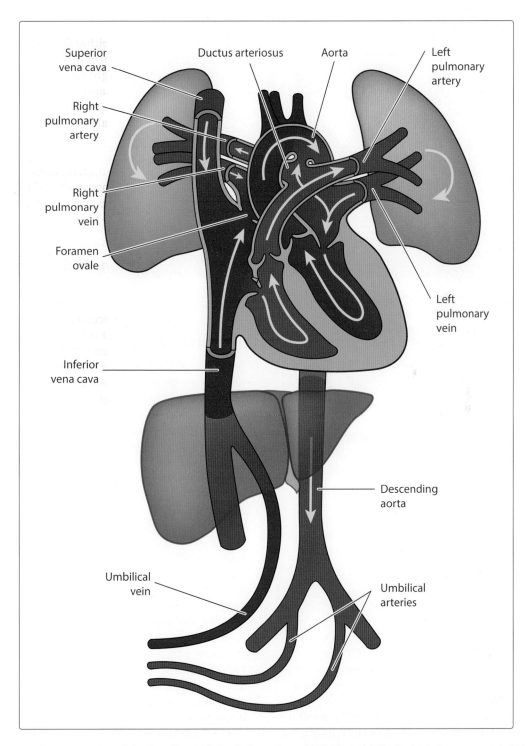

Figure 1.2 Representation of the foetal central circulation prior to birth. The umbilical veins bring oxygenated blood to the sinus venosus and right atrium. Much of the flow passes through the foramen ovale to the left heart then largely to the cerebral circulation. The rest passes into the right ventricle and through the pulmonary artery and ductus arteriosus to the aorta and the rest of the body. Venous return from the foetus passes back to the placenta.

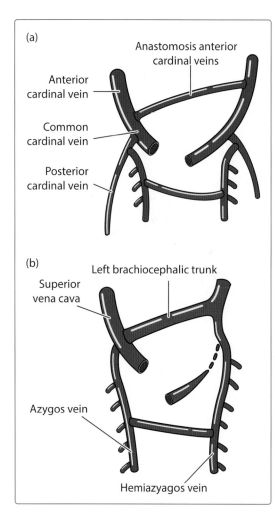

Figure 1.3 Antero-posterior view showing development of the superior vena cava and left brachiocephalic trunk. (a) Early in development before eight weeks. (b) Later in development, showing involution of the left superior vena cava.

vein. The superior vena cava consists of three segments, the right anterior cardinal vein beyond the brachiocephalic junction, right common cardinal vein and right horn of the sinus venosus.

- Venous plexuses along the ulnar border of the upper limb fuse to form the basilic, axillary then subclavian vein which opens into the internal jugular vein. Veins along the radial border form the cephalic vein which joins the axillary vein.

1.2 Developmental abnormalities of the superior vena cava

- A left or double superior vena cava is seen in about 0.5% of the normal population and 5% of subjects with congenital heart disease. Most are asymptomatic, the abnormality only being identified on screening for conditions such as atrial septal defect. They result from persistence of the left anterior and common cardinal veins (Figure 1.4). Duplication is more common than just a left-sided vein. A persistent left-sided superior vena cava usually joins the right atrium either directly or through the coronary sinus, but joins the left atrium in about 10%.

Veins in the trunk

- Veins on the left side partly disappear while veins on the right side persist as the major veins. Posterior cardinal veins are gradually replaced by three sets of veins:
  - Subcardinal veins drain the kidneys and gonads.
  - Supracardinal veins drain the body wall.
  - Sacrocardinal veins drain the lower extremities.
- A connecting vein between the two posterior cardinal veins forms the left renal vein, and this usually passes in front of the aorta. An anastomosis between the sacrocardinal veins becomes the left common iliac vein.
- The left posterior cardinal vein below the left renal vein disappears, the left supracardinal vein becomes the hemiazygos veins and the right supracardinal vein becomes the azygos veins which open into the right anterior cardinal vein.
- The inferior vena cava has several segments of different origin (Figure 1.5). From cephalad to caudal these are:
  - Suprahepatic from the proximal right vitelline vein.
  - Hepatic from an anastomosis between the right vitelline and right subcardinal veins beyond the developing liver.

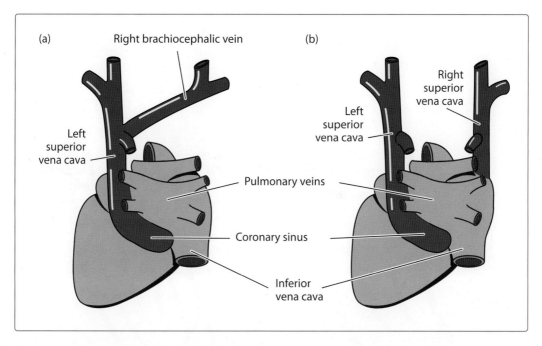

Figure 1.4 Posterior view showing anomalies of the superior vena cava. (a) Left superior vena cava draining into the right atrium through the coronary sinus. (b) Double superior vena cava due to failure of the communicating vein between the two anterior cardinal veins (left brachiocephalic trunk) to develop.

- Renal from a segment of the right subcardinal vein.
- A junctional segment formed through an anastomosis between the right subcardinal and right supracardinal vein.

- Infrarenal from the right supracardinal vein.
- The distal segment that connects the right supracardinal and most distal part of the bilateral posterior cardinal veins.

1.3 Developmental abnormalities of the inferior vena cava

- Congenital anomalies of the inferior vena cava are present in some 0.5% of adult subjects. The most common congenital abnormalities are duplication and retro-aortic left renal vein. Deep vein thrombosis may occur in about 5% of these subjects.
- Agenesis of the inferior vena cava occurs if the right subcardinal vein has failed to develop so that blood reaches the heart through the azygos vein and superior vena cava.
- Duplication of the inferior vena cava is present in up to 3% of subjects and occurs if the left sacrocardinal vein has failed to lose its connection with the left subcardinal vein (Figure 1.6). A left inferior vena cava can occur if the right supracardinal vein also disappears. There is a persistent communication between the left common iliac vein and the left renal vein which then typically crosses anterior to the aorta to join the right inferior vena cava. Though asymptomatic, double or left inferior vena cava can have important implications for interventional radiology or vascular surgery.
- Membranous occlusion of the suprahepatic inferior vena cava can be a cause of primary Budd–Chiari syndrome (see Chapter 17).

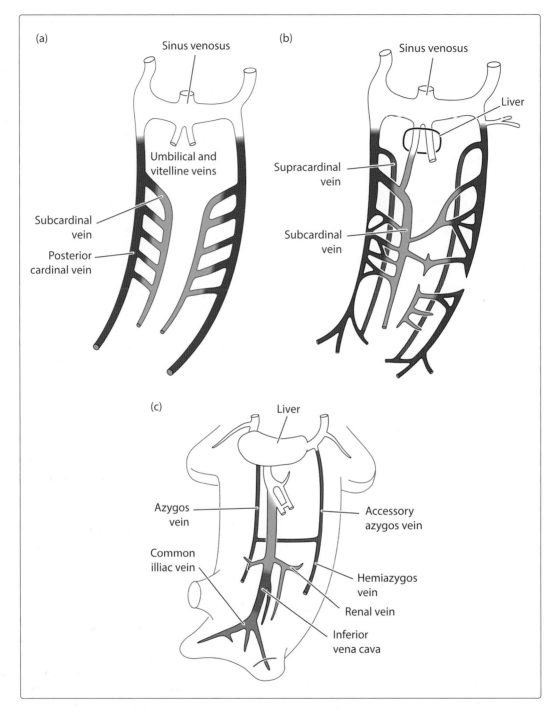

Figure 1.5 Development of the inferior vena cava over the first eight weeks. (a) Antero-posterior view of the posterior cardinal veins showing the subcardinal veins that drains the abdomen. (b) development of the supracardinal veins draining the retroperitoneum and retropleural areas. (c) Later, as the supracardinal veins become the azygous veins, the sacrocardinal veins drain the lower limbs, the left side regresses to allow the right sacrocardinal vein to join the right posterior cardinal vein to form the inferior vena cava.

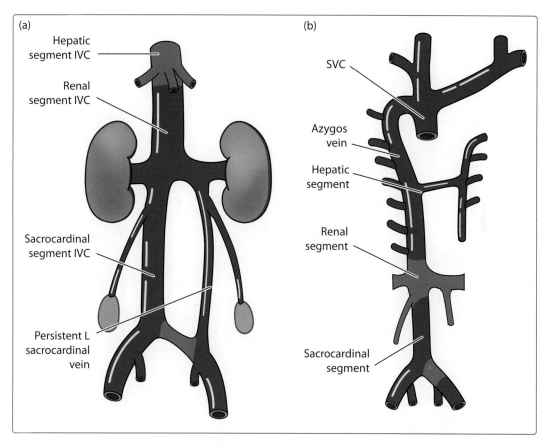

Figure 1.6 Anomalies of the inferior vena cava (IVC). (a) Double inferior vena cava due to persistence of the left sacrocardinal vein. (b) Agenesis of the most cephalad segment of the inferior vena cava with flow diverted to the azygos vein.

Veins in the lower limbs

- Neurovascular structures develop in three groups: preaxial – initially facing in the cranial direction and later rotating to be medial, axial – deep in the limb, and postaxial – facing caudal then lateral.
- It is postulated that development of lower limb veins from the posterior cardinal veins is under the control of growth factors produced by three 'angio-guiding nerves' (Figure 1.7).[4,5]
  - Femoral nerve in the preaxial plane.
  - Sciatic nerve in the axial plane.
  - Posterior femoral cutaneous nerve in the postaxial plane.
- Three venous plexuses develop along these angio-guiding nerves by about the eighth week.
- Veins in the postaxial plane form the small saphenous vein and thigh extension.
- Veins in the axial plane become the deep femoral veins.
- Veins in the preaxial plane become the femoral and great saphenous veins.
- Superficial veins appear before deep veins. Flow from the lower limb through the posterior cardinal vein forms a primitive sciatic vein and fibular vein. Flow is progressively transferred from postaxial to preaxial veins, which then form the main connection between limb and pelvic veins. If the fibular vein persists then it forms an abnormal lateral marginal vein. If the sciatic vein persists then it continues to form the main drainage system from the lower limb.

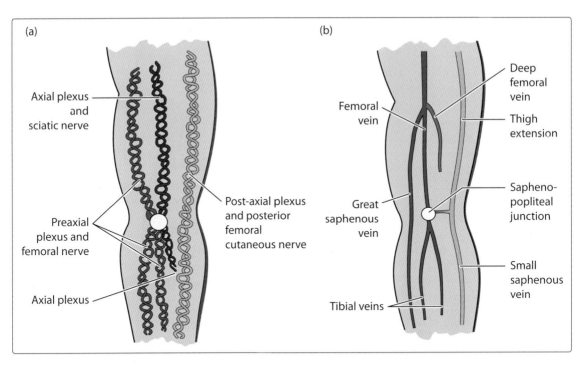

Figure 1.7 Development of veins in the lower limbs associated with the three 'angio-guiding nerves'. (a) Foetus: Preaxial femoral nerve and venous plexus (blue). Axial sciatic nerve and venous plexus (red) that give rise to the sciatic vein. Postaxial posterior femoral cutaneous nerve and venous plexus (yellow). (b) Adult: Preaxial plexus forms the femoral vein and great saphenous vein (blue). Axial plexus normally disappears. Postaxial plexus forms the small saphenous vein and thigh extension (yellow). An axio-preaxial anastomosis forms the deep femoral vein (green). An axio-postaxial anastomosis forms the terminal small saphenous vein (green) leading to the sapheno-popliteal junction (white). (From Creton D. *Phlebolymphology* 2005;48:347–54.)

- Anastomoses develop between the three venous systems to form connections:[6,7]
  - Axial veins below-knee to preaxial veins above-knee form the popliteal vein.
  - Axial to postaxial veins at the knee become the sapheno-popliteal junction, which is variable as to its presence and position.
  - Preaxial to postaxial veins above knee form the vein of Giacomini.

The lymphatic system

- Dilations of lymphatic channels form six primary lymph sacs at six to nine weeks. There are two jugular lymph sacs near the anterior cardinal veins, two iliac lymph sacs near the posterior cardinal veins, one retroperitoneal lymph sac in the root of the mesentery on the posterior abdominal wall and one that becomes the cisterna chyli dorsal to the retroperitoneal lymph sac at the level of the adrenal glands.
- Lymphatic vessels grow from these lymph sacs along the major veins to the head, neck, and arms from the jugular sacs, to the lower trunk and legs from the iliac sacs, and from the retroperitoneal and cisternal sacs to the gut.
- The cisterna chyli is initially connected to the jugular lymph sacs by two large channels, the right and left thoracic ducts. The final thoracic duct is formed by the caudal portion of the right thoracic duct, an anastomosis between the two thoracic ducts and the cranial portion of the left thoracic duct. Each lymphatic duct joins the venous system at the junction of the subclavian and internal jugular veins at the base of the neck (Figure 1.8).

1.4 Developmental abnormalities of lower limb veins

- A persistent lateral marginal vein or persistent sciatic vein are collectively referred to as persistent embryonic veins.[8–10] They occur in about 1% of the general population but are present in almost 20% of limbs with the Klippel–Trenaunay syndrome (see Chapter 26).
- A persistent lateral marginal vein refers to superficial veins that extend from the dorsal venous arch of the foot to the lateral thigh. These are connected to tributaries of the great and small saphenous veins and to deeper veins.
- A persistent sciatic vein is a deep vein lying along the midline of the posterior thigh on the medial side of the sciatic nerve. It represents the main trunk of the primordial deep venous system. It can be:
  - Complete, commencing from the terminal small saphenous vein or popliteal vein, sometimes with an anastomosis with the medial circumflex thigh vein, draining into the internal iliac, inferior gluteal or deep femoral veins.
  - A proximal or superior vein that emerges in the proximal thigh and passes through the buttock to end in the pelvis.
  - A distal or inferior vein found in the inferior medial thigh.
- The most common variant of the persistent sciatic vein is for axial veins to persist as small arcades that communicate with the deep femoral vein; persistence as the major outflow tract for the lower limb is rare.
- Aplasia of the femoral vein can occur with collateral drainage to the common femoral vein, into the internal iliac vein or even into the azygos vein depending on whether it involves the femoral vein only or common femoral vein as well. Aplasia of the great saphenous vein has been reported. Aplasia of valves in the deep veins is not rare and later leads to clinical features of deep venous reflux.

- Except for the sac from which the cisterna chyli develops, all lymph sacs are converted into groups of lymph nodes at about the third month. Mesenchymal cells invade each sac and break them up into lymphatic sinuses with supporting connective tissue. Lymphocytes come to the nodes from the thymus gland just before birth. Other lymphatic tissues that develop are the spleen and tonsils.

History[11]

- Hippocrates (460–370 BC) believed in *preformationism*–that humans were fully formed in miniature inside germ cells, a belief in keeping with theological teaching and accepted for the next 1300 years.
- Aristotle (384–322 BC) studied human embryos and argued that semen supplied the form to embryos and mothers menstrual blood supplied substance to aid in development.
- Galen of Pergamon (129–200) proposed that the umbilical cord was necessary for respiration.
- Albertus Magnus (1200–1280), also known as Saint Albert the Great and referred to as the greatest German philosopher of the Middle Ages, challenged long-held theological views with scientific observations to propose the 'interactions between male and female seeds'.
- The Italian biologist Marcello Malpighi (1628–1694) supported *preformationism*, describing embryo development as a simple unfolding of an already miniature adult organism. This was finally challenged by the scientist Antonie van Leeuwenhoek (1632–1723), philosopher Gottfried Wilhelm Leibniz (1646–1716) and physiologist and embryologist Caspar Wolff (1733–1794) who proposed *epigenesis* in line with modern understanding of development, although this took a further 100 years to be fully accepted.
- By the end of the eighteenth century, the mammalian egg was finally seen and recognized

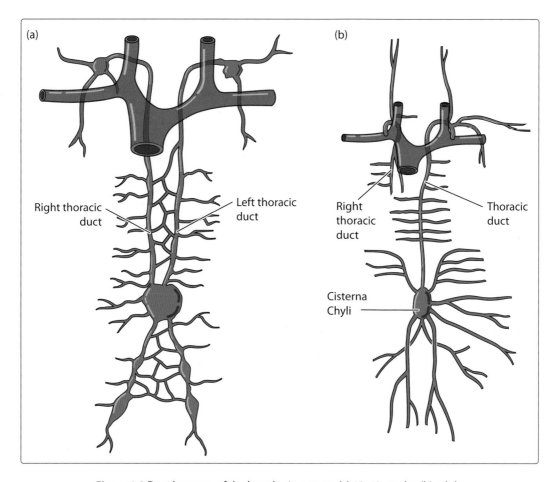

(a)

Right thoracic duct

Left thoracic duct

(b)

Right thoracic duct

Thoracic duct

Cisterna Chyli

Figure 1.8 Development of the lymphatic system, (a) 10–12 weeks, (b) adult.

as a single cell, and the surgeon John Hunter (1728–1793) showed that the maternal and foetal circulations were distinct and separate.

References

1. Uhl J-F. Focus on embryogenesis of the human lower limb. *Phlebolymphology* 2015;22:55–63. http://www.phlebolymphology.org/focus-venous-embryogenesis-human-lower-limbs/

2. Lee BB. Venous embryology: The key to understanding anomalous venous conditions. *Phlebolymphology* 2012;19:170–81. http://www.phlebolymphology.org/venous-embryology-the-key-to-understanding-anomalous-venous-conditions/

3. Caggiati A. The venous valves of the lower limbs. *Phlebolymphology* 2013;20:87–95. http://www.phlebolymphology.org/the-venous-valves-of-the-lower-limbs/

4. Uhl J-F, Gillot, LCP. Relationship between the small saphenous vein and nerves: Implications for the management of chronic venous disease. *Phlebolymphology* 2006;13:22–27. http://www.phlebolymphology.org/relationship-between-the-small-saphenous-vein-and-nerves-implications-for-the-management-of-chronic-venous-disease/

5. Gillot C. Dispositifs veineux poplités: Hypothèses et certitudes. *Phlébologie* 1998;51:65–74. Referred to in: http://www.veinsurg.com/en/references/25-chirurgie/97-saphenopopliteal-junctions-are-significantly-lower-when-incompetent-embryological-hypothesis-and-surgical-implications

6. Creton D. Saphenopopliteal junctions are significantly lower when incompetent. Embryological hypothesis and surgical implications. *Phlebolymphology* 2005;48:347–54. http://www.veinsurg.com/en/references/25-chirurgie/97-saphenopopliteal-junctions-are-significantly-lower-when-incompetent-embryological-hypothesis-and-surgical-implications

7. Uhl J-F, Gillot C. Anatomy and embryology of the small saphenous vein: Nerve relationships and implications for treatment. *Phlebology* 2013;28:4–15. https://www.ncbi.nlm.nih.gov/pubmed/23256200

8. Oduber CE, Young-Afat DA, van der Wal AC, van Steensel MA, Hennekam RC, van der Horst CM. The persistent embryonic vein in Klippel-Trenaunay syndrome. *Vasc Med* 2013;18:185–91. https://www.ncbi.nlm.nih.gov/pubmed/23966121

9. Cherry KJ, Gloviczki P, Stanson AW. Persistent sciatic vein: Diagnosis and treatment of a rare condition. *J Vasc Surg* 1996;23:490–97. https://www.ncbi.nlm.nih.gov/pubmed/8601893

10. Gillot C. Le prolongement post-axial de la petite veine saphène. Étude anatomique. Considérations fonctionnelles. *Intérêt pathologique. Phlébologie* 2000;53:295–25.

11. Wellner K. A history of embryology, by Joseph Needham. 2010. The Embryo Project Encyclopedia. https://embryo.asu.edu/pages/history-embryology-1959-joseph-needham

Anatomy of veins and lymphatics

The section for anatomy of lower limb veins is based on a consensus from experts at a meeting of the Union Internationale de Phlebologie held in San Diego.[1,2]

Information gained from anatomical dissections has been supplemented in recent years by ultrasound studies for veins[1-4] and dye studies for lymphatics.[5]

Skin histology

Epidermis

- The epidermis is a stratified squamous epithelium with five layers from the surface (Figure 2.1):
  - Stratum corneum – cornified layer
  - Stratum lucidum – clear translucent layer
  - Stratum granulosum – granular layer
  - Stratum spinosum – spinous layer
  - Stratum basale/germinativum – basal or germinal layer

The stratum malpighii (Malpighian layer) refers to both the spinous and basal layers.

- The epidermis is maintained by cell division within the basal layer. Differentiating cells move towards the surface through the other layers, lose their nuclei, fuse to form squamous sheets in the stratum corneum then desquamate. While nuclei are disintegrating, cells are secreting keratin and lamellar bodies containing lipids and proteins to maintain the skin's water barrier. Cell production equals loss in normal skin, taking about two weeks to travel from the basal layer to the top of the granular layer and a further four weeks to cross the stratum corneum.
- The epidermis contains inflammatory and other cells including melanocytes, Langerhans (antigen-presenting) cells and Merkel (light touch-receptor) cells.

Dermis

- The superficial papillary dermis has projections into the epidermis and deep to this is the reticular dermis. The dermis contains collagen, elastin fibres and extracellular matrix.

Skin circulation

- The epidermis is avascular and nourished by diffusion from the dermis. There are several interconnecting vascular networks – the sub-papillary and sub-dermal cutaneous networks, superficial, middle and deep subcutaneous networks, and a plexus lying on the deep fascia (Figure 2.2).[5]
- The sub-papillary plexus lies at the epidermal-dermal junction, gives off dermal papillary loops, and is involved in thermoregulation. The sub-dermal plexus is at the junction of dermis and subcutaneous tissues and is responsible for skin nutrition. Blood flows through a series of ascending arterioles towards the skin, innervated pre-capillary sphincters regulate flow from arterioles to capillaries, and blood flows directly from arterioles to venules through arteriovenous anastomoses when the sphincters are closed. Sub-dermal collecting venules drain into subcutaneous venules and then to veins that form a large capacitance reservoir.

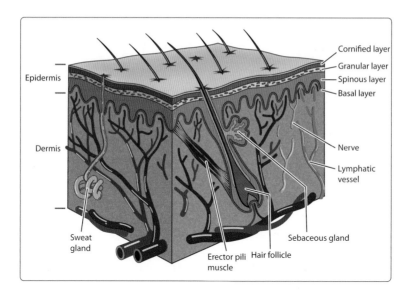

Figure 2.1 Histology of the skin to show the morphological layers of the epidermis, dermis and subcutaneous fat with adnexae.

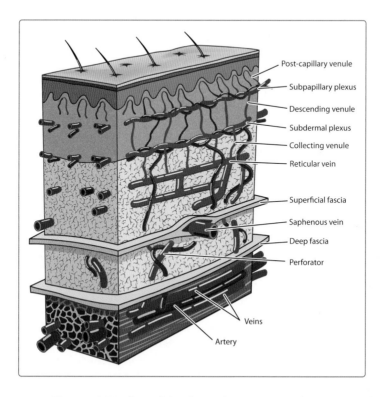

Figure 2.2 Histology of the skin to show microcirculation.

- Post-capillary venules are 12–35 μ diameter and collecting venules are 40–60 μ in the upper and mid dermis, enlarging to 100–400 μ in deeper tissues. Venules larger than 20 μ diameter have an endothelium and collagen fibres, smooth muscle cells appear by 45 μ and a full muscle layer is visible by 200 μ. Valves are seen in venules greater than 40 μ diameter.

Vascular histology

Vein wall

- Veins have thinner walls than arteries with less muscle and elastin but considerably more collagen. The blood supply for the wall is through vasa vasorum. There is an increasing proportion of smooth muscle to other components moving from large proximal to small distal veins, which allows peripheral veins to better counter hydrostatic pressure. There are several types of collagen throughout the body characterized as types I–XII, and about 90% of collagen in veins is of type I, some 10% is of type III and there are small amounts of type V.

Intima

- A single layer of fusiform endothelial cells sits on a sub-endothelial layer of fine connective tissue and a poorly-developed fenestrated internal elastic membrane. The endothelium is covered by a semi-permeable layer termed the glycocalyx, which is a network of proteoglycans and glycoproteins about 10 μ thick.

Media and adventitia

- The media has proportionately less muscle or elastin and more collagen compared to arteries. The media has concentric lamellar layers of elastic fibres and smooth muscle cells that produce collagen and elastin together with microfibrils and ground substance. The adventitia mostly consists of collagen which comes from fibroblasts and is the thickest layer.

Venous valves

- Valve anatomy is complex.[6,7] They are usually bicuspid thin avascular half-moon folds of collagen covered by endothelium with smooth muscle at their base. The attachment of cusp to vein wall is the *limbus* or *agger*, the space between the cusp and vein wall is the *sinus* and where the two cusps meet is the *commissure*.

Microcirculation

- The microcirculation consists of arterioles, metarterioles, precapillary sphincters, capillaries, arteriovenous connections and venules. Post-capillary venules have only an endothelial intima, lack a smooth muscle media and are surrounded by undifferentiated mesenchyme.

Veins of the upper limbs, head, neck and chest

Deep veins of the upper limb

- Paired ulnar and radial venae comitantes join at the elbow to become the brachial veins. On each side, these become the axillary vein at the inferior border of the teres major muscle, and the axillary vein becomes the subclavian vein at the first rib. Each subclavian vein joins the internal jugular vein to become the brachiocephalic trunk (innominate vein) just behind the sternal end of the clavicle (Figure 2.3).

Superficial veins of the upper limb

- Interconnected superficial veins form a dorsal venous arch at the base of the back of the hand. Veins in the palm form palmar arches (Figure 2.3).
- The basilic vein arises from the ulnar side of the dorsal or palmar arches of the hand and passes along the ulnar side of the forearm and medial arm. It either joins the brachial veins in the upper half of the arm or axillary vein higher up.
- The cephalic vein arises from the radial end of the dorsal venous arch of the hand to pass

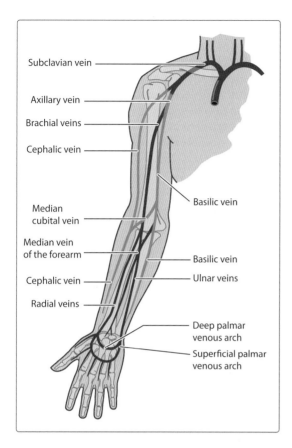

Figure 2.3 Deep and superficial veins of the upper limb (deep veins – dark blue, superficial veins – light blue).

along the radial aspect of the forearm, then along the arm to dive between the deltoid and pectoralis major muscles to join the subclavian vein.

- Veins pass up the anterior forearm to form the median vein of the forearm which joins either the basilic or median cubital vein. The median cubital vein in the antecubital fossa is the largest connection between cephalic and basilic veins. Numerous perforating veins direct flow from superficial to deep.

The thoracic outlet

- There are three consecutive spaces between the base of neck and upper arm where the subclavian vein, subclavian artery or brachial plexus (C5–T1 nerve roots) can be compressed (see Chapter 16) (Figure 2.4).

- The interscalene triangle is located at the base of neck.
  - The boundaries are the scalenus anterior muscle in front, scalenus medius muscle behind and first rib at the base.
  - The lower brachial plexus and subclavian artery can be compressed as they lie behind the scalenus anterior.
  - The subclavian vein cannot be compressed as it lies in front of the scalenus anterior.
- The costoclavicular space is inferolateral to the clavicle.
  - The boundaries are the clavicle, first rib, costoclavicular ligament and edge of scalenus medius.
  - This is the most common site for neurovascular compression.
- The coracopectoral space is the most distal.
  - It is situated between the pectoralis minor muscle, coracoid process and ribs.
  - This is the least likely space for compression to occur.

Cerebral veins

- Veins of the cerebrum form superficial and deep groups which on leaving the brain run in the subarachnoid space and pierce the meninges to drain into dural venous sinuses. These drain the central nervous system, face and scalp to the internal jugular veins (Figure 2.5).
- The superficial system of superior, superficial middle and inferior cerebral veins drains the cerebral cortex to the midline superior sagittal sinus. The deep system drains to the midline great cerebral vein of Galen which joins the inferior sagittal sinus to form the straight sinus. The cavernous sinus drains the ophthalmic veins and lies on either side of the sella turcica, and from here blood returns to the internal jugular vein through the superior and inferior petrosal sinuses, then the transverse sinus.
- The confluence of the superior sagittal and straight sinuses forms a transverse then sigmoid sinus on each side to become the internal jugular veins leaving the skull though the jugular foraminae.

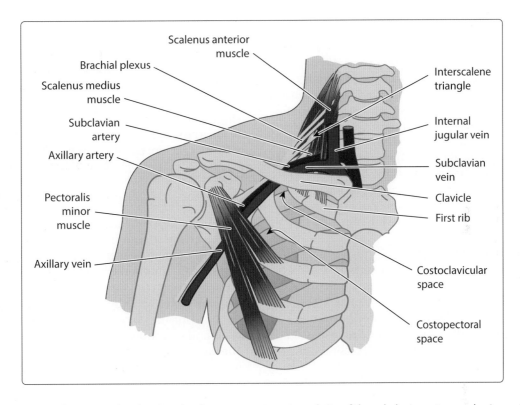

Figure 2.4 The thoracic outlet showing the three compartments and site of the subclavian artery and vein, and the brachial plexus.

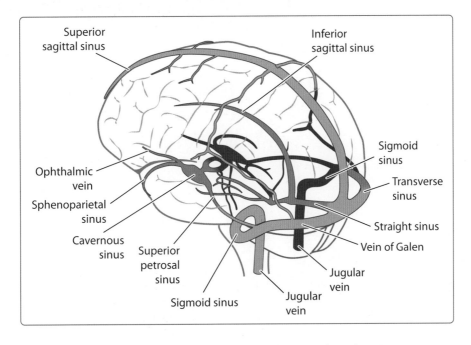

Figure 2.5 Cerebral sinuses draining to the internal jugular veins.

Jugular veins

- The internal jugular vein leaves the base of the skull posterior to the carotid artery, then spirals around the artery to become anterior as it joins the subclavian vein to form the brachiocephalic trunk. It lies between the two heads of sternomastoid in the mid portion and posterior to the clavicular head at the base of the neck. The brachiocephalic trunks join on the right side of the neck to become the superior vena cava. The external jugular vein begins at the angle of the mandible and courses posterior to the sternomastoid to join the subclavian vein.

Vertebral veins

- A complex interconnecting series of valveless longitudinal veins form anterior and posterior intraspinal and extraspinal vertebral venous plexuses. The anterior intraspinal veins carry the most flow and are responsible for a considerable amount of cerebral drainage when the subject is erect.

- The vertebral veins receive blood from the base of the brain then leave the skull to enter a foramen in the transverse process of the atlas. They descend with the vertebral artery in a canal formed by the transverse foramina of the cervical vertebrae and emerge as a single trunk below the sixth cervical vertebra to join the subclavian or internal jugular veins or brachiocephalic trunk.

Facial veins

Veins of the forehead, nose, and orbit

- Flow from the forehead is through the supratrochlear and supraorbital veins which join to form the angular vein at the side of the nose (Figure 2.6). The supraorbital vein sends a branch through the supraorbital notch that communicates with the ophthalmic vein to establish an anastomosis between the facial veins and cavernous sinus.
- The angular vein runs down the side of the nose to become the anterior facial vein.

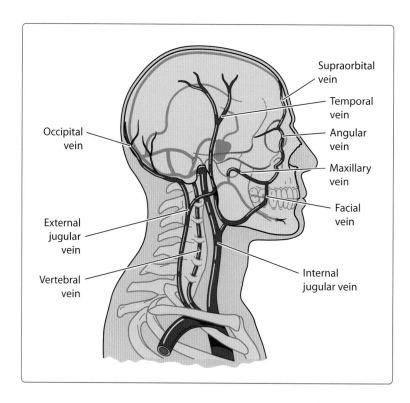

Figure 2.6 Veins of the face.

Pre-tarsal and post-tarsal veins of the eyelids drain to the superficial temporal, angular and facial veins.

Veins of the cheek and lip

- The facial vein connects to the deep facial vein and joins the pterygoid plexus medial to the upper ramus of the mandible, then crosses superficial to the submandibular gland to join the internal jugular vein.

Veins of the temple and ear

- Veins on the side and top of skull unite above the zygomatic arch to form the superficial temporal vein which drains the scalp and forehead. It enters the parotid gland and joins the internal maxillary vein to become the posterior facial vein which joins the internal jugular vein.
- The posterior auricular vein descends behind the ear to join the posterior division of the posterior facial vein to form the external jugular vein.
- The occipital vein begins at the back of skull and joins the deep cervical and vertebral veins, or ends in the internal or external jugular veins. There are connections with the superior sagittal and transverse sinuses within the skull.

Azygos and hemiazygos veins

- The azygos vein is unpaired and usually passes up in the posterior mediastinum on the right side beside the vertebral column (Figure 2.7). It drains blood from the posterior thoracic and abdominal wall to the superior vena cava, and communicates with the vertebral venous plexuses.
- The hemiazygos vein usually continues from the left ascending lumbar vein, and passes up through the left crus of the diaphragm to ascend on the left side of the vertebral column. It passes to the right across the vertebral column behind the aorta, oesophagus and thoracic duct at about the level of the ninth thoracic vertebra, to end in the azygos vein. The hemiazygos vein may be connected above to the accessory hemiazygos vein, the two of them being a mirror of the azygos vein on the right side.

2.1 Clinical relevance of veins of the upper limbs and face

- The basilic vein has no accompanying artery so that it is a safe entry point for a peripherally inserted central cannula (PICC) line.
- Surgery is performed for haemodialysis to treat renal failure by direct anastomosis or an interposition vein or synthetic graft between an artery and a vein in the upper limb (see Chapter 17).
- The internal jugular and subclavian veins provide a good point of access for percutaneous transvenous procedures such as ovarian coil embolization.
- The axillary vein is at danger for iatrogenic injury with local anaesthetic nerve blocks or interventional radiology for the upper or lower extremity.
- The azygos vein connects the superior and inferior vena cava systems to provide an alternative pathway for flow to the right atrium if either vena cava is occluded.

- The thoracic duct can be damaged by surgery in the neck on the left side.
- Compromise of the thoracic outlet by anatomical variations or past bony trauma can compress the subclavian vein as well as nerves and the subclavian artery to cause thoracic outlet syndrome.
- The 'dangerous triangle of the face' involves the upper lip and paranasal area as a site for communications between the facial vein and cavernous sinus, either directly through the ophthalmic vein or indirectly through the pterygoid plexus. It is a potential site for the spread of infection, and in theory could pose a danger for passage of sclerosant during treatment with a possible risk of cavernous sinus thrombosis, although this does not seem to pose a threat in practice.

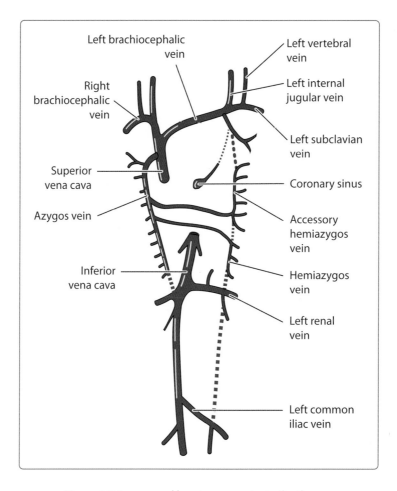

Figure 2.7 Azygos and hemiazygos veins in the thorax.

Veins of the abdomen

Hepato-portal venous system

Splanchnic and portal veins

- The portal venous system comprises all veins draining the abdominal part of the digestive tract including the lower oesophagus but excluding the lower anal canal. The portal vein results from the confluence of the superior mesenteric and splenic veins behind the neck of pancreas. Further tributaries are the left and right gastric, paraumbilical and cystic veins (Figure 2.8).
- The portal vein is about 7cm long and lies in front of the inferior vena cava and superior mesenteric artery. It divides into right

and left portal veins at the porta hepatis to accompany hepatic artery branches into the liver. The right portal vein gives branches to the caudate lobe then divides into anterior and posterior branches which subdivide into superior and inferior segmental branches to supply the right lobe of liver. The left portal vein supplies the lateral segments of the left lobe.

Hepatic veins

- The right, left and middle hepatic veins pass from the back of the liver to the inferior vena cava immediately below the diaphragm. The most common pattern is a right hepatic vein and a common trunk for the middle

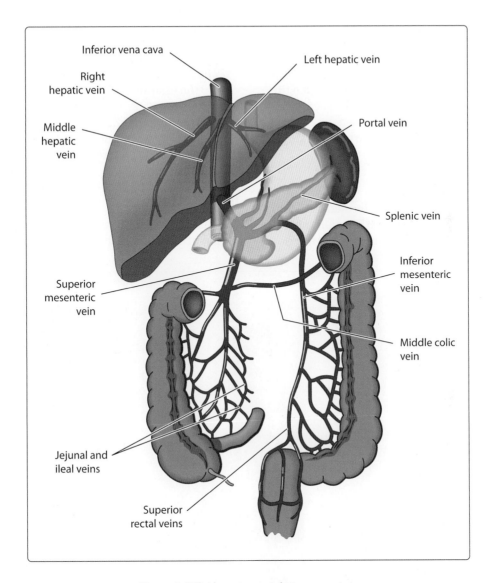

Figure 2.8 The hepato-portal venous system.

and left hepatic veins, but all three may join as a common trunk or the three may drain independently. The middle hepatic vein lies in the interlobar fissure separating the right and left lobes of liver. Two to three caudate veins drain separately into the inferior vena cava below the main hepatic veins.

Congenital anomalies

- The portal vein may be double. A pre-pancreatic portal vein is associated with situs inversus. The portal vein or its branches may be absent, often in association with agenesis of corresponding liver lobes, and this leads to periportal collaterals and cavernous transformation of the portal vein.
- Abnormal portal vein branching occurs in approximately 20% of subjects, with trifurcation of the main portal vein, right posterior segmental branch arising from the main portal vein, or right anterior segmental branch arising from the left portal vein.
- Hepatic vein variations include a small right hepatic vein and large right inferior or middle

hepatic vein, or accessory vein from the left or middle hepatic vein.

- Communication between a portal and hepatic vein is uncommon, though intrahepatic porto-systemic shunting between the right portal vein and inferior vena cava can occur. Intrahepatic arterio-venous connections between the hepatic artery, portal vein, and hepatic veins are rare.

Renal veins

- Each renal vein is usually formed from four divisions at the hilum and is usually singular, but can be duplicated. Because the inferior

vena cava is on the right side, the left renal vein usually receives the left inferior phrenic, suprarenal, gonadal and second lumbar veins, whereas these veins drain directly into the inferior vena cava on the right side (Figure 2.9).

- Renal veins enter the inferior vena cava at approximately the lower third of the first lumbar vertebra, the left renal vein slightly higher than the right.

Inferior vena cava

- The inferior vena cava is formed by the junction of the common iliac veins, usually at the

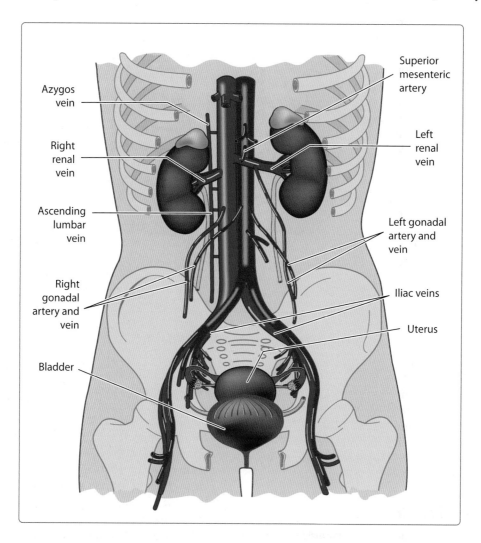

Figure 2.9 The inferior vena cava and renal veins, and the common and external iliac veins.

fifth lumbar vertebra. It passes retroperitoneal to the right of the aorta to leave the abdomen through the diaphragmatic caval hiatus at the T8 level. After passing up behind the liver, it has a short intrathoracic course before draining into the right atrium. There are no valves in the inferior vena cava (Figure 2.9).

2.2 Clinical relevance of abdominal veins

- The portal venous system is remarkable in that it has no valves and begins and ends in capillaries. There are multiple connections between the portal and systemic venous systems which can open to decompress portal hypertension in patients with liver disease (see Chapter 17).
- Transjugular intrahepatic porto-systemic shunt (TIPS) involves percutaneous insertion of a stent between a large branch of the hepatic and portal venous systems within the liver. This allows portal venous drainage to the systemic venous circulation to relieve portal hypertension (see Chapter 17).
- The left renal vein normally lies in front of the aorta, but it may pass behind the aorta instead as a retro-aortic left renal vein, or there may be veins in front and behind the aorta, as circum-aortic renal veins (see Chapter 1).
- The inferior vena cava can be duplicated (see Chapter 1).

Veins of the pelvis

A consensus document under the auspices of the Federative International Committee on Anatomical Terminology and International Federation of Associations of Anatomists has clarified nomenclature and drainage patterns of pelvic veins.[8]

Common iliac vein

- Each common iliac vein is formed by the junction of internal and external iliac veins in front of the sacroiliac joints, and extend to the right side of the fifth lumbar vertebra, where they join to form the inferior vena cava. The right common iliac vein is shorter and runs almost perpendicular, lying behind and lateral to the right common iliac artery. The left common iliac vein is longer and runs more obliquely, first medial to the left common iliac artery, then posterior to the right common iliac artery (Figure 2.9).
- An ascending lumbar vein passes upwards from each common iliac vein to form the origin of the azygos vein on the right and hemiazygos vein on the left side, connecting the inferior and superior vena cavae.

External iliac vein

- The external iliac vein ascends along the brim of the lesser pelvis and joins the internal iliac vein. The right-sided vein lies medial to the external iliac artery, then moves behind the artery, while the left-sided vein lies medial to the artery in its whole course (Figure 2.10).
- The deep circumflex iliac vein joins the external iliac vein approximately 2cm proximal to the inguinal ligament, and has large communications with tributaries of the iliolumbar veins and veins of the anterior abdominal wall.
- The inferior epigastric vein joins the external iliac vein approximately 1–2 cm proximal to the inguinal ligament and collects blood from the deep anterior abdominal wall. Anastomoses with the superior epigastric vein in the abdominal muscles provides a further connection between the inferior and superior vena cavae. The superficial epigastric vein drains the external abdominal wall to the common femoral vein just distal to the inguinal ligament. Suprapubic veins join the left and right inferior epigastric veins.

Internal iliac vein

- The internal iliac vein commences where the inferior gluteal and internal pudendal veins join at the greater sciatic foramen and receives parietal and visceral tributaries.

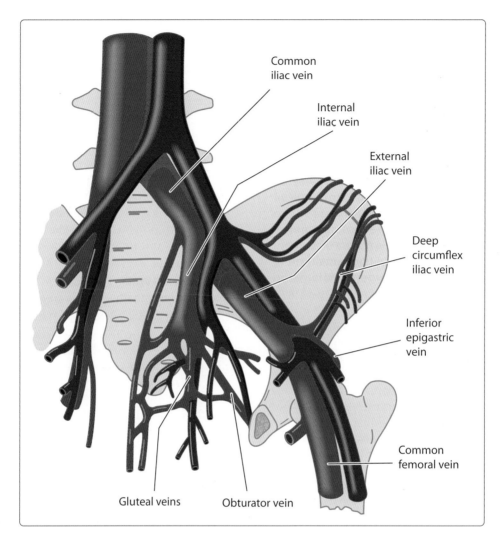

Figure 2.10 The internal iliac venous circulation in a female.

It ascends behind and lateral to the corresponding artery to join the external iliac vein. It is duplicated in some 30% of subjects, and if so then one trunk receives blood from visceral tributaries and the other from parietal tributaries (Figure 2.10).

- Parietal tributaries from outside the pelvis are the superior and inferior gluteal veins that drain gluteal muscles, and the obturator vein that drains medial thigh muscles. The obturator vein may be replaced by an accessory obturator vein that joins the external iliac vein.

- Parietal tributaries from the walls of the pelvis form the sacral venous plexus behind the rectum, which drains blood from spinal veins through the medial sacral veins into the left common iliac vein, iliolumbar vein into the common iliac veins and lateral sacral vein into the internal iliac veins.

- Visceral tributaries arise in the rectal, vesical and pudendal plexuses, and the vaginal and uterine or prostatic plexuses. There are extensive connections between the plexuses and, through them, between the inferior and superior vena cavae.

- External and internal rectal venous plexuses lie within the rectal wall. The internal rectal plexus forms the haemorrhoidal plexus and drains both cranially through the superior rectal veins to the inferior mesenteric vein in the portal circulation, and through the middle rectal veins and internal pudendal vein to the internal iliac vein in the systemic venous circulation.
- The pudendal plexus lies behind the pubic symphysis in front of the bladder and connects with the internal pudendal vein and is commonly known as the plexus of Santorini.
- In the female, the uterine plexuses lie along the sides and superior angles of the uterus between the two layers of the broad ligament, the vaginal plexuses are placed at the sides of the vagina, and the ovarian plexuses surround the ovaries. These form a major connection between pelvic veins and the pubic, suprapubic, obturator, inferior epigastric and deep circumflex iliac veins passing to veins in the lower limbs.
- In the male, the superficial dorsal vein of the penis drains the prepuce and skin of the penis and opens into the external pudendal veins, tributaries of the great saphenous vein. The deep dorsal vein of the penis drains the glans penis and corpora cavernosa and passes to the pudendal plexus behind the symphysis pubis and in front of the bladder and prostate and then to the internal pudendal vein.

Valves in the iliac veins

- These veins usually have no valves with an occasional valve as follows:[6,7]
  - Common iliac vein – one (usually incomplete) in 1%–5%.
  - Internal iliac vein and tributaries – one in 5%–10%.
  - External iliac vein – one in approximately 25%.

Gonadal veins

- Evolution of gonadal veins is separate to iliac veins. They pass upwards on the posterior abdominal wall in front of the ureter and

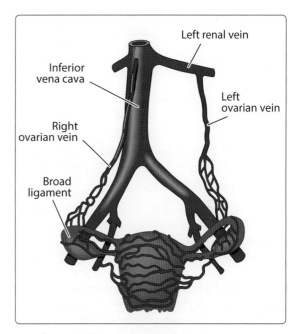

Figure 2.11 Ovarian veins and veins across the broad ligaments.

psoas major muscle. Their termination in 80% of subjects is for the right gonadal vein to join the inferior vena cava directly at the level of the second lumbar vertebra and for the left gonadal vein to join the left renal vein (Figure 2.11), as would be expected from evolutionary development of the inferior vena cava (see Chapter 1). There are variations in 20%, with two veins and, rarely, three veins, and a duplicated vein may join the inferior vena cava directly at a more distal level. Gonadal veins contain valves in 60% on the left side and 50% on the right, with a terminal ostial vein in about 80% of these. They have connections both with veins draining to the internal iliac veins and to veins of the lower limbs.

- Ovarian veins commence in the plexus within the upper part of the broad ligament of the uterus and uterine venous plexus.
- Testicular veins emerge from the posterior aspect of testis collecting blood from the epididymis, and fuse to form the pampiniform plexus which twines around the testicular artery, ascends with the ductus deferens in

the spermatic cord, then forms three to four veins that pass through the inguinal canal into the abdomen.

Vulvar and vaginal veins[9]

- These drain anteriorly through the external pudendal veins at the sapheno-femoral junction to the external iliac system, and posteriorly by the internal pudendal veins to the internal iliac vein. Thus, vulvar veins anastomose between the pelvic wall veins and the veins of the pelvic viscera, between the internal and external iliac systems, and with the circulation of the medial aspect of the thigh.

2.3 Clinical relevance of pelvic veins

- The left common iliac vein can be compressed where it is crossed by the right common iliac artery to potentially cause the May–Thurner syndrome (see Chapter 16) although such compression can be demonstrated in some 25% of asymptomatic healthy volunteers. Iliac veins can also be compressed by the left common iliac artery or internal iliac arteries.
- There are potential anastomoses between the inferior and superior vena cavae through the ascending lumbar vein between the common iliac and azygos veins on the right, and hemiazygos vein on the left, through the inferior and superior epigastric veins in abdominal wall muscles, and through visceral and vertebral venous plexuses.
- There are three sites for communication also known as 'leak points' between pelvic veins and veins in the lower limb.
  - The superficial inguinal ring, where the veins of the round ligament meet the superficial veins of the anterior abdominal wall to connect uterine and ovarian systems with those of external pudendal veins, genital veins and veins of the anterior abdominal wall.
- The obturator canal, where deep veins of the proximal medial thigh muscles and the obturator vein empty into the proximal internal iliac vein.
- The gluteal region, where thigh veins join the inferior gluteal vein.
- Connections from the internal rectal plexus through the superior rectal veins to the inferior mesenteric vein in the portal circulation and through the middle rectal veins and internal pudendal vein to the internal iliac vein in the systemic venous circulation can serve as a porto-caval anastomosis in the pathological state of portal hypertension (see Chapter 17).
- The ovarian veins enlarge greatly during pregnancy, and a period of venous stasis occurs following childbirth. Reflux in the ovarian veins can cause symptoms of pelvic congestion (see Chapter 17).
- The right-angle junction of left testicular and left renal veins probably explains why most varicoceles occur on the left side.
- Vulvar varices on the labia majora and minora affect 10% of pregnant women, most often in the fifth month of a second pregnancy.

Veins of the lower limbs

- Descriptive names are preferred to eponymous nomenclature. Some veins have been renamed (Figure 2.12).[1,2]
  - Femoral vein – previously superficial femoral vein.
  - Deep femoral vein – previously profunda femoris vein,
- Great saphenous vein – previously also called the long, greater or internal saphenous vein.
- Anterior and posterior thigh circumflex veins – previously anterior and posterior thigh veins.
- Small saphenous vein – previously also called the short, lesser or external saphenous vein.

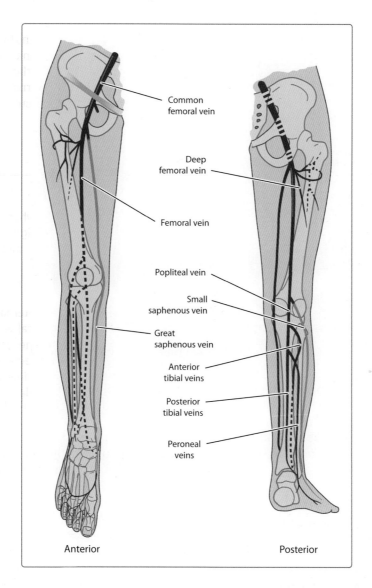

Figure 2.12 Deep and superficial veins of the lower limb (deep veins – dark blue, superficial veins – light blue).

Veins of the foot

- The deep plantar venous arch runs from the proximal end of the first interosseous space to the base of the fifth metatarsal. The medial plantar vein is a thin short vein that is usually duplicated, and runs along the medial border of the sole from the medial end of the plantar arch to the medial malleolus. The lateral plantar vein located between the two muscle layers of the sole of the foot is large and duplicated, and extends from the lateral end of the plantar venous arch across the sole to join the medial plantar vein and form the posterior tibial veins (Figure 2.13).[10]

- A superficial dorsal plexus is in continuity with superficial veins of the leg. Marginal veins and a dorsal arch are separated from the superficial dorsal plexus by a fascial layer corresponding to that covering the

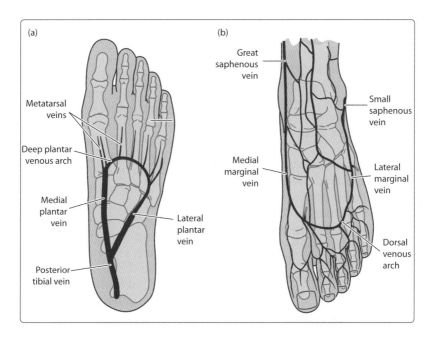

Figure 2.13 Veins of the foot. (a) Plantar aspect. (b) Dorsal aspect.

saphenous veins. The medial marginal vein arises from the perforator of the first metatarsal interspace and is contiguous with the great saphenous vein. The lateral marginal vein becomes the small saphenous vein.

Deep veins at and below the knee

- The anterior tibial, posterior tibial and peroneal veins, collectively termed crural veins, are usually duplicated and they join to form the popliteal vein (Figure 2.14).
- The posterior tibial veins arise from the medial and lateral plantar veins and drain the posterior compartment of the leg and plantar surface of the foot. Peroneal veins drain the deep compartment. Anterior tibial veins arise from dorsal veins of the foot and pass along the anterior compartment of the leg and through the proximal interosseous membrane below the knee.
- Gastrocnemius veins are paired or multiple, and the medial are larger than the lateral veins. They commence as a plexus in each muscle and form trunks 1–5 cm long that pass across the popliteal fossa to terminate

in the popliteal vein or, less often, in the posterior tibial, peroneal or small saphenous veins.

- Soleus veins commence in each muscle belly as a plexus, then form a single channel to pass to the posterior tibial or peroneal veins.
- The popliteal vein is formed at the lower border of the popliteus muscle on the medial side of the popliteal artery. As it ascends, it crosses behind the artery to lie on its lateral side. It then passes through the adductor magnus foramen to become the femoral vein. Some 20% of popliteal veins are duplicated.

Deep veins above knee

- Their course is relatively constant. The femoral vein lies posterolateral to the artery in the thigh, moving medial approaching the groin.[11] Some 10% of femoral veins are duplicated, but this is usually segmental, and only 2%–3% of veins are duplicated in their full length. The deep femoral vein joins the femoral vein 4–9 cm below the inguinal ligament to form the common femoral vein.

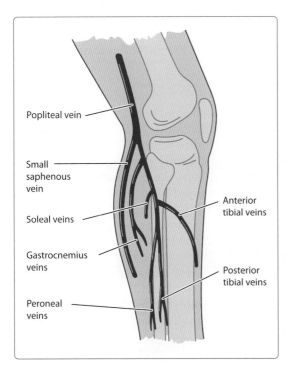

Figure 2.14 Veins at the region of the knee.

The common femoral vein lies medial to the corresponding artery and nerve.

Sapheno-femoral junction

- In many countries, this is known as the *crosse* (shepherd's crook) (Figure 2.15). The great saphenous vein passes through the fossa ovalis (saphenous opening) in the fascia lata of the thigh to join the common femoral vein 3–4 cm below and lateral to the pubic tubercle. Tributaries to the great saphenous vein near the sapheno-femoral junction are the superficial external pudendal, deep external pudendal, superficial inferior epigastric and superficial circumflex iliac veins, as well as the anterior and posterior thigh circumflex veins (Figure 2.13).
- Anatomical variations are common.[12] The median number of sapheno-femoral junction tributaries is four and at least one tributary drains directly into the common femoral vein in almost one-half of subjects, commonly the deep external pudendal vein.

Great and accessory saphenous veins

- The great saphenous vein passes from in front of the medial malleolus to terminate in the groin. It lies within a superficial compartment formed by the deep and superficial fascias – the 'saphenous eye' or ultrasound image of the 'Egyptian eye' (see Chapter 10) (Figure 2.16). There are variations of the great saphenous vein in the thigh and calf (Figure 2.17).
- Great saphenous tributaries include the anterior and posterior thigh circumflex veins, inter-saphenous veins and an occasional lateral venous system which represents the remnant of the embryonic lateral marginal vein. Inter-saphenous veins connect the great and small saphenous veins above and below the knee. Two main saphenous tributaries are usually present in the calf, an anterior branch and the posterior arch vein, which begins behind the medial malleolus and joins the great saphenous vein just distal to the knee. All tributaries lie superficial to the superficial fascia.
- The anterior and posterior accessory saphenous veins lie in individual saphenous compartments near their proximal ends. The anterior accessory saphenous vein is present in at least 50% of limbs and lies anterior and lateral to the great saphenous vein and anterior to the femoral vein, forming the alignment sign seen on ultrasound (see Chapter 10). There are variations of the origin of the anterior accessory saphenous vein (Figure 2.18).

Sapheno-popliteal junction

- The small saphenous vein terminates directly or indirectly into deep veins in approximately 75% of limbs, but passes up as the thigh extension with no junction in 25%.
- The level at which the small saphenous vein joins a deep vein is variable. It is within the popliteal fossa in approximately two-thirds, usually 2–4 cm above the knee crease, but higher than this in some 25%, with the small saphenous joining the femoral, deep femoral or great saphenous veins. The junction

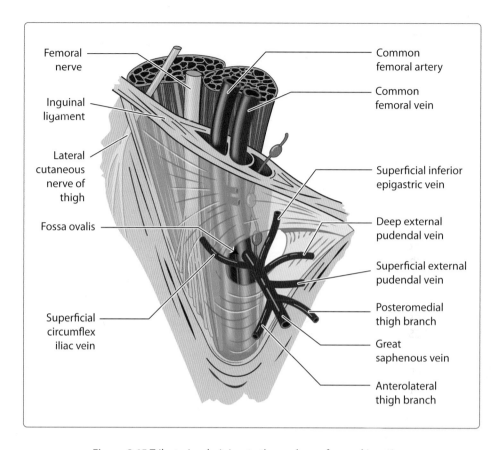

Figure 2.15 Tributaries draining to the sapheno-femoral junction.

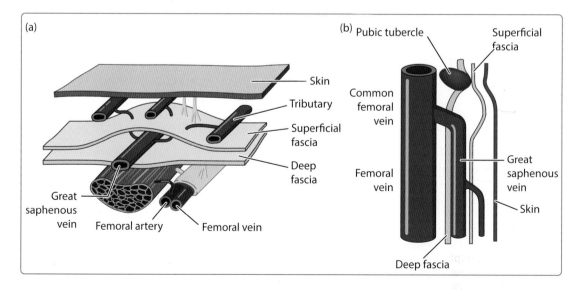

Figure 2.16 Relation of the great saphenous vein to the superficial fascia showing it in the saphenous compartment. (a) tangential view (b) anterior view.

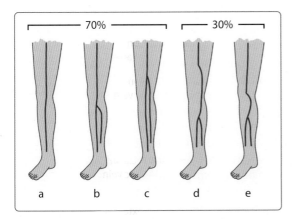

Figure 2.17 Variations of the great saphenous vein (GSV) in the distal thigh and calf. GSV present at the knee (70%): (a) no major tributaries; (b) major tributaries below the knee; (c) major tributary above the knee. GSV not present at the knee (30%); (d) absence of considerable length of GSV above the knee; (e) absence of short length of GSV at and below the knee.

is below the knee crease in <10%, usually joining the great saphenous or gastrocnemius veins.

- The small saphenous vein most often terminates on the posterior or postero-lateral

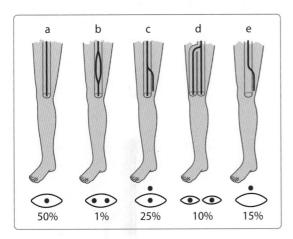

Figure 2.18 Variations of the great saphenous vein (GSV) in the thigh. GSV present to the knee: (a) no major tributaries; (b) GSV duplicated – one compartment – very uncommon; (c) major tributary that joins above the knee; (d) GSV duplicated – two compartments. GSV not present at the knee: (e) absence of variable length of GSV above knee.

aspect of the popliteal vein, but may terminate on either side or, rarely, at the front of the deep vein. It can terminate into a gastrocnemius vein.

Small saphenous vein

- The small saphenous vein begins behind the lateral malleolus as a continuation of the lateral marginal foot vein and passes to the popliteal fossa. It moves from a subcutaneous plane to become sub-fascial in a saphenous compartment at about mid-calf in most limbs. Duplication is very uncommon.
- A small saphenous artery is adjacent and usually posterolateral, but at varying positions in relation to the small saphenous vein, and it is at risk of being injected during treatment.

Thigh extension and vein of Giacomini*

- A thigh extension is the continuation of the small saphenous vein and is present in 95% of limbs.[13,14] It has its own fascial compartment and lies between the semitendinosus muscle medially and long head of biceps muscle laterally.
- There are various terminations of the thigh extension. It may:
  - continue straight up into the gluteal area as a single vein or divided into many deep and superficial tributaries
  - join the deep femoral vein as a posterior or posterolateral thigh perforator
  - divide into many muscular or subcutaneous branches on the posterior thigh
  - connect to the posterior thigh circumflex vein which then passes up to the great saphenous vein in the medial thigh, this complex of veins has been termed the vein of Giacomini
  - be a combination of the above terminations

---

* Carlo Giacomini (1840–1898), Professor of Anatomy, University of Turin, Italy.

Vein of the popliteal fossa

- The vein of the popliteal fossa or lateral popliteal perforator is a large tortuous vein coursing over the back of the knee and upper calf separate to the great or small saphenous veins.[15] It perforates the deep popliteal fascia and joins the popliteal vein above the sapheno-popliteal junction. Ultrasound shows it to be present in about 3%–5% of subjects and commonly affected by varicose disease.[16]

Perforating veins of the lower limb

- Perforators pass through the deep fascia to connect deep and superficial veins. Valves direct flow from superficial to deep, although some may allow bidirectional flow, or they may be absent.[4] There are 100 or more perforating veins in the lower limbs but only a few are clinically important. They are grouped into those of the thigh, knee, leg, ankle and foot.
- Thigh perforators are medial, anterior, lateral or posterior. Medial thigh perforators usually pass from the great saphenous to the femoral vein.
- Calf perforators are medial, anterior, lateral or posterior, and may join the great saphenous vein or the posterior arch vein, a posterior tributary previously called Leonardo's vein. Medial calf perforators connect to the great saphenous vein or major tributaries, pass deep to connect to tibial veins or to calf muscle venous plexuses, and are the most likely to be involved by disease.
- Foot perforators are dorsal, medial, lateral and planter. They are valveless or contain valves oriented from deep to superficial. The perforator of the first metatarsal interspace generally has a large diameter, is without valves, connects the dorsal venous arch with the deep plantar system, and is the true starting point of all venous networks in the foot. Medial marginal perforators open into the medial marginal vein to form plantar and dorsal veins. Lateral marginal perforators join the lateral marginal vein at a peri-malleolar plexus.

- Eponymous nomenclature is now discouraged, but time-honoured names for specific lower limb perforators are:
  - Hunterian – upper femoral canal
  - Dodd – lower femoral canal
  - Boyd – upper para-tibial
  - Cockett – lower posterior tibial
  - Sherman – lower para-tibial
  - Hach – posterolateral thigh
  - May – intergemellar
  - Bassi – para-Achilles
  - Gillot – medial gastrocnemial
  - Thierry – popliteal fossa

Valves in lower limb veins

- The presence and number of valves in veins of the lower limbs are:[5,6]
  - Common femoral vein – one or two in ≈70%.
  - Femoral vein – most often three, the most constant just below the junction with the deep femoral vein.
  - Popliteal vein – most often one to three.
  - Anterior tibial and peroneal veins – approximately 10 each.
  - Posterior tibial vein – up to 20.
  - Great saphenous vein – ≈5–10 evenly distributed above- and below-knee, with a terminal valve in 98%–99% and pre-terminal valve in 70%–85%, so that there are no valves at its termination in about 2%.
  - Small saphenous vein – ≈7–10, with a terminal valve in 95% and pre-terminal valve in only 64% of limbs with a sapheno-popliteal junction.
  - Perforating veins – one to five, with no valves in 25% in the leg and most in the foot, and all valves deep to the deep fascia.

Nerves related to lower limb veins[17]

- The femoral nerve lies well lateral to the common femoral vein and is at little risk of injury during treatment.
- The saphenous nerve branches from the femoral nerve in the femoral triangle then passes between the sartorius and gracilis muscles with the great saphenous vein down the thigh, then down the medial border of

tibia. It lies anterior to the great saphenous vein with a shared adventitia in the middle third of the leg in 60% of limbs and in the lower third in 85%.

- The common peroneal and posterior tibial nerves descend from the bifurcation of the sciatic nerve at the apex of the popliteal fossa or higher. The posterior tibial nerve supplies muscles of the posterior flexor compartment of the leg and the intrinsic plantar muscles of the foot, as well as sensation through the sural nerve. The common peroneal nerve supplies the extensor and peroneal muscle groups, as well as sensation from the front of the leg and the dorsum of the foot.
- The common peroneal nerve winds around the neck of the fibula where it is prone to injury. The average shortest distance between the small saphenous vein and nerves in the popliteal fossa is <5 mm to the posterior tibial and <15 mm to the common peroneal nerve, but either nerve can be as close as 1mm from the vein. The posterior tibial nerve can pass in front of or behind the small saphenous vein as it dives into the sapheno-politeal junction, and is very closely related to the gastrocnemius veins. These nerves are at high risk of injury during treatment for small saphenous disease, particularly behind the knee.
- The sural nerve is responsible for sensation from the posterolateral lower third of the calf and lateral side of the foot and fifth toe. It has a variable relation to the small saphenous vein, separated by fascia in the upper leg, but closely apposed distally. In approximately 60% of limbs, the vein is superficial to the nerve proximally, medial to the nerve in the middle third and lateral in the distal third of the leg. In some 30%, the vein is medial to the nerve throughout and in 10% it is lateral to the nerve. The distance between the small saphenous vein and sural nerve is <5 mm in 70% of limbs in the proximal one-third and <5 mm in 90% in the distal one-third. Thus, the nerve is at risk of damage during treatment, particularly for the distal vein.

2.4 Clinical relevance of lower limb veins

- The many variations in the presence and position of major superficial veins in the lower limbs makes it essential to map these prior to any intervention for treating venous disease.
- The position of the sapheno-femoral junction is reasonably constant, but the presence and position of the sapheno-popliteal junction is variable, requiring mapping by ultrasound prior to surgical intervention.
- Femoral vein duplication is often associated with deep venous reflux.
- The proximity of the common peroneal and posterior tibial nerves to the small saphenous vein behind the knee makes it essential to detect their position and protect them during endovenous or open surgical treatment. The proximity of the sural nerve to the small saphenous vein makes it essential to separate the two during endovenous thermal ablation.

Lymphatic system

Lymphatics

- Lymphatics commence in the superficial dermis but are not present in the epidermis (Figure 2.19). They form a network of blind-ended avalvular capillaries with diameters 20–70 μ, especially rich over the palm and fingers and the sole and toes. Lymphatics lie beneath mucosa and the serosal lining of body cavities and major organs. They absorb interstitial fluid through a porous endothelium.
- They drain to pre-collectors that are up to 300 μ diameter, and these contain valves, have some smooth muscle cells in their wall and drain to the subcutaneous plane.
- Subcutaneous lymph collecting vessels have a smooth muscle layer and are the vessels commonly identified as lymphatics. They are found in nearly every part of the body that contains blood vessels. Their intima consists

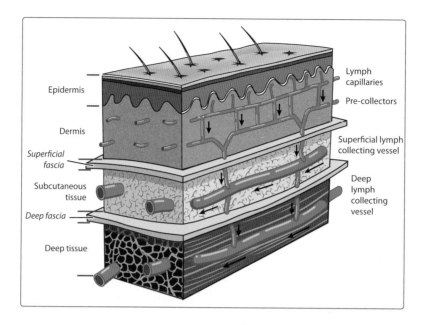

Figure 2.19 Schematic diagram of the relationship between the lymph capillaries, pre-collectors and lymph collecting vessels. Perforating lymphatics pass across the deep fascia allowing drainage to either superficial or deep lymph nodes.

of elongated endothelial cells supported on an elastic membrane, the media is composed of transverse smooth muscle and fine elastic fibers, and the adventitia consists of connective tissue intermixed with smooth muscle cells, fine blood vessels and a fine nerve plexus.

- Superficial lymphatic vessels in the limbs are situated immediately beneath the skin accompanying superficial veins. Perforators pass to deep lymphatic vessels through the deep fascia. Deep lymphatics are fewer in number but larger than superficial vessels, and they accompany deep blood vessels. Visceral lymphatics lie in the submucous areolar tissue throughout the length of the digestive, respiratory, genito-urinary tracts, subserous tissue of the thoracic and abdominal lining and even in the brain.
- Valves in lymphatic vessels resemble those in veins, though are closer together. A lymphatic vessel is dilated just distal to a valve giving it a beaded appearance, and the segments between valves are called lymphangions.
- The thoracic duct has a more complex structure tending towards that of an artery.

Lymph nodes

- A lymph node is normally <2 cm long and largely consists of lymphoid follicles through which lymph is filtered. There are some 500–600 lymph nodes, grouped in the inguinal region, pelvis, para-aortic space, mediastinum, axilla and neck.
- A lymph node has a capsule that leads to trabeculae dividing the node into follicles which contain sinusoids. A node has a cortex to which afferent lymphatics drain and a medulla that contains lymphoid tissue and which extends to the hilum, where efferent lymphatics leave. Blood vessels enter and leave at the hilum, but arterioles, capillaries and venules remain separate from lymph passing through sinusoids within the node.

Lower limb lymphatics and lymph nodes

- Superficial lower limb lymphatics consist of a larger medial group that follow the great saphenous vein and a smaller lateral group that follow the small saphenous vein.

- Deep lower limb lymphatics are just two or three vessels that run with each of the deep veins in the calf and femoral vein in the thigh. Deep lymphatics of the buttock follow gluteal blood vessels.
- Lower limb lymph nodes are a single anterior tibial node, six or seven popliteal nodes in the popliteal fossa, and 12–20 inguinal nodes in the femoral triangle. At a more proximal level are collections of iliac and para-aortic nodes.
- Lower limb lymphatics form a right and left lumbar lymphatic trunk, while vessels from the viscera form an intestinal lymphatic trunk, and these join to enter the cisterna chyli.

Cisterna chyli

- The cisterna chyli is situated to the right and behind the aorta at the right crus of the diaphragm. It is formed by the junction of the right and left lumbar and intestinal lymphatic trunks. It receives all lymph from the body except for that from the right upper quadrant, which goes to the right thoracic duct. Lumbar trunks are formed by the union of efferent vessels from the lateral aortic lymph glands. They receive lymph from the lower limbs, walls and viscera of the pelvis, kidneys and suprarenal glands and deep lymphatics from the abdominal wall. The intestinal trunk receives lymph from the stomach and intestine, pancreas and spleen, and lower and front part of the liver.

Thoracic duct

- The thoracic duct is 38–45 cm long in an adult and extends from the second lumbar vertebra to the base of neck (Figure 2.20). It passes through the aortic hiatus of the diaphragm and ascends through the posterior mediastinum between the aorta and azygos vein, lying on the vertebral column and behind the oesophagus.
- At the fifth thoracic vertebra, it inclines toward the left to pass through the superior mediastinum and behind the aortic arch and thoracic part of the left subclavian artery to enter the neck. It then arches just above the clavicle to cross anterior to the left subclavian artery to end by joining the junction of the left subclavian and internal jugular veins. It can comprise two vessels of unequal size and there may be variations in its termination. It is joined by the left jugular, subclavian and broncho-mediastinal trunks and receives several subsidiary trunks.

Right lymphatic duct

- The right lymphatic duct is about 1.5 cm long, courses along the medial border of the right scalenus anterior muscle at the base of neck and ends in the right subclavian vein at its angle of junction with the right internal jugular vein. It receives several subsidiary trunks which frequently open separately into the vein.
- The right lymphatic duct receives lymph from the right side of head and neck through the right jugular trunk, right upper extremity through the right subclavian trunk, right side of the thorax, right lung, right side of the heart and part of the convex surface of the liver through a brachio-cephalic trunk.

2.5 Clinical relevance of lymphatics

- Perforating lymphatics carry some lymph directly from superficial to deep lymphatics so that drainage can be to both superficial and deep lymph nodes. Tumour cells from a breast cancer can metastasize to internal mammary nodes rather than to the axillary sentinel node, resulting in false negative sentinel node biopsies.
- Indocyanine green lymphography (IGG) allows definition of lymphatic pathways prior to direct lymphatic surgery or to plan construction of plastic surgical flaps.
- Indocyanine green lymphography may also allow future mapping of lymphatic pathways to allow surgeons to better avoid damaging them by dissection during operations, for example in the inguinal or axillary regions.

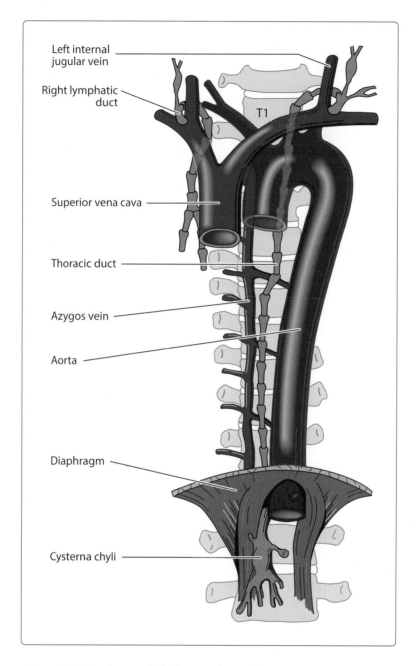

Figure 2.20 The cisterna chyli, thoracic duct and its termination in the neck.

History

- The Greek anatomists Erasistratus (304–250 BC) and Herophilos (335–280 BC) working in Alexandria carried out anatomical dissections to demonstrate the valves of the heart, to distinguish veins from arteries and to identify lymphatics.
- Hippocrates (460–370 BC) was one of the first to refer to lymph nodes, a Roman physician Rufus of Ephesus identified lymph nodes and the thymus in the late 1st century AD

and the Greek physician Galen (129–200) described the lacteals and mesenteric lymph nodes.

- The Persian philosopher Avicenna (980–1037) was one of the most influential figures of the Islamic Golden Age and wrote some 40 texts, including *The Book of Healing* and *The Canon of Medicine*. Included was a description of the saphenous vein from the Arabic 'safin' meaning 'deep or embedded'. Alternative explanations are from the Hebrew 'safoon' meaning 'hidden or covered' or Greek 'saphaina' meaning 'manifest or to be clearly seen'.

- Some of the first accurate drawings of venous anatomy were by Leonardo da Vinci (1452–1519), despite the absence of the posterior arch vein that was later to bear his name.

- Andreas Vesalius (1514–1564) from Brussels was the author of the influential book 'De Humani Corporis Fabrica' (*On the Fabric of the Human Body*) which included many observations regarding vascular anatomy, including venous valves.

- Venous valves were described by Giovanni Canano in 1540, Ludovicus Vassaeus in *Anatomen Corporis Humani Tabulae Quatuor* published in 1544 and by Sylvius Ambianis in 1555. Their function was identified by Andrea Cesalpino in *De re anatomica* in 1559: 'certain membranes placed at the openings of the vessels prevent the blood from returning'.[4]

- Gabriele Falloppio (1523–1562) described what are now known as lacteals; an Italian physician Gaspare Aselli (1581–1626) identified lacteals and the thoracic duct in dogs in 1622 and Johannes Veslingius (1598–1649) drew the earliest sketches of lacteals in humans in 1647. The Italian professor of anatomy Bartolomeo Eustachi (1513–1574) described the thoracic duct and azygos vein. A Swedish scientist Olaus Rudbeck (1630–1702) and Danish physician Thomas Bartholin (1616–1680) presented their descriptions of lymphatic vessels at about the same time.

- The Italian biologist and physician Marcello Malpighi (1628–1694), who invented the microscope while working in Bologna, was the first to demonstrate capillaries and show the link between arteries and veins that had eluded William Harvey.

References

1. Coleridge-Smith P, Labropoulos N, Partsch H, Myers K, Nicolaides A, Cavezzi A. Duplex ultrasound investigation of the veins in chronic venous disease of the lower limbs–UIP consensus document. Part I. Basic principles. *Eur J Vasc Endovasc Surg* 2006;31:83–92. http://www.ejves.com/article/S1078-5884(05)00540-X/fulltext

2. Cavezzi A, Labropoulos N, Partsch H, Ricci S, Caggiati A, Myers K, Nicolaides A, Smith PC. Duplex ultrasound investigation of the veins in chronic venous disease of the lower limbs--UIP consensus document. Part II. Anatomy. *Eur J Vasc Endovasc Surg* 2006;31:288–99. http://www.ejves.com/article/S1078-5884(05)00539-3/fulltext

3. Parsi K. Anatomy for the phlebologist. http://www.conferencematters.co.nz/pdf/ParsiAnatomy%20and%20physiology%202007.pdf

4. Suami H. Lymphosome concept: Anatomical study of the lymphatic system. *J Surg Oncol* 2017;115:13–17. https://www.ncbi.nlm.nih.gov/pubmed/27334241

5. Caggiati A. The venous valves of the lower limbs. *Phlebolymphology* 2013;20:87–95. http://www.phlebolymphology.org/the-venous-valves-of-the-lower-limbs/

6. Meissner MH. Lower extremity venous anatomy. *Semin Intervent Radiol* 2005;22;147–56. http://www.ncbi.nlm.nih.gov/pmc/articles/PMC3036282/

7. Kachlik D, Pechacek V, Musil V, Baca V. The venous system of the pelvis: New nomenclature. *Phlebology* 2010;25:162–73. https://www.researchgate.net/publication/45287854_The_venous_system_of_the_pelvis_New_nomenclature

8. Van Cleef J-F. Treatment of vulvar and perineal varicose veins. *Phlebolymphology* 2011;18:38–43. http://www.phlebolymphology.org/treatment-of-vulvar-and-perineal-varicose-veins/

9. Parsi K. Dermatological manifestations of venous disease. *Part II. Aust NZ J Phlebol* 2008;11:11–42. http://www.sydneyskinandvein.com.au/PDF_Uploads/42_DermManPart2.pdf

10. Ricci S. The venous system of the foot: Anatomy, physiology, and clinical aspects. *Phlebolymphology* 2015;22:64–75. http://www.phlebolymphology.org/the-venous-system-of-the-foot-anatomy-physiology-and-clinical-aspects/

11. Uhl JF, Gillot C, Chahim M. Anatomical variations of the femoral vein. *J Vasc Surg* 2010;52:714–9. https://www.researchgate.net/publication/45089610_Anatomical_variations_of_the_femoral_vein

12. Souroullas P, Barnes R, Smith G, Nandhra S, Carradice D, Chetter I. The classic sapheno-femoral junction and its anatomical variations. *Phlebology* 2016;27. Epub http://www.ncbi.nlm.nih.gov/pubmed/26924361

13. Georgiev M, Myers KA, Belcaro G. The thigh extension of the lesser saphenous vein: From Giacomini's observations to ultrasound scan imaging. *J Vasc Surg* 2003;37:558–63. http://www.ncbi.nlm.nih.gov/pubmed/12618692

14. Georgiev M, Myers KA, Belcaro G. Giacomini's observations on the superficial veins of the abdominal limb and principally the external saphenous. *Int Angiol* 2001;20:225–33. https://www.ncbi.nlm.nih.gov/pubmed/?term=Giacomini%27s+observations+on+the+superficial+veins+of+the+abdominal+limb+and+principally+the+external+saphenous

15. Delis KT, Knaggs AL, Hobbs JT, Vandendriessche MA. The nonsaphenous vein of the popliteal fossa: Prevalence, patterns of reflux, hemodynamic quantification, and clinical significance. *J Vasc Surg* 2006;44:611–9. http://www.ncbi.nlm.nih.gov/pubmed/16950443

16. Uhl JF, Gillot C. Anatomy and embryology of the small saphenous vein: Nerve relationships and implications for treatment. *Phlebology* 2013;28:4–15. https://www.ncbi.nlm.nih.gov/pubmed/23256200

3 Physiology of veins and lymphatics

> This chapter refers to an evaluation of venous haemodynamics prepared on behalf of the Union Internationale de Phlebologie.[1]

The chapter will discuss fluid hydrodynamics, venous physiology in general, and lower limb veins, the vein wall, lymphatics and the microcirculation.

Ideal flow in a rigid hollow tube

- Laws relating to flow in a tube have been extensively studied.[2] In general, they assume that the tube is rigid, flow velocity is constant with no energy loss along its length, and fluid is incompressible and has constant viscosity relative to flow (Newtonian*). This is very different to blood flow in veins, with their branching network of pliable vessels joining at random angles. However, the laws of hydrodynamics form a starting point to understanding vascular physiology.

Steady state laminar flow in a tube

- Flow is proportional to cross-sectional area or radius such that

$$Q = v \cdot A \text{ or } v = \frac{Q}{A} = \frac{Q}{\pi r^2}$$

where Q is the flow (mL/s), A is the cross-sectional area (cm^2), v is the velocity (cm/s) and r is the internal radius (cm).

- Resistance to flow is given by Poiseuille's equation[†]

$$R = \frac{\Delta P}{Q} = \frac{(8\eta L)}{(\pi r^4)}$$

where ΔP is the pressure gradient between two points, Q is the flow (mL/s), R is resistance, η is the coefficient of viscosity (poise), L is the length (cm) and r is the radius (cm).

Energy and pressure for flow in a tube

- The driving force for flow is determined by its potential energy (PE) and kinetic energy (KE).
- PE is the latent capacity to do work and results in pressure variations depending on the position of the part in relation to the effect of gravity (Figure 3.1):

$$PE = \rho g h$$

where ρ is the fluid density, g is the acceleration due to gravity and h is the height of the tube.
- KE is energy resulting from the fact that fluid is flowing and that flow increases where a tube narrows

$$KE = \frac{1}{2}mv^2$$

where m is mass and v is the flow velocity.

---

* Sir Isaac Newton (1642–1726), English physicist and mathematician.

† Jean-Louis-Marie Poiseuille (1799–1869), French physician and physiologist.

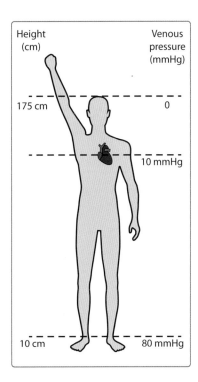

Figure 3.1 Potential energy. Fluid flows from a low pressure (high PE) at the heart to a high pressure (low PE) at the feet. 1 mmHg = 1.36 cm water.

- Assuming conservation of energy, pressures at two points (1 and 2) along a tube are indicated by Bernoulli's equation*

$$P_1 + \rho g h_1 + \frac{1}{2}\rho v_1^2 = P_2 + \rho g h_2 + \frac{1}{2}\rho v_2^2 \text{ or}$$

$$\Delta P = \rho g(h_2 - h_1) + \frac{1}{2}\rho(v_2^2 - v_1^2)$$

- The pressure (p – kPa) within a cylindrical tube results from tension in the wall as determined by the Laplace equation†

$$P = \frac{\gamma}{r}$$

where γ is the wall tension (kg/cm²) and r is the radius (mm).

---

* Daniel Bernoulli (1700–1782), a second-generation member of a Swiss family of 12 eminent mathematicians.
† Pierre-Simon, Marquis de Laplace (1749–1827), French scholar.

Turbulence within a tube

- Disturbed flow at a high velocity causes turbulence with chaotic fluid movements, considerable energy loss and fall in pressure that is not regained. The point at which flow breaks up is defined by Reynold's number‡ (R_e)

$$R_e = \frac{v d \rho}{\eta}$$

where d is the diameter (cm), v is the velocity (cm/s), ρ is the fluid density (gm/cm³ = 1.056 for blood) and η is the coefficient of viscosity (poise). Laminar flow transitions to turbulent flow in rigid tubes with Reynolds numbers between 2000 and 4000.

Blood flow in veins

- The venous system acts as a reservoir with variable capacity and normally holds about 60% of the total resting blood volume. Veins provide passive conduits for blood flow at low pressure and velocity.

Distribution of venous volume

- On standing, 300 mL or more of blood shifts to the abdomen and lower limbs. Within seconds, pressure receptors in the heart, lungs, carotid sinus and aortic arch mediate a sympathetic response to cause vasoconstriction of capacitance and arteriolar vessels and increased cardiac output. This normally stabilizes the circulation within about 60 seconds with a heart rate increased by about 10–15 beats/min, diastolic pressure increased by about 10 mmHg and with little change in systolic pressure.[3]

Regulation of venous pressure

- Several energy sources provide the pressure to cause blood to return from the periphery to the heart. The pressure within the lumen acts against the tone of the vein wall and pressure in surrounding tissues so that forward flow

---

‡ Osborne Reynolds (1842–1912), British engineer and physicist.

occurs against the hydrostatic pressure due to gravity, particularly when standing.

Vis a tergo and vis a fronte

- The *vis a tergo* (force acting from the rear) is the pressure exerted through the capillary circulation which is 12–18 mmHg on the venous side of the capillary. This acts against the *vis a fronte* (right atrial pressure) which is 4–7 mmHg, resulting in a weak pressure gradient for venous return. Normally, the result is constant forward flow, with any tendency to reflux being prevented by venous valves.
- Pulsatile right atrial contractions cause transient increase in venous pressure and arrest of flow which is restored as the atrium relaxes, although the effect is only observed in central veins.

Vein wall tension

- Intrinsic vein wall tension depends on both its passive rigidity and active vein wall tone. Venous smooth muscle tone is controlled by sympathetic adrenergic nerve activity, circulating vasoactive substances and local metabolites. Flow in superficial veins is increased by vasodilatation with heat or exercise and reduced by vasoconstriction caused by cold.
- Large veins form a capacitance system and can store blood with little change in transmural pressure. This reservoir of blood can be mobilized when needed by increasing tone in the venous wall. Smaller veins express more variable tone, with transmural pressure controlled by intrinsic and extrinsic neuro-humoral responses.
- The resultant intraluminal lateral (parietal) pressure is determined by the volume of blood within the veins.

Hydrostatic pressure

- If all valves are open, then the hydrostatic pressure at any point results from the weight of the column of blood from the level of the right atrium above the point, and varies according to the body's shape and position. The difference between the actual venous

pressure and hydrostatic pressure is the *hydraulic pressure*.
- If valves close, then the column is broken up into segments with lower hydrostatic pressure in each. Because there are many connections between veins with low resistance to flow, the venous pressure at rest is identical in all veins in the same horizontal plane.

Interstitial pressure

- Interstitial pressure is normally low. However, an increase in interstitial fluid volume causes variable increase in interstitial pressure, depending on how rigidly the structure is enclosed. For example, pressure increases rapidly in the brain or kidney but less so in most soft tissues. The deep fascia in the limbs restricts expansion of deep tissues and veins so that injury or any other cause of inflammatory swelling can compromise the circulation by causing a 'compartment syndrome'.

Thoraco-abdominal pressure

- In a steady state, intra-thoracic pressure at rest is lower and intra-abdominal pressure is higher than atmospheric pressure, and both can have a profound effect on venous flow. There are phasic variations of flow with respiration in proximal veins in the limbs, but this is usually lost in distal veins.
- Intra-thoracic pressure changes with respiration causing opposite effects in the upper and lower limbs. Inspiration decreases intra-thoracic pressure increasing the pressure gradient and venous drainage from veins and lymphatics of the upper limbs to central veins. However, as the diaphragm descends, it increases the intra-abdominal pressure causing flow from veins and lymphatics in the lower limbs to slow. The reverse occurs during expiration, when lower limb flow increases.
- Obesity results in an increased intra-abdominal pressure by up to 20 mmHg. Straining or the Valsalva manoeuvre[*] increases the

---

[*] Antonio Maria Valsalva (1666–1723), Professor of Anatomy at Bologna, Italy.

intra-abdominal pressure by up to 50 mmHg, sufficient for venous and lymphatic flow from all limbs to slow or stop.

3.1 Determinants of venous pressure

- Vis a tergo and vis a fronte
- Venous tone
- Hydrostatic pressure
- Interstitial pressure
- Thoraco-abdominal pressure.

Venous compliance and resistance

- Volume and pressure in veins changes under different conditions which can be plotted as a graph (Figure 3.2). Veins collapse at a low transmural pressure to form an ellipse and there is minimal stretch of the vein wall so that large changes in venous volume result in only small increments in transmural pressure. As the vein fills, the venous cross-section becomes circular and the wall stretches, so that small changes in volume eventually result in a considerable increase in venous pressure.
- The compliance is the slope of a tangent at any point on the pressure–volume curve.

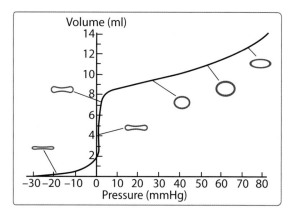

Figure 3.2 Pressure/volume relationships in a vein. There is minimal change in pressure in the initial stage of filling until the vein becomes elliptical, but the pressure then progressively rises as the vein fills and becomes circular.

Resistance to flow is low at high pressure when the veins are distended.
- After emptying veins with passive or active movement, it normally takes three to five minutes for arterial inflow to refill them. After exertion stops, valves float open and the column of blood again becomes continuous.

Venous blood flow

- Flow velocity in a vein is inversely proportional to the cross-sectional area (the Castelli equation[*]), and at rest is greatest in large veins such as the vena cava and, at times, non-existent in smaller veins of the limbs. This makes small veins in the dependent lower limbs more susceptible to venous thrombosis at rest, though muscle contraction quickly reverses this situation.
- Flow velocity and direction in any vein are affected by the Venturi effect[†], with increased pressures causing forward flow in some and lower pressures leading to retrograde flow in others.

Venous valves

- Venous valves are present in peripheral superficial and deep veins and in most perforating veins, and become more numerous as the distance from the central circulation increases. 'Micro-valves' in collecting venules and small veins act to prevent reflux to the capillary bed.
- Valves are not just passive flaps but also actively control flow by smooth muscle contraction at the base of the cusps. Opening and closing of valves influence venous blood flow.[4] The opening phase lasts approximately 0.25 s, but the cusps stop at about 65% open, causing flow to accelerate and form a jet. There is then an equilibrium phase of approximately 0.65 s, and flow splits into two streams at each valve cusp, with part directed into the valve sinus, forming

---

[*] Benedetto Castelli (1578–1643), an Italian physicist who worked in Pisa and Rome.
[†] Giovanni Battista Venturi (1746–1822), an Italian physicist working at the University of Modena.

a vortex along and behind the valve cusp which helps to prevent stagnation inside the valve pocket.

- Valve closure normally occurs in <0.5 s, so that there is a brief physiological reflux as pressure within the sinus forces the leaflets of the valve back together.

Lower limb veins

- Valves are open most of the time, both in normal subjects and in those with venous disease. Blood is usually flowing in a cephalad direction at rest and when there is skeletal muscle contraction, but not during extreme straining when there is an increased intra-abdominal pressure. Pressure at the foot is 80–100 mmHg when standing in the resting position, and the pressure at the groin is 30–40 mmHg in an individual of average height.
- When lying, sitting or standing still, veins gradually fill from below, all valves are open so that there is a continuous column of blood, valves do not interfere with the hydrostatic pressure and blood velocity is often less than 1 cm/s.
- A veno-arteriolar reflex results in arteriolar vasoconstriction if the local venous pressure is increased by 40 mmHg or more, which helps to minimize oedema.

3.2 Normal ankle venous pressures

- Supine – 10–12 mmHg
- Sitting – 50–60 mmHg
- Standing – 80–90 mm Hg
- Walking – 20–30 mm Hg

Venous pumps

- Lower limb skeletal muscular contraction during walking causes compression of veins in the foot, calf and thigh in sequence to act as a 'second heart'.[5] This results from direct compression of intramuscular veins or pressure on axial veins against adjacent rigid structures such as bone. Lower limb muscle contraction can be referred to as *muscle systole* and relaxation as *muscle diastole*.

Foot and distal calf pump

- The venous foot pump is activated during each step by compression caused by body weight and by plantar muscle contraction (Figure 3.3). The lateral plantar veins contain 20–30 mL of blood. During walking, the foot is in contact with the ground for 60% of the time with weight taken on the metatarsal heads, heel and lateral plantar surface, but not on the medial part, except in subjects with flat feet. The tarsal arch is flattened, veins are stretched and blood ejected as a high-speed jet from the lateral plantar veins to the smaller diameter distal posterior tibial veins. Muscles also contract as the toes curl contributing to emptying of the veins. Veins refill when the foot is off the ground.
- A small volume is expelled from marginal veins into the great saphenous vein and connecting peroneal and anterior tibial veins and this is significantly increased if the calf deep veins are overloaded.

Calf muscle pump

- As the leg is lifted, the ankle dorsiflexes, the calf muscles and Achilles tendon are stretched and the muscles descend within the deep fascia like a piston, and this empties blood from the distal posterior tibial and peroneal veins towards the popliteal vein (Figure 3.4). As the foot again strikes the ground, weight-bearing activates the foot pump to refill the veins.
- Calf muscle pumping is activated by plantar-flexion as the foot comes up on its toes. Gastrocnemius and soleus muscles contract to empty the extensive intramuscular venous sinuses. Muscle contraction also squeezes the axial calf veins to propel blood upwards. The pressure gradient closes the closest distal valve during muscle systole. This is the most active component of the venous pump and intramuscular pressures

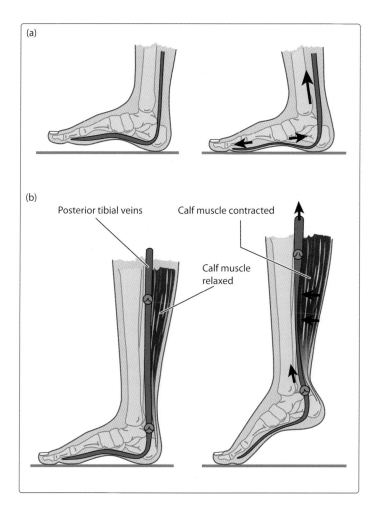

Figure 3.3 The pumping mechanism from foot and distal calf veins with walking. (a) Taking a step empties blood into the distal calf veins. (b) Calf muscle contraction forces the muscles distally in a piston fashion to propel blood up into proximal calf veins.

rise to more than 200 mmHg with a strong contraction to empty some 60–150 mL of blood from the calf to the thigh.

- Relaxation as the other leg takes its step allows venous pressure to fall in the deep calf veins, but less so in superficial veins and very little in the popliteal vein. Blood flows from superficial to deep calf veins through perforators. The pressure gradient closes the closest proximal valve during muscle diastole.

Thigh muscle pump

- Contraction of the semimembranosus muscle in particular pumps blood from the deep femoral vein into the common femoral vein, the amount depending on the intra-abdominal pressure.

Volume and pressure changes after exercise

- Volume changes in lower limb veins can be measured after moderate exercise using air plethysmography (see Chapter 10). Continuing exercise empties some two-thirds of the resting venous volume.
- Exercise causes the venous pressure in a dorsal foot vein to decrease by approximately 60 mmHg to reach a steady state after about

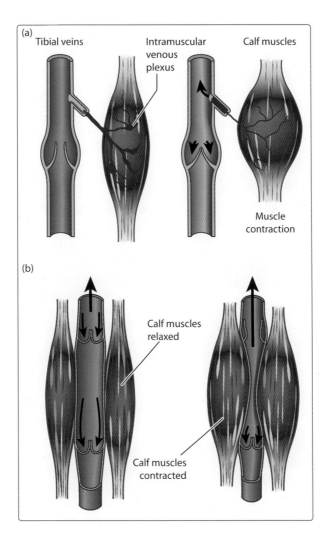

Figure 3.4 The pumping mechanism from calf veins with walking. (a) Calf muscle contraction squeezes blood out of calf muscle sinuses into axial calf veins. (b) These are compressed in turn to propel blood out of the limb, with reflux prevented by distal valve closure.

3–12 steps depending on the walking speed. This reduces the hydrostatic pressure from 80–90 mmHg to 25–30 mmHg (see Chapter 10). Pressure normally returns to the resting level within about 30 seconds after exercise has ended.

The vein wall and circulating mediators

- From inside to outside, the vein wall consists of endothelium, sub-endothelial basement membrane, media and adventitia, and each contains extracellular matrix.

Endothelium

- Transport mechanisms carry essential metabolites across endothelial cells.[6] Small molecules such as water and electrolytes cross the capillary membrane through pores, larger molecules such as proteins are taken up and transferred through intimal cells by pino-cytosis, and larger macromolecules readily pass through 80–100 μ gaps called fenestrae. Otherwise, the endothelium is a barrier to free passage of macromolecules and cells from blood to the underlying interstitium.

- The glycocalyx is a layer on the surface of endothelial cells approximately 10μ thick which produces many chemical factors responsible for regulating thrombosis and fibrinolysis, angiogenesis, vasomotor function and vascular repair, and which provides a barrier to filtration of larger molecules.
- The endothelium produces and reacts to:
  - Vasodilator and vasoconstrictor factors involved in regulation of vascular tone.
  - Agents involved in inflammation and immunity.
  - Procoagulant and antithrombotic factors that regulate haemostasis (see Chapter 20).

Smooth muscle and vasomotor function

- Vascular smooth muscle function is controlled by humoral and sympathetic nervous mechanisms.[7] Local neural sympathomimetic control through noradrenergic receptors can be over-ridden by central or presynaptic control. Smooth muscle cell vasomotor function is mediated by $\alpha 1$ and $\alpha 2$ adrenergic receptors.
- Smooth muscle cell contraction is stimulated through surface receptors to release Ca^{2+} from the intracellular sarcoplasmic reticulum. This initiates activation of the contractile proteins myosin and actin through several enzymes including myosin phosphatase. Ca^{2+} enters the cells through Ca^{2+} ion channels to replenish the stores. There is underlying baseline vasoconstrictor tone. Agonists such as noradrenaline, angiotensin II and endothelin bind to surface receptors to initiate enzymatic activation and contraction. Smooth muscle relaxation results from removal of the contractile stimulus or by an agent that stimulates inhibition of the contractile mechanism, by decreased intracellular Ca^{2+} or increased myosin phosphatase activity.

Adventitia

- The vascular adventitia is composed of various cells including fibroblasts, immunomodulatory dendritic cells and macrophages, progenitor cells, vasa vasorum endothelial cells and pericytes, and adrenergic nerves.[8] Even adventitial cells influence smooth muscle function and control inflammation in the media in response to vascular stress or injury.

Extracellular matrix

- The extracellular matrix (ECM) is present in each layer of the wall and forms more than one-half of the vein wall mass.[9] It contains a complex of glycoproteins embedded in a ground substance of glycosaminoglycans and proteoglycans. Glycoproteins consist of carbohydrate chains joined to polypeptide side-chains by glycosylation. Glycosaminoglycans are long unbranched polysaccharides and attract water to form a lubricant in the extracellular matrix. Proteoglycans are heavily glycosylated proteins that contribute to the bulk of the ECM. Fibronectin is a glycoprotein produced by SMCs and fibroblasts, and it plays a role in cell migration, growth, differentiation and adhesion, controls other matrix proteins including collagen-I and collagen-III, and is involved in coagulation.
- The ECM contains collagen and elastin. Mature elastin is an insoluble protein that is the most durable element of ECM, with a half-life of some 40 years, but fibres degrade and fragment with age leading to increased stiffness of the wall. Elastin inhibits SMC migration and proliferation.

Adhesion molecules

- Protein adhesion molecules on cell surfaces bind cells together or to the extracellular matrix. Integrins mediate cell interactions with collagen, fibrinogen, fibronectin and vitronectin in the ECM and influence cell apoptosis, differentiation and survival. Selectins bind carbohydrates such as mucins and are endothelial- (E-selectin), leukocyte- (L-selectin) or platelet- (P-selectin) derived.

Inflammatory mediators

- Many agents influence inflammation at the vessel wall. Plasma-derived mediators include bradykinin, the complement system and coagulation factors. Cell-derived mediators include leukotrienes which are synthesized in white cells from arachidonic acid, as are prostaglandins, and interleukin, which is produced by macrophages and endothelial cells.

Integrins

- Matrix receptors termed integrins detect changes in matrix rigidity and composition and are responsible for tissue remodelling. They control SMCs and fibroblasts to maintain cell numbers and activities through collagen and fibronectin but not elastin. In contrast, interstitial matrix proteins such as collagen-I, collagen-III, fibronectin and osteopontin enhance SMC growth. Inhibiting the integrins that bind to these interstitial matrix proteins blocks SMC proliferation occurring in response to growth factors.

Matrix metalloproteinases

- Matrix metalloproteinases (MMPs) are a group of enzymes that break down constituents in the ECM, as well as affect smooth muscle and endothelial cells. Some 14 MMPs have been identified in blood vessels. They are produced in a relatively inactive form and are normally controlled by their endogenous tissue inhibitors (TIMPs) to result in connective tissue homeostasis. An MMP/TIMP imbalance can result in breakdown of elastin and collagen.

Cytokines

- Cytokines are proteins released predominantly by helper T-cells and macrophages. They have a specific effect on interactions between cells to modulate immune reactions, particularly B-cells, T-cells, macrophages, mast cells, neutrophils, basophils and eosinophils. They act through receptors and normally control the balance between humoral and cell-based immune responses, and regulate the development of different cell populations. They are different to hormones and growth factors.
- Cytokines are either anti- or pro-inflammatory. Anti-inflammatory cytokines promote healing and reduce inflammation, whereas pro-inflammatory cytokines, though necessary for healing, generally make disease worse and can cause auto-immune conditions.
    - Anti-inflammatory cytokines that regulate this response include interleukin (IL)-1 receptor antagonist, IL-4, IL-10, IL-11, and IL-13.
    - Pro-inflammatory cytokines include interleukins (IL-1β, IL-6) and tumour necrosis factor (TNF-α). IL-1β is released primarily by monocytes, macrophages, fibroblasts and endothelial cells during cell injury, infection and inflammation. Once released, they induce a cascade of further cytokine production.
    - Various cytokines termed chemokines induce activation and migration of leukocytes. They include monocyte chemoattractant protein (MCP-1), monocyte inflammatory protein (MIP-1α, MIP-1β) and growth related oncogene (GRO/KC).
- TNFα, IFN-γ enhance cellular immune response while IL-4, IL-10 and IL-13 enhance antibody responses.

Growth factors

- Growth factors are produced from endothelial and smooth muscle cells. Vascular endothelial growth factors (VEGF) promote angiogenesis, attract leukocytes and cause vasodilation. Platelet-derived growth factors (PDGF) and fibroblast growth factors (FGF) are also involved.
- Reduced shear stress with venous stasis at the vein wall produces transforming growth factor beta (TGF-β), which is multifunctional. TGF-β1 is a key factor in vascular remodelling by decreasing protease activity while increasing protease inhibitor activity and collagen synthesis.

Microcirculation

- Arterioles contain vascular smooth muscle and are the major site for control of systemic vascular resistance. Meta-arterioles and precapillary sphincters determine whether a capillary is open or closed. Smooth muscle in their walls contract and relax regularly, termed vaso-motion, resulting in variable capillary flow. In resting skeletal muscle, the smooth musculature causes many capillaries to be closed until they open in response to local changes and stimuli, such as the release of vasodilator metabolites with exercise. This offers the potential for a large reserve capacity for additional flow.

Diffusion

- Very large volumes of water containing small molecules diffuse in both directions across capillary membranes. Diffusion is defined by Fick's law*. *Flux* across a membrane is directly proportional to the concentration difference $(C_2 - C_1)$ and surface area (A) of the membrane and inversely proportional to its thickness (t), with a constant of proportionality (k) as a measure of membrane permeability

$$Flux = \frac{k \cdot A(C_2 - C_1)}{t}$$

Filtration

- Smaller volumes of water pass through the capillary wall by filtration due to a difference between the balance of hydrostatic pressure exerted on the capillary wall by the interstitial fluid and blood volume, and the balance of the opposing oncotic pressures on either side of the capillary wall caused by plasma proteins in the blood and the interstitium.
- These pressures change along the capillary causing net outward flow at the arterial end and net inward flow at the venous end. This is based on Starling's law.† The forces are:

- hydrostatic pressures in the capillary (P_c) and interstitium (P_i)
- oncotic pressures in the capillary (p_c) and interstitium(P_i)
- The net fluid *flux* depends on:
  - a reflection coefficient – (k_1)
  - a filtration coefficient – (k_2)

so that

$$Flux = k_1(P_c - P_i) - k_2(p_c - p_i)$$

- Starling's Law is a convenient tool, but it assumes semipermeable membranes and does not account for active transport, fenestrae and the nature of the glycocalyx. The glycocalyx results in an increase in interstitial fluid plasma protein concentration and lower than expected lymph formation.[10]

Viscosity

- A fluid is 'Newtonian' if its viscosity is constant for different rates of shear, whereas the viscosity of a non-Newtonian fluid varies with the rate of shear. Non-Newtonian fluids that become thinner and less viscous as they are stirred are termed thixotropic. Water is Newtonian but blood is non-Newtonian and thixotropic.
- Blood viscosity is determined by plasma viscosity, haematocrit and the mechanical properties of red blood cells. Plasma viscosity is determined by plasma protein concentration and types. Haematocrit has the strongest impact on whole blood viscosity, and an increase to 60%–70%, as occurs in polycythaemia, can cause blood viscosity to become ten times that of water, causing greatly increased resistance to flow and decreased oxygen delivery. High concentrations of leukocytes, platelets or fibrinogen increase the viscosity.

Lymphatic drainage

- Plasma consisting of fluid and proteins is filtered from blood in capillaries into the interstitium.[11] For the whole body, there is outward filtration of some 20 L and inward shift of some 17 L per day. The remaining 3 L

---

* Adolf Eugen Fick (1821–1901), German Physiologist, Universities of Zurich and Wurzburg.
† Ernest Henry Starling (1866–1927), Professor of Physiology, University College, London.

stays in the interstitium and is drained by the lymphatic system. Failure to remove excess or increased outward filtration results in oedema. Lymph resembles blood plasma, but is more dilute, with a specific gravity of about 1.015, due to lack of fibrinogens and globulins.

- The lymphatic system has no central pump. However, collecting lymphangions are able to contract due to smooth muscle in their wall, with flow aided by adjacent muscle contraction, arterial pulsations, changes in abdominal and thoracic pressures with the respiratory cycle, and changes in posture. Smooth muscle in conducting lymphatics usually contract at 6–10 cycles per minute in sequence so that when one lymphangion contracts the next most proximal one dilates. Lymph flows at around 125 ml/hour, and this rate may be increased ten-fold during exercise and through infections. Numerous valves at about 1 mm intervals ensure centripetal lymph flow with no reflux. However, lymphatics can fail for similar reasons to veins.

- Lymphatics transport tissue fluid together with proteins, adipogenic and inflammatory signaling molecules, antigens, antigen-presenting cells, bacteria and particulate matter through regional lymph nodes. Small intestinal lacteals pass to lymphatics in the mesentery to transport longer-chain fatty acids and fats as chyle from the digestive system.

Immunology

- Protection against foreign substances and organisms is provided by both the innate and adaptive or acquired immune systems.

- The innate immune system is non-specific in its response, which involves antimicrobial peptides, complement activation, antigen presentation and recruitment of leukocytes to remove foreign substances using cytokines. The complement cascade is a series of activated proteins which trigger pathogen opsonization and lysis, inflammatory cell recruitment and neutralization of antigen-antibody complexes.

- The adaptive or acquired immune system relies on lymphocyte memory of prior antigen exposure to generate both cellular and humoral responses. T-lymphocytes are activated when an antigen is presented to a major histocompatibility complex receptor, while B-lymphocytes already have the antibody to such an antigen on their surface. The commonest antigen-presenting cells are dendritic cells, macrophages and B-cells. T-helper cells are crucial for activating and regulating the immune response.

- Basic testing of immune function typically involves a white blood cell count and T-lymphocyte count, HIV screening, serum protein and immuno-electrophoresis for immunoglobulin levels. Complement testing can be used to help diagnose the cause of recurrent microbial infections, angioedema and autoimmune diseases such as collagen diseases, glomerulonephritis, serum sickness and vasculitis.

History

- An early reference to the human circulation is from documents attributed to Indian scholars from about 400 BC, one stating that 'The blood [Rasa] is first ejected out of the heart, it is then distributed to all parts of the body, and thereafter it returns back to the heart through the blood vessels [Sirah]'.

- The philosopher Empedocles of Agrigentum in Sicily (490–430 BC) proposed that the heart was the centre of the circulation, although Hippocrates (460–370 BC) considered that all veins arose in the liver.

- Galen (129–216) believed in two different types of blood flow: venous blood generated in the liver from ingested food then carried from the right ventricle to the lesser organs where it is consumed and converted into body mass, and arterial blood that originates from the left ventricle and is infused with air from the lungs then carried to the higher organs such as the brain.

- Andreas Rhazes (854–925), a Persian physician and philosopher, refuted the traditional concept of circulating humours. Haly Abbas (died 982–994), also a Persian physician most famous for the *Complete Book of the Medical Art*, provided a rudimentary concept of the capillary system.

- Andrea Cesalpino (1519–1603), a physician and philosopher working in Rome, identified the function of valves, centripetal flow in veins and the probable presence of capillaries.
- Ibn al-Nafis, a physician in Damascus in the 12th century, was the first to describe the pulmonary circulation. The Spaniard Michael Servetus (1511–1553) also described the pulmonary circulation, which contributed to his being burnt to death for heresy.
- William Harvey (1578–1657) in *De Motu Cordis* ('On the Motion of the Heart and Blood') was the first to completely describe the systemic circulation and properties of blood being pumped to the brain and body by the heart. His experiments indicated the possible existence of capillaries, despite not being able to see them due to technical limitations. It was not until the 1800s that his work gained wide acceptance.
- Richard Lower (1631–1691), an English physician known for his works on the function of the cardiopulmonary system (*Tractatus de Corde*), described *vis a tergo* in 1670. The Italian anatomist Antonio Maria Valsalva (1666–1723) described the changes in blood flow in the limbs resulting from respiration causing *vis a fronte* in 1710.
- Alexander Monro (1733–1817) of the University of Edinburgh Medical School was the first to describe the function of the lymphatic system in detail.

References

1. Lee BB, Nicolaides AN, Myers K, Meissner M, Kalodiki E, Allegra C, Antignani PL. Venous hemodynamic changes in lower limb venous disease: The UIP consensus according to scientific evidence. *Int Angiol* 2016;35:236–352. http://www.ncbi.nlm.nih.gov/pubmed/27013029

2. Braithwaite J. An introduction to hydrodynamics. 2011 https://astro.uni-bonn.de/~jonathan/misc/hydro_notes.pdf

3. Lamarre-Cliché M, Cusson J. The fainting patient: Value of the head-upright tilt-table test in adult patients with orthostatic intolerance. *CMAJ* 2001;164:372–376. http://www.ncbi.nlm.nih.gov/pmc/articles/PMC80733/

4. Lurie F, Kistner RL, Eklof B, Kessler D. Mechanism of venous valve closure and role of the valve in circulation: A new concept. *J Vasc Surg* 2003;38:955–961. http://www.jvascsurg.org/article/S0741-5214(03)00711-0/abstract

5. Ricci S. The venous system of the foot: Anatomy, physiology, and clinical aspects. *Phlebolymphology* 2015;22:64–75. http://www.phlebolymphology.org/the-venous-system-of-the-foot-anatomy-physiology-and-clinical-aspects/

6. Galley HF, Webster NR. Physiology of the endothelium. *Br J Anaes* 2004;93:105–113. https://academic.oup.com/bja/article/93/1/105/265701/Physiology-of-the-endothelium

7. Webb RC. Smooth muscle contraction and relaxation. *Advances Physiol Educ* 2003;27:201–206. http://advan.physiology.org/content/27/4/201

8. Stenmark KR, Yeager ME, El Kasmi KC, Nozik-Grayck E, Gerasimovskaya EV, Li M, Riddle SR, Frid MG. The adventitia: Essential regulator of vascular wall structure and function. *Annu Rev Physiol* 2013;75:23–47. https://www.ncbi.nlm.nih.gov/pubmed/23216413

9. Xu J, Shib GP. Vascular wall extracellular matrix proteins and vascular diseases. *Biochim Biophys Acta* 2014;1842:2106–2119. http://www.sciencedirect.com/science/article/pii/S0925443914002191

10. Levick JR, Michel CC. Microvascular fluid exchange and the revised Starling principle. *Cardiovasc Res* 2010;87:198–210. https://academic.oup.com/cardiovascres/article/87/2/198/442215/Microvascular-fluid-exchange-and-the-revised

11. Stücker O, Pons-Himbert C, Laemmel E. Towards a better understanding of lymph circulation. *Phlebolymphology* 2008;15:31–36. http://www.phlebolymphology.org/towards-a-better-understanding-of-lymph-circulation/

Application of these principles will be discussed in later chapters.

Ultrasound

- Sound waves consist of alternating cycles of compression and rarefaction in a medium (Figure 4.1).[1-4] The *frequency* is the number of cycles per second (1 Hertz (Hz) = 1 cycle/second). The range of human hearing is from about 20 Hz to 20 kHz. Ultrasound is high-frequency sound >20 kHz and the frequencies used for clinical diagnosis are 2–20 MHz.
- Other characteristics of sound waves are:
  - *Period* – time for one cycle (s).
  - *Wavelength* – length of one cycle (mm).
  - *Velocity* – speed of sound wave propagation (cm/s).
  - *Amplitude* – peak amount of energy in a sound wave.
  - *Power* – rate of energy transfer (watts (W)).
  - *Intensity* – power/area (W/m^2).

Behaviour of ultrasound waves

- All modes for diagnostic ultrasound are based on the *pulse–echo principle*. A transducer generates ultrasound pulses which are transmitted into tissues and echoes are detected as they return to the transducer. The amplitude of a detected echo relates to the tissues examined. The depth of tissue producing each echo is determined by measuring the time between pulse transmission and echo detection.
- Properties of ultrasound are:
  - *Propagation velocity* – average in soft tissue = 1540 m/s.

- *Acoustic impedance* – resistance to transmission through a tissue – average in soft tissue = $1.6 \, kg/m^2/s$ (Rayls).
- *Interface* – junction between tissues of different acoustic impedances.
- *Reflection* when ultrasound strikes an interface larger than the wavelength at angles approaching 90°. A 'strong reflector' is one where impedances on each side of the interface are considerably different.
  - Most soft tissues and blood – reflections are weak compared to those from solid tissues.
  - Skin:air – >99% reflected so that coupling gel is required between transducer and skin.
  - Soft tissue:bone – ~40% reflected.
- *Refraction* occurs when ultrasound strikes an interface at an angle less than 90°. Part of the beam is reflected and the remainder continues to be transmitted but at a different angle.
- *Scattering* occurs as ultrasound strikes particles or a rough surface, the degree depending on the ultrasound frequency and angle of insonation. Small particles such as blood cells scatter equally in all directions termed *Rayleigh scattering*.[*]
- *Interference* – several sound waves with different frequencies pass through a tissue and enhance or compete.
- *Absorption* – conversion of ultrasound energy to heat as it travels through tissues.
- *Attenuation* – loss of ultrasound energy as it passes through tissues, proportional

---

[*] John William Strutt, 3rd Baron Rayleigh (1842–1919), English Physicist.

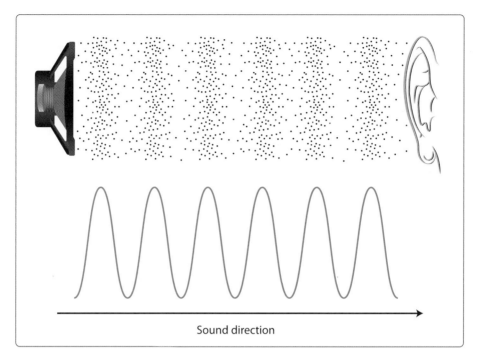

Figure 4.1 The sinusoidal wave of energy passing through a medium causes alternating compression and expansion, producing sound.

to the ultrasound frequency, distance from the transducer to study site and tissue density. Only a minute fraction of the transmitted ultrasound energy returns to the transducer.

The Doppler effect

- Sound waves emitted from a source are reflected by objects in their path. The frequency of reflected sound increases if the object is moving towards the source or decreases if it is moving away, and the change in frequency is the Doppler shift*. Ultrasound from a stationary probe directed towards flowing blood detects a Doppler shift (f_d) from red blood cells that is proportional to blood flow velocity (Figure 4.2). If f_o = ultrasound frequency transmitted from the probe, v = velocity of moving blood, θ = angle between the direction of blood flow and axis

of insonation, and c = velocity of ultrasound in tissue ($\sim$1540 m/s)

$$f_d = \frac{2f_o \cdot v \cdot \cos\theta}{c} \quad \text{or} \quad v = \frac{f_d \cdot c}{2f_o \cdot \cos\theta}$$

- The Doppler shift is very small compared to the ultrasound frequency, and the resultant signals when processed produce sounds in the kHz range that are well within the human audible range. The Doppler shift can be converted to a spectral signal, colour or sound. The faster the flow, the greater the shift and the higher the amplitude of the signal or tone of the audible signal.
- Ultrasound machines calculate Doppler shifts for any incident angle.

If $\theta = 90°$ then $\cos\theta = 0$ and no flow signal will register. The maximum shift occurs when $\cos\theta = 90°$, and this is used to scan for perforators. In general use, the optimal angle is $\theta \approx 60°$. Errors in measuring θ cause larger errors in velocity calculation as θ increases and it is best to avoid

---

* Christian Andreas Doppler (1803–1853), an Austrian Mathematician and Physicist.

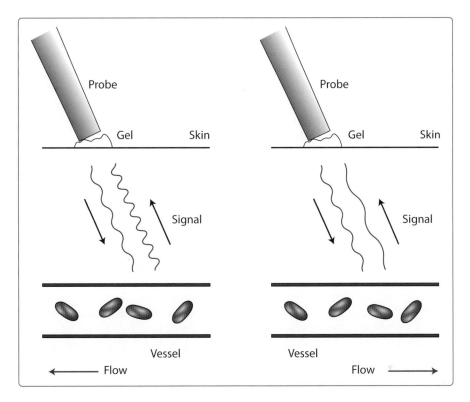

Figure 4.2 Doppler shift. (a) Blood moving towards the probe produces a positive Doppler shift. (b) Blood moving away from the probe produces a negative Doppler shift.

$\theta > 60°$. For example, a 5% error for $\theta = 30°$ results in a 5% error for velocity whereas 5% error for $\theta = 70°$ results in a 20% error for velocity.

Transducers

- Sound is generated and detected by piezo-electric crystals in the transducer. An alternating current applied to a crystal causes it to expand and contract to generate sound waves at a known frequency, and conversely is compressed or stretched by a returning sound wave to generate an alternating current which is then processed to form an image.
- Modern transducers are constructed with a row of piezoelectric crystal elements known as the *array*, with a backing to dampen resonance. The shape of the transducer surface is the *footprint* and the area covered by the beam is the *field of view*. The main pulsed ultrasound beam is three-dimensional and projected in a certain direction. Each reflected echo is represented by a pixel assigned brightness or colour depending on the ultrasound mode, and many pixels together make an image. Modern transducers use broadband piezoelectric crystals that generate variable frequencies, which allow different modes to appear to be operating simultaneously.
- Image quality is determined by:
  - *Pulse repetition frequency* (PRF) – the frequency for pulses emitted by the transducer (kHz). In B-mode this is fixed to a maximum to allow echo return for the selected depth. In colour mode, it is adjustable and many machines simply refer to this as 'the scale'.
  - *Depth of view.* This depends on the ultrasound frequency, power of the signals and tissue type.
  - *Time gain compensation* (TGC). Echoes from numerous depths can be suppressed or enhanced to provide an even signal

throughout, with deeper reflections enhanced to appear equal to superficial signals.

- *Dynamic range.* This allows the operator to increase or reduce the range of echo brightness and contrast.
- *Compression curves.* These manipulate how echo brightness is stored and assigned shades of grey on the display.
- *Field of view and lines of sight.* These determine the extent of image displayed on the screen and number of lines forming the image.
- *Frame rate.* The image is erased when the process has completed a field of view and the screen is refreshed with a new image to produce what appears to be continuous real-time scanning. The display can be frozen at any time.
- *Persistence.* This averages brightness or colour allocated to each pixel over more than one frame. Increased persistence smooths the appearance of real-time images but sacrifices temporal resolution, which can cause blurring of movement.
- An ultrasound beam is focused by an acoustic lens, and steered by varying the sequence for activating piezoelectric crystals in the array so that each is pulsed at different times.
- Axial resolution is the ability to resolve two echoes from different depths along a beam, lateral resolution is the ability to resolve two echoes slightly apart at the same depth across a beam and temporal resolution is the ability to resolve events at different times.

Types of array transducers

Linear array transducer

- Characteristics are:
  - Footprint – straight row of 128–512 elements.
  - Field of view and lines of sight – rectangular with parallel lines of sight.
  - Resolution – even throughout depth due to parallel lines of sight.
  - Beam production – it never involves the entire array at any one time as the elements are excited in sequence.

- Frequencies – medium to high (commonly 5–12 MHz) to provide good superficial resolution though poor penetration.
- Steering of the beam by progressive element activation from one side to the other – possible with some machines.
- Focussing by sequential element firing – possible.

Curvilinear (curved) array transducer

- Characteristics are:
  - Footprint – long curved row of 128–512 piezo-elements.
  - Field of view and lines of sight – larger field of view than for linear array transducers because of radial lines of sight, although this makes probe angling more difficult.
  - Resolution – decreased resolution at the edges due to decreased numbers of elements forming the beam, and worse resolution in the deeper field of view due to diverging lines of sight. Resolution is poorer than for a linear array transducer but better than a phased array transducer.
  - Angle of insonation – perpendicular to the transducer for both B-mode and Doppler, with groups of elements used together as for the linear array transducer.
  - Beam production – same as for the linear transducer.
  - Frequencies – low to medium (2–7 MHz) used for deep studies.
  - Steering – not possible.
  - Focussing – possible.

Phased array transducer

- Characteristics are:
  - Footprint – small with a short straight row of 64–128 piezoelectric crystals. This makes it easy to manoeuvre where angling is difficult in tight locations.
  - Field of view and lines of sight – larger field of view than for linear array transducers because of radial lines of sight.
  - Resolution – decreased resolution at the edges due to a smaller number of elements forming the beam, and worse resolution in the deeper field of view due to radial lines of sight.

- Frequencies – lower than for the other transducers (2–4 MHz) providing good penetration for deep vessels.
- Steering and beam production – electronic throughout the field of view, with all elements within the array used together to form a single group for B-mode, and separate elements steered to collect all Doppler shifts.
- Focussing – possible.

Image modes – duplex ultrasound

- Machines combine pulsed B-mode (brightness) and Doppler modalities. Pulsed-Doppler can be viewed as spectral or colour Doppler. The same transducer is used for both and the machine can switch between them at great speed to give an illusion of real-time imaging for each. Lower frequencies are required for Doppler than B-mode to pick up slow flow causing low Doppler shifts.

B-mode ultrasound

- B-mode provides two-dimensional real-time grey-scale images that relate to the depth, direction and brightness of each echo.
- Echogenicity represents the acoustic impedance mismatch at interfaces, and echoes range from bright to dark depending on the amount of reflection. A structure that returns echoes is *echoic* and if no echoes are returned then the area is *anechoic*. A strong reflector is *hyperechoic* and a weak reflector is *hypoechoic*. An area in the image that shows reflections is *echogenic* and an area that shows absent reflections is *echolucent*. A structure that has a relatively uniform echogenicity is *homogeneous*, whether it be echogenic or hypoechoic, and a structure with variable echogenicity is *heterogeneous*, containing both echogenic and hypoechoic areas or echoes of varying brightness.
- Tissue characteristics that affect echogenicity are reflection and scattering at acoustic interfaces, attenuation and absorption, and depth of the reflector. Technical considerations that determine echogenicity are the gain setting, transducer frequency and dynamic range.

Spectral Doppler

- Spectral Doppler has a gate to provide a sample volume that can be placed into any selected area in the B-mode image to determine the interval after emission that returning signals are received and, therefore, the depth from which the sample is taken. Larger gates are used for venous applications to allow greater sensitivity to flow.
- Spectral analysis shows a quantitative Doppler shift spectrum and direction, usually displayed as the maximum velocity rather than frequency. The maximum possible PRF and maximum recordable Doppler shift are dependent on the sample depth, since the next ultrasound pulse should not be emitted before all information from the previous pulse is received. The upper limit for the Doppler shift that can be measured without range ambiguity is the Nyquist limit, which is $\leq$PRF/2 – otherwise echoes would be returning while signals are being transmitted.

Colour Doppler

- Colour Doppler is displayed in a box in the B-mode image that can be changed in size or direction. Each pixel represents a Doppler shift from the position where the echo originated. Mean frequencies and flow directions are assigned colours to display qualitative information in real-time shown in terms of flow direction, mean Doppler shift and variance. Multiple transducer elements produce the colour profile, typically 8–20 pulses per line of sight to obtain frequency shift information for each pixel, termed the ensemble length or packet size. A large colour box slows processing speeds and prolongs temporal resolution.

Computed tomography (CT)

- Helical CT scanning acquires data about a volume of tissue. A voxel is a three-dimensional unit of image, comparable to the two-dimensional pixel of ultrasound. CT voxels are currently well under 1 mm diameter in all planes, so images can be viewed in any plane with equal resolution.

- Images are usually viewed in axial, coronal and sagittal planes and can be rendered in three-dimensional pictures. Contrast can be used to add vessel tracking images. Data presented on the screen can be expressed in Hounsfield Units (HU) where air = −1000, water = 0 and cortical bone is 1000. This makes soft tissues = 10–60 HU, fat = −50–120 HU and bone = 700–3000 HU. Contrast containing iodine within a blood vessel may lift the density of a vessel to 350 HU.
- Much more volumetric information is available to the operator on a computer workstation than is recorded on CT slices on film, so that contrast can be adjusted and the scan moved through multiple planes, analogous to the difference between performing an ultrasound and viewing the recorded images.
- Current CT is so fast that contrast protocols allow an abdomen to be scanned in the arterial phase to demonstrate the aorta and branches, the portal venous phase to show a portal vein thrombus and in the venous phase to display a compressed iliac vein.
- The advantages of CT are that it is ubiquitous and relatively inexpensive compared with MRI, has high spacial resolution providing contrast is adequate, and allows rapid acquisition of data. Disadvantages are the use of ionising radiation, potential complications of iodine contrast and limited soft tissue discrimination.

Magnetic resonance imaging (MRI)

- MRI has great ability to differentiate between tissues and can show very fine anatomical detail. The physics of MRI is very complicated, and physicists are constantly working for major manufacturers to create new or improved scanning sequences. There should be a low threshold for discussing a planned scan with the radiologist.
- In a magnetic field, charged particles like hydrogen spin and are excited by pulses of electromagnetic energy. As they relax, they give off an electromagnetic signal which is acquired by the scanner. Different sequences utilize differences in tissue characteristics to acquire information to distinguish tissues on the basis of their chemical makeup.
- Sequence acquisition – T1, T2, proton density, diffusion, fat saturation – may take five minutes each as the particles are repeatedly excited, and so a complete scan may take 45 minutes. Apart from claustrophobia, patient movement including respiration is a limiting factor.
- T1 sequences show fat as white, water as black and soft tissues in between with very good spatial resolution, consequently showing excellent anatomy. T2 sequences show both fat and water as white and are sensitive to oedema, which is prominent in pathological inflammation.
- Angiographic sequences, even without contrast, can utilize excited blood that has flowed out of or flowed into the examined region. Gadolinium contrast can also be used to highlight vessels providing three-dimensional angiographic sequences with arterial, capillary and venous phases, similar to traditional angiograms with sub-second temporal resolution.

Laser

- LASER is light amplification by stimulated emission of radiation.
- The electromagnetic spectrum (Figure 4.3) consists of light with wavelengths measured in nanometers (nm – one billionth of a meter), ranging from:
  - Gamma rays: < 0.1 nm
  - X-rays: 0.1–10 nm
  - Ultraviolet: 10–400 nm
  - Visible: 440–760 nm
  - Near-infrared: 700–1400 nm
  - Mid-infrared: 1400–20,000 nm
  - Far-infrared: 15,000-1,000,000 nm
  - Microwaves and radiowaves: >1,000,000 nm or 1 mm-100 km
- Laser can produce light in the range of ultraviolet 160 nm to infrared rays up to 20,000 nm

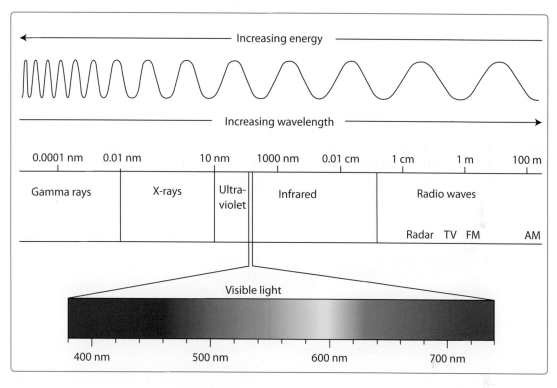

Figure 4.3 The electromagnetic spectrum.

Laser systems

- A laser system consists of a gain medium, a power source supplied as an electric current or another light and a resonant chamber with mirrors. Applied energy causes electrons to become excited and move to higher orbitals. As electrons return from the excited back to a ground state, they spontaneously emit photons some of which are absorbed by other atoms causing them to achieve a high-energy state. As this process is repeated, an increasing amount of energy is produced – amplification of stimulated emission. Eventually, stimulated emission becomes the primary source of energy within the chamber, with more atoms in a high-energy than in a low-energy state. Energy is reflected between mirrors in the resonant chamber and some energy is allowed to escape as a beam of light (Figure 4.4). This is monochromatic – same wavelength, coherent-waves are in phase in time and space, and collimated – nearly parallel. Laser light is captured, delivered through a flexible optical fibre and focused to a small spot.
- The active medium contains the atoms that produce the electromagnetic radiation with different wavelengths (Figure 4.5). The type of active medium gives the laser its name, and for medical applications includes gas, solid crystalline materials, semiconductor materials or liquid dye solutions.
- Continuous-wave lasers have been largely replaced by pulsed lasers to reduce the risk of overheating. Power output of short-pulse lasers is in the megawatt range, causing rapid heating. Different methods of pulse generation produce pulses of varying duration, energy and repetition rate.

Tissue interactions

- When the laser beam interacts with tissues, it is either reflected, scattered, absorbed or transmitted. Absorbing molecules in a tissue are termed chromophores. In the skin, these can be melanin, haemoglobin, water or exogenous pigment

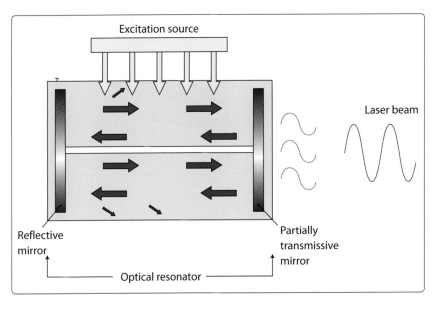

Figure 4.4 Components of the laser generating system.

such as a tattoo. Haemoglobin is the most commonly selected skin chromophore and it has several absorption peaks.

- The optical window of skin is the range of wavelengths that produce maximal penetration, and wavelengths below 620 nm are mostly absorbed by haemoglobin and melanin, while wavelengths above 1200 nm are predominantly absorbed by water in the epidermis and superficial dermis (Figure 4.6). Within a vein, these are absorbed by haemoglobin and water in the lumen.

- The longer the wavelength, the deeper the penetration into tissues to cause damage (Figure 4.7). As tissue temperatures rise, enzyme activity and cell function ceases at >50°C, proteins denature with collagen disruption at 60°C, membrane permeability is lost at 80°C and water molecules vaporize, gas bubbles disrupt cells and tissues decompose at >100°C.

- The aim is to cause selective photothermolysis with permanent thermal damage to targeted structures but no damage to adjacent tissues. The thermal relaxation time is the

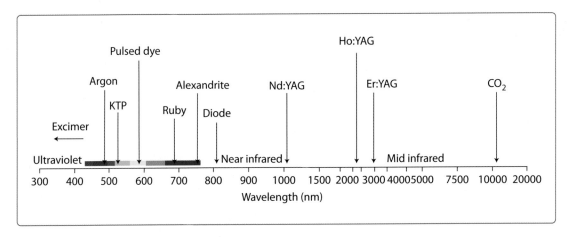

Figure 4.5 The range of wavelengths for laser light determined by the exciting medium.

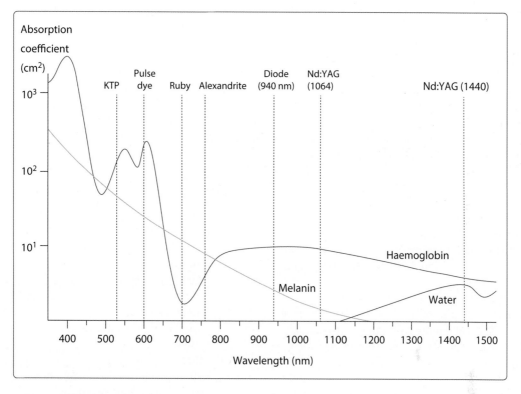

Figure 4.6 Absorption of laser light by various components in the skin and blood.

time taken for a target chromophore to lose 50% of generated heat to surrounding tissue, and is tissue specific, chromophore specific and varies depending on the size of the target. The thermal relaxation time is about 1 ms for a 50 μ telangiectasis but about 1.5 s for a 2 mm diameter vein. The laser pulse duration is selected to provide optimal selective photothermolysis through the thermal relaxation time.

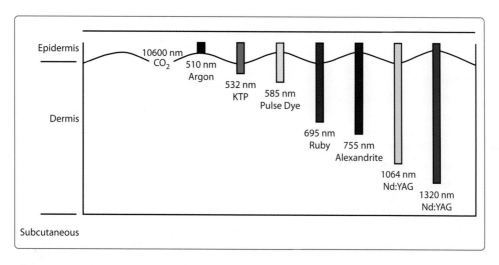

Figure 4.7 Depth of penetration through the skin for various laser frequencies determined by the medium used.

Wavelength

- The laser wavelength is chosen to be near the maximum absorption of the target chromophore, long enough to penetrate to the depth of the target and away from the target range of competing chromophores. Longer wavelengths penetrate more deeply with less scattering. Low scattering is good for cutting while high scattering effects good photocoagulation.

Pulse duration

- Optimal pulse duration depends on the time needed for the tissue temperature to return to baseline after heating the target chromophore (thermal relaxation time). If a tissue is heated for less than or equal to its thermal relaxation time, then accumulated heat and subsequent damage is confined to the target object, whereas heat conduction can lead to damage to surrounding structures if it is heated for a longer duration.

Spot size

- Spot size is the diameter of the beam emitted from the laser as it strikes the tissue surface. Energy entering the target tissue is attenuated more rapidly with a small spot size compared to a larger spot size, because scattering is greater.

Energy delivery

- Energy is measured in Joules (J). The linear endovenous energy density (LEED – J/cm) and fluence (J/cm^2) can be calculated, where cm is the length of vein treated.

Power density

- Power density is the power transmitted per unit area of cross-section of a laser beam (W/cm^2) and is inversely proportional to the square of the diameter of the spot size. Low power density produces slow heating that coagulates tissue, while high power density heats tissue quickly and can vaporize it. At extremely high power density, heating is so rapid that the target tissue disintegrates from photomechanical disruption rather than from vaporization.

Superficial laser

- Surface transcutaneous laser can be used to treat telangiectases and reticular veins. Surface laser is less effective than sclerotherapy for lower limb telangiectasias, requires more treatment sessions and is more expensive. Different laser settings are used according to blood vessel diameters, depth and skin type.
- Laser systems most commonly used for vascular lesions are:
  - Solid:
    - KTP – (potassium titanyl phosphate – 532 nm) widely used for telangiectasia,
    - Alexandrite (755 nm),
    - Nd:YAG (neodymium-doped yttrium aluminium garnet – 1064 nm), a longer wave-length system allowing deeper penetration to target larger coarse capillaries and facial venules, larger venous lakes, vascular malformations and port wine stains.
  - Liquid:
    - PDL (Pulsed dye laser – 585 nm and 595 nm) which have a fluorescent organic dye in a liquid solution, emit yellow light which corresponds to the second oxyhemoglobin peak and are particularly used for facial telangiectases and smaller venous lakes.
  - Gas:
    - CO_2, which provides an excellent cutting instrument because scattering is minimal, absorption in water is good, soft tissue vaporization is rapid and surrounding tissue damage is negligible.
    - Argon (488–514 nm) which produces blue–green light and is used to coagulate blood vessels in dermatology, ophthalmology, and liver surgery.
    - The excimer laser, which has an active medium composed of argon, krypton or xenon with fluorine or chlorine. It emits ultraviolet radiation with enough energy to break chemical bonds between molecules, but with little thermal damage, and is used to remove surface material from the skin.

- Good comparative studies between light modalities are lacking, though it appears that Nd:YAG is better for larger veins and for darker skins, though it is more painful with a higher pigmentation risk than shorter wavelengths. PDL may be better for fine telangiectases. Pre-injecting indocyanine green to enhance 810 nm laser is a promising technology.[5]

Laser hazards

- Beam hazards include those related to direct or incidental impact, fire, burns and ocular damage. Non-beam hazards include plume, and electrical or mechanical faults. Eye hazards are related to the wavelength. CO_2 lasers are absorbed in water and can cause a corneal burn. Nd:YAG, argon, KTP and diode pass through water and other clear structures to focus at the retina to cause a burn and permanent loss of retinal function. All personnel, including the patient, must wear safety goggles with optical density for the wavelength being used whenever the laser is being operated, and must never stare directly into the laser beam. Secure the doors, hang danger signs and shade the windows.

Intense pulsed light

- Intense pulsed light (IPL) uses a filtered flash lamp device that emits radiation between 420 and 1300 nm. Ideal indications for its use include diffuse telangiectasia, lentigines, poikiloderma and essential progressive telangiectasia.
- Unlike lasers, intense pulse light systems are polychromatic with a band of wavelengths, non-coherent with waves that are not in phase, and divergent (non-collimated).

Radio frequency

- Radio frequency (RF) is in the spectrum of electromagnetic energy waves in the radio and microwave range, from wavelengths 1 cm to 100 km. RF ablation devices typically operate in a range of 350–500 kHz. This produces local heat by an electrode to destroy tissue at the site of delivery. Surgical diathermy works at a higher frequency.
- Electric currents that oscillate at radio frequencies have different properties to direct or alternating current of lower frequencies and do not cause electric shock.
- There are at least two commercial systems used for venous ablation. A widely-used system employs a catheter that heats the vein in short 7 cm or 3 cm segments with treatment cycles. It is considered that this allows for rapid and uniform heating of the vein and eliminates the variability associated with a continuous pull-back technology. Power typically starts at 18 W and then drops to 10 W within 10 s.
- The system has continuous intra-operative feedback from the radio frequency generator, which helps provide a consistent, effective treatment temperature-controlled energy delivery. The feedback mechanism monitors intravascular heat parameters in real time to deliver optimal therapeutic power.
- Heat penetrates for about 1.5 mm from the probe, requiring dilute local anaesthetic surrounding the vein to avoid damage to local tissues. The operating temperature is 120°C and this achieves an appropriate temperature of 80–100°C at the inner vein wall to cause adequate damage.

History

- The first ultrasonic device was the dog whistle invented in 1876 by Sir Francis Galton. The maximum upper range of human hearing is about 20 kHz for children, declining to 15–17 kHz for middle-aged adults. The top end of a dog's hearing range is about 45 kHz, while a cat's is 64 kHz and the frequency of the dog whistle is 23–54 kHz.
- The piezoelectric effect was described by the French chemist Pierre Curie in 1880.
- Ultrasound produced by rapid vibration was introduced by the French physicist and human rights activist, Paul Langevin in 1917, to detect submarines. By the Second World War, this had been perfected as SONAR (SOund NAvigation and Ranging) distance.

- Shigeo Satomura working in Osaka, Japan, implemented the Doppler effect to monitor the heart and peripheral blood vessels in 1955.[6]
- Donald Baker, Eugene Strandness and Wayne Johnson working with Robert Rushmer at the University of Washington in Seattle, developed pulse Doppler technology to study vascular physiology and disease in 1967.[7]
- The 1979 Nobel Prize in Physiology or Medicine was awarded to Allan Cormack and Godfrey Hounsfield 'for the development of computer assisted tomography'. Hounsfield was working for EMI, who were able to provide financial support due to their success sponsoring the Beatles.
- The 2003 Nobel Prize in Physiology or Medicine was awarded to Paul Lauterbur of the University of Illinois and to Sir Peter Mansfield of the University of Nottingham for 'discoveries concerning magnetic resonance imaging'. Research leading to the prize had been commenced by Lauterbur some 30 years before.
- The theoretical foundations for laser were established by Albert Einstein in 1917 in a paper *Zur Quantentheorie der Strahlung (On the Quantum Theory of Radiation)* using Max Planck's law of radiation. Charles Townes, Nikolay Basov and Aleksandr Prokhorov shared the Nobel Prize in Physics in 1964 'for fundamental work in the field of quantum electronics which has led to the construction of oscillators and amplifiers based on the maser–laser principle'.
- Serbian–American Nikola Tesla (1856–1943) first postulated the application of radiofrequency to medicine in 1891. French physician Jacques-Arsène d'Arsonval (1851–1940) discovered that frequencies above 10 kHz did not cause electric shock. German physician Karl Franz Nagelschmidt introduced diathermy in 1907.

References

1. Coleridge-Smith P, Labropoulos N, Partsch H, Myers K, Nicolaides A, Cavezzi A. Duplex ultrasound investigation of the veins in chronic venous disease of the lower limbs–UIP consensus document. Part I. Basic principles. *Eur J Vasc Endovasc Surg* 2006;31:83–92. http://www.ncbi.nlm.nih.gov/pubmed/16226898
2. Cavezzi A, Labropoulos N, Partsch H, Ricci S, Caggiati A, Myers K, Nicolaides A, Smith PC. Duplex ultrasound investigation of the veins in chronic venous disease of the lower limbs–UIP consensus document. Part II. Anatomy. *Eur J Vasc Endovasc Surg* 2006;31:288–99. http://www.ncbi.nlm.nih.gov/pubmed/16230038
3. Myers KA, Clough A. *Practical Vascular Ultrasound. An Illustrated Guide.* 2014; CRC Press. https://www.crcpress.com/Practical-Vascular-Ultrasound-An-Illustrated-Guide/Myers-Clough/p/book/9781444181180
4. Zygmunt J, Pichot O, Dauplaise T. *Practical Phlebology: Venous Ultrasound.* 2013; CRC Press. https://www.crcpress.com/Practical-Phlebology-Venous-Ultrasound/Zygmunt-Pichot-Dauplaise/p/book/9781853159480
5. Meesters AA, Pitassi LH, Campos V, Wolkerstorfer A, Dierickx CC. Transcutaneous laser treatment of leg veins. *Lasers Med Sci* 2014;29:481–92. https://www.ncbi.nlm.nih.gov/pubmed/24220848
6. Satomura S. Ultrasonic Doppler method for the inspection of cardiac function. *J. Acoust. Soc. Am.* 1957;29:1181–85. http://www.ob-ultrasound.net/satomura.html
7. Rushmer RF, Baker DW, Johnson WL, Strandness DE. Clinical applications of a transcutaneous ultrasonic flow detector. *JAMA* 1967;199:326–8. http://www.ncbi.nlm.nih.gov/pubmed/?term=Rushmer+RF%2C+Baker+DW%2C+Johnson+WL%2C+Strandness+DE.+Clinical

5 Pharmacology for venous and lymphatic diseases

Pharmacodynamics and pharmacokinetics

- *Pharmacodynamics* refers to how a drug affects a patient. It studies the relationship between drug concentration at its site of action and resulting effects, for both its time-course and intensity of therapeutic and adverse actions.
- *Pharmacokinetics* refers to how a patient deals with a drug. It is the study of the time-course of drug absorption, distribution, metabolism and excretion.
- *Administration* and *absorption* refer to how a medication can enter the body to liberate its active ingredients by the topical, oral or parenteral route. Absorption after oral intake is affected by a drug's interaction with food, and oral administration is ineffective if the drug is destroyed by digestion. Intramuscular injection or intravenous infusion are necessary if the drug or patient's condition does not allow oral administration or if a rapid effect is required.
- *Distribution* determines where a medication passes to in interstitial and intracellular fluids and where it is expected to exert an effect. Drugs may be free in the plasma, plasma protein-bound or sequestered in fat depots and non-target tissues (Figure 5.1). The volume distributed is the amount of drug as a proportion of the concentration in plasma. Biochemical tests can be used to measure drug concentration in plasma or to measure its metabolic effects.

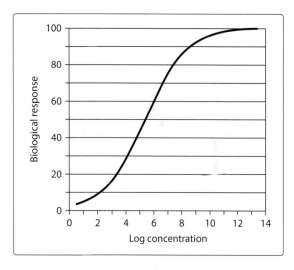

Figure 5.1 Dose-response curve.

- It is necessary to know whether a drug can cross the placenta or enter breast milk because of potential harm that it may cause to a foetus or infant. Smaller molecules cross the placenta more easily, but placental transmission also involves active secretory pathways.
- *Metabolism* refers to how a medication is broken down, particularly as it passes through the liver. *Excretion* refers to how a medication is removed, generally in urine and faeces. Drug dosage needs to be reduced in patients with renal or hepatic disease. Typical drug metabolism involves oxidation by liver cytochrome P450 then glucuronidation to render metabolites water-soluble, with subsequent renal excretion.

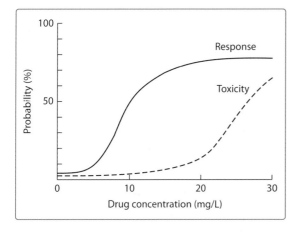

Figure 5.2 Drug toxicity.

- The *half-life* for action refers to the time taken to remove 50% of a medication's concentration by metabolism and excretion. However, metabolites from some drugs remain active. *Potency* can be measured by the concentration at which 50% of a drug's maximum effect is achieved, referred to as the 50% effective concentration or EC_{50}. The *dose–response* relationship describes change in effect on a patient caused by differing doses over time, which determines what is a safe level for dosage.
- *Toxicity* is the degree to which a medication can do harm to a patient. It hopefully develops above the therapeutic range (Figure 5.2). The effect of a drug varies between patients, some can cause hypersensitivity syndromes in part due to pharmacogenetics, and most cause toxicity in large doses, while there is cross-reactivity between multiple drugs administered, thus altering their effects. The LD_{50} is a population-based estimate of a dose that is 50% of that likely to cause death.

Sclerosants

Action of sclerosants

- Sclerosants can be detergent, osmotic or chemical irritant agents. They cause endothelial cell death, disrupt intercellular cement

and cause an inflammatory response which leads to fibrosis that hopefully obliterates the vein. Thrombus formation invariably follows endothelial damage, and excessive thrombosis is detrimental because it may allow the vein to recanalize.

Detergent sclerosants

- Two detergent drugs, sodium tetradecyl sulphate and polidocanol, are the most commonly-used agents. Manufacturers' product information is shown in Table 5.1.

Sodium tetradecyl sulphate (STS)

- Sodium tetradecyl sulphate (Fibrovein, Sotradecol, Trombovar) – sodium 1-isobutyl-4-ethyloctyl sulphate – is an anionic synthetic long chain fatty acid (Figure 5.3).
- Fibrovein is manufactured as a sterile solution in 0.2%, 0.5%, 1% and 3% concentrations buffered to pH7.6. Additives in commercial preparations include 2% benzyl alcohol, sodium and potassium phosphate and sodium hydroxide. The recommended maximum daily dose is 4 mL of 3%.
- It was developed in the 1940s. It causes a delayed burning sensation with extravasation rather than pain. A higher incidence of allergic reaction is thought to result from repeated treatment, and may occur with an interval of several years between sessions. The incidence of allergy has decreased in recent decades due to better production methods with less carbitol contamination. A test dose of 0.25–0.5 mL should be given up to 24 hours before treatment where special caution is indicated, although this in itself could sensitize the patient.
- It has not been established whether it is safe to use in pregnancy, but is category B2 due to toxicity in animal studies (see below). It is not known if it passes into human milk.

Polidocanol

- Polidocanol or Laureth-9 (Aethoxysklerol, Asclera) – polyethylene glycol monododecyl ether – is a non-ionic detergent (Figure 5.4).

Table 5.1 Part product information for STS and polidocanol

	STS	Polidocanol
pH	7.6	6.5–8.0
Presence of alcohol	2% benzyl alcohol	5% ethanol
Storage	Protect from light	<25°C
Recommended maximum dose	4 mls 3%	2 mg/kg (5 mls of 3% in 75 kg person)
LD_{50} (in mice)	90 mg/kg	1200mg/kg
Negative cardiac inotropy (rats)	No	Yes (increased if use with lignocaine)
Pregnancy category	B2 (inadequate animal studies)	B3 (rabbit mutagenesis)
Contraindicated in asthma?	Yes	If poorly controlled
Ulcers with intradermal injection	>0.5% concentration	if >1% concentration

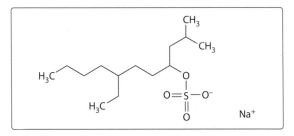

Figure 5.3 Sodium tetradecyl sulphate has an 11-carbon backbone (undecanyl) with a methyl and an ethyl side-chain plus a sulphate ion in the 4-position.

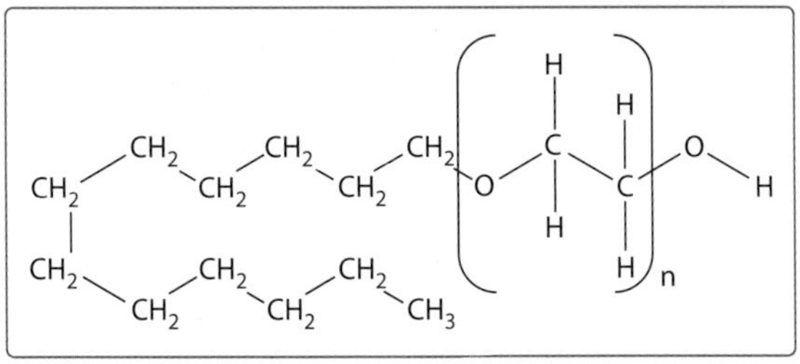

Figure 5.4 Polidocanol is a 12-carbon alcohol (dodecanol) with a variable number of ethoxy ($O–C_2H_4–$) groups in the chain.

- It is available as a sterile solution in 0.5%, 1%, 2%, 3% and 5% concentrations buffered to pH6.5–8.0. Additives in the commercial preparation include 5% ethanol and sodium and potassium phosphate. There is 90% elimination from the blood in 12 hours due to excretion in the urine and faeces. The recommended maximum daily dose is 2 mg/kg, equivalent to 5 mL of 3% in a 75 kg person.

- It was introduced as a local anaesthetic agent then as a sclerosant in the 1960s. It has a very low incidence of allergic reactions. Injection can be painful, especially if there is extravasation before the local anaesthetic effect takes place.
- It does not cross the blood–brain barrier but does cross the placenta, should not be used in early pregnancy and is category B3. It is not known if it is excreted into human milk.

Action of detergent sclerosants

- Detergent sclerosants are surfactants normally used for reducing surface tension.[1-5] They are adsorbed at the cell membrane to disrupt the normal architecture of the lipid surface causing it to desquamate in sheets. They are amphiphilic organic compounds with a hydrophilic head end which is attracted to water and a hydrophobic tail end away from water. At a certain concentration, they clump into spheres called *micelles* and this is termed the critical micelle concentration. An ionic surfactant such as STS has a critical temperature termed the *Krafft temperature* below which it does not form micelles and above which solubility increases greatly as large amounts of surfactant can be incorporated into micelles. A non-ionic surfactant such as polidocanol does not have a Krafft point but exhibits a *cloud point* which is the temperature above which its solubility decreases so that it precipitates as a 'cloud'.

Because of this, some practitioners add small quantities of STS to polidocanol to improve its micellar function, as addition of an ionic to a non-ionic surfactant will raise its cloud point. However, the biological activity of surfactants is now known to be due to monomers in solution, with micelles functioning as a reservoir to replenish surfactant adsorbed from solution.

- STS is an anionic detergent that denatures proteins including clotting factors, whereas polidocanol is non-ionic and has no effect on proteins. Both sclerosants cause endothelial and blood cell damage in lower concentrations and cell lysis in higher concentrations, with platelets being the most and erythrocytes the least vulnerable.
- They release pro-inflammatory and angiogenic mediators from circulating blood cells including interferon-γ, tumour necrosis factor-α, interleukins 1α, 1β, 6, 8 and 17, vascular endothelial growth factor and fibroblast growth factor. They break up platelets into platelet microparticles, retaining much of their activity, though they do not aggregate due to suppression of GP IIb/IIIa receptors. Both cause some dehydration of the vein wall, and back pressure on the capillaries causes intravascular fluid loss.
- Both sclerosants interfere with clotting factor activities, procoagulant phospholipids and platelet-derived microparticles, and both inhibit fibrinolysis. In low concentrations, sclerosants are procoagulant, cause damage to the platelet membrane that induces platelet lysis and subsequent release of microparticles that possess procoagulant phospholipid activity. In high concentrations, both sclerosants are anticoagulant, STS more than polidocanol, and they destroy both platelets and microparticles, resulting in decreased procoagulant phospholipid. Strong clots are formed at low sclerosant concentrations (0.1%), weak clots prone to lysis are formed at mid-range concentrations (STS 0.15%, polidocanol 0.15%–0.3%), and clot formation is inhibited at higher concentrations (STS > 0.3% and polidocanol >0.6%). Dilution at a distance from the injection site results in a procoagulant effect for both detergents at about 5–15 cm from the injection site which disappears by about 45 cm away. Fibrinolysis results in elevated D-dimer levels at one hour which persists for more than one week.

- Both circulating red cell membranes and albumin compete for sclerosant binding, and there is enough plasma protein in 1 ml of blood to neutralise 0.2 mL of 3% STS and 0.4 mL of 3% polidocanol. Detergent sclerosants are consumed in whole blood compared with plasma and saline controls beyond the neutralizing effects of plasma proteins, so that the sclerosant lytic activity on endothelial cells is increased 23-fold for STS and 59-fold for polidocanol in a saline environment compared to whole blood, a reason to consider flushing the vein with saline before injection.

5.1 Comparison of STS and polidocanol

- STS is anionic, destroys protein clotting factors and is procoagulant only at 0.1% or lesser strengths.
- Polidocanol is non-ionic, only damages platelets and not coagulant factors and is procoagulant up to 0.6%.
- STS is two to three times as potent as polidocanol.
- Polidocanol probably causes more local urticarial reaction at injection points, and STS can cause haemoglobinuria.
- There are similar complications at equivalent doses, except that tissue necrosis with extravasation is probably more common with STS.
- The lethal volume after intravenous injection in rats is four to six times as high for STS as polidocanol in equivalent concentrations.
- Both produce allergic/anaphylactic reactions but with historically decreasing incidence, and with fewer cases from polidocanol.
- There is no cross allergy between polidocanol and STS.

Other detergent sclerosants

- *Sodium morrhuate* (Scleromate®) is made from fatty acids of cod liver oil, but has problems of anaphylaxis and extensive necrosis with perivascular leakage. *Ethanolamine oleate* (Ethamolin®) can cause local ulcers and pulmonary and renal toxicity. Both have fallen out of favour due to their side-effects.

Osmotic sclerosants

- *Hypertonic saline* is a widely-used osmotic agent. Suggested hypertonic saline concentrations are 23.4% for reticular veins and 11.7% for telangiectases. Hypertonic solutions probably cause osmotic dehydration of endothelial cells, but these do not appear to be desquamated as with detergent sclerosants. Their action is considerably slower and more localized than for detergent sclerosants. Hypertonic saline carries no risk of allergic reactions and is useful in patients with an allergy history. However, injection is painful, side-effects include extravasation necrosis, haemosiderin staining, muscle cramping and salt load, and it is associated with a higher litigation risk.
- *Sodium chloride solution with dextrose* (Sclerodex) has been used. Other hypertonic solutions are sodium salicylate 10%–40%, sodium chloride 10% + sodium salicylate 30%, invert sugar 75%, saccharose 5%, phenol 1%, dextrose 66%, sodium chloride 20% and sodium salicylate 30%.

Chemical sclerosants

- *Sodium iodide* as 4% poly-iodinated ions (Variglobin®) also acts directly on endothelial cells to produce endosclerosis, in part related to dissolution of intercellular cement which occurs after about 30 seconds of exposure.
- *Alcohol* (95% or 100%) is the most potent sclerosant. It injures vascular endothelium and denatured blood protein, and is used for arteriovenous and lymphatic malformations and arterio-venous fistulae. It can be associated with adjacent nerve and soft tissue injury and pulmonary toxicity in high doses.

- *Chromated glycerine* – 72% (Scleremo®) is a very weak chemical irritant and has been used to treat fine telangiectases since 1925. Advantages are that it rarely causes post-treatment hyperpigmentation, telangiectatic matting or tissue necrosis. However, it is very viscous, and causes pain with injection, requiring dilution with lignocaine before injection.

Foamed sclerosants

- Foamed detergent sclerosants were introduced to increase exposure of drugs to the vein wall and enhance their effect. Although few practitioners use foam for direct vision sclerotherapy, most prefer foam for larger veins. STS or polidocanol can be mixed in a syringe with air or a biocompatible gas such as 30% O_2 with 70% CO_2, or 100% CO_2. Varisolve® is a CO_2/polidocanol proprietary mix.
- Foam has several potential advantages.
  - It is more viscous than liquid and does not readily mix with blood but instead displaces it so that the sclerosant is less diluted and stays in contact with the endothelium for longer. This effect becomes less relevant for small vessels such as telangiectases.
  - The active surface area of sclerosant increases exponentially with reduction in bubble diameter so that the large surface area of fine bubbles results in increased contact between sclerosant and endothelium. This leads to a more prolonged and effective damage to the vein lining, allowing sclerotherapy for larger diameter veins.
  - Foam is readily visible on ultrasound due to acoustic shadowing.
- However, there are concerns about the finding that foam escapes from the treated site into the general circulation to cause a risk of damage to other organs. There have been no fatal cases of anaphylaxis reported with foam, but there may be increased incidence of deep vein thrombosis and central nervous system disturbances. There is very rapid chemical denaturation of sclerosant contained in the bubbles when contacting blood, and this may

explain the very low incidence of consequent systemic adverse effects.

- The Tessari technique uses two 5 mL syringes connected via a three-way stopcock to pump air or gas in one and sclerosant in the other back and forth some 20 times.[6] A mixture of 2 mL or 2.5 mL of air with 0.5 mL of sclerosant gives a ratio of 1:4 or 1:5. If the relative volume fraction of liquid is less than 5%, the foam is classified as drier, whereas if it is more than 5%, it is classified as wetter. Wetter foams (e.g. Tessari's) have maximum stability. Uniform bubble diameter also provides more stability because smaller bubbles empty into larger bubbles. There is no evidence for bacterial contamination from making foam using room air.

- The average bubble radius for Tessari foam using air is approximately 20 μ after 10 seconds and 35–40 μ after 60 seconds, but it is strictly dependent on variables such as type of gas, sclerosant, drug concentration and type of syringe. Bubble sizes for foam prepared with CO_2 are 25%–30% smaller though combined 70% CO_2/30% O_2 bubbles are only 15%–20% smaller.

- Duration of effectiveness before the fine bubbles coalesce and the gas and liquid separate is 30–90 seconds and even faster with pure CO_2, but passing the mixture through a 5 μ filter delays bubble coalescence, resulting in a more consistent size and longer-lasting denser foam. Foam half-life is also dependent on the different variables referred to above. The time of persistence for microbubbles is proportional to rd/DSf, where r is the radius of the bubbles, d is the density of the gas inside the microbubble, D is the diffusibility of the gas through the microbubble membrane and Sf is the saturation factor of the gas in blood.

- Diffusion into the bubble membrane and vein wall is 50 times greater for CO_2 than nitrogen, so that CO_2 alone would be very short-acting and the more inert nitrogen prolongs the action. Further, a bubble of CO_2 that passes through a patent foramen ovale to the cerebral circulation would be expected to be absorbed much faster than

an air bubble mostly containing nitrogen. Foam has 10^5 times the viscosity of liquid, resulting in less systemic washout. Foam lasts longer horizontally and at 4°C; polidocanol POL foam is less stable than STS at room temperature, but they are equally stable at 4°C.

- Syringes containing no silicon in the plunger produce a longer-lasting foam with smaller bubble size. Very small 27–30 g needles may disrupt foam bubbles leading to a more-liquid and less-viscous foam, with a shorter half-life.

Cyanoacrylates

- Cyanoacrylates can be used to occlude vessels, including embolization of high-flow arterio-venous malformations and, recently, for closure of saphenous veins and tributaries.[7,8]

- The cyanoacrylate molecule has a two-carbon ethylene group, a B-carbon which has two hydrogens attached which contribute to its electric activity, and an A-carbon which has a cyano-group and an ester function called a carbonyl (Figure 5.5a). Various hydrocarbons perform the carbonyl function and provide its name, such as n-butyl cyanoacrylate, ethyl-2-cyanoacrylate, methyl 2-cyanoacrylate and 2-octyl cyanoacrylate.

- A cyanoacrylate cannot form a bond with a dry surface but undergoes a chemical reaction within seconds on contact with an anion

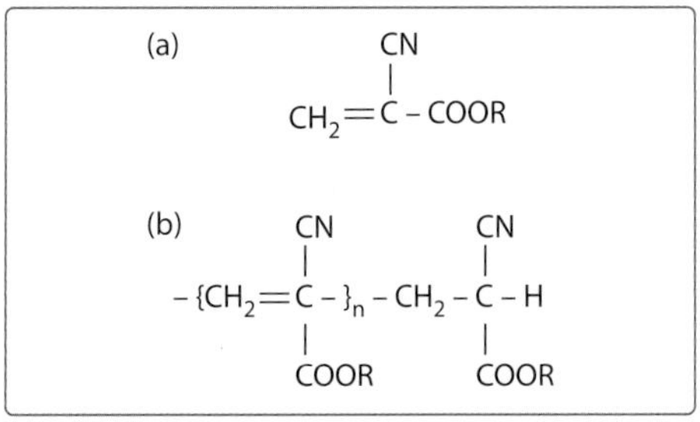

Figure 5.5 (a) Basic structure of a cyanoacrylate monomer. (b) Polymerization in the presence of a hydroxy or free electron to produce a stable but highly reactive molecule.

such as the hydroxyl moiety in water or various anions in blood. Anions bond to the B-carbon, and the A-carbon becomes negatively charged and contributes further negative charge to adjacent B-carbons initiating polymerization (Figure 5.5b). The longer the attached hydrocarbon, the slower the rate of polymerization, the less heat released and the lower the histotoxicity.

- Cyanoacrylates are clear, colourless, low-viscosity liquids that spread rapidly and polymerize quickly upon contact with negatively-charged anions. They have household, industrial, medical and veterinary uses. Ethyl-2-cyanoacrylate is sold under trade names such as 'Super Glue.' Others have been used since the 1970s for closure of vascular malformations, wound closure, haemostasis and control of bleeding gastric varices.
- The proprietary adhesive used for vascular closure is n-butyl-2-cyanoacrylate. Various additives to make these agents radiopaque and to delay polymerization within the delivery catheters have been used for embolization of malformations. The reaction in a blood vessel causes acute inflammation in the wall and surrounding tissues, which progresses to a chronic granulomatous process with foreign body giant cells, fibrosis after about one month and variable capillary ingrowth. Incomplete occlusion can allow isobutyl 2-cyanoacrylate to dissipate on long-term follow-up, resulting in recanalization.
- Cyanoacrylates have varying degrees of tissue toxicity based on release of formaldehyde during polymerization. Smaller side-chain esters such as methyl and ethyl cyanoacrylates are more toxic than are the longer side-chain esters such as isobutyl and butyl cyanoacrylates. However, the United States National Toxicology Program and the United Kingdom Health and Safety Executive concluded that cyanoacrylate is safe. The technique for venous closure has been approved by the Food and Drug Administration in the USA and the Therapeutics Goods Administration in Australia. Cyanoacrylates are bacteriostatic.

Local anaesthetic agents
Mechanism of action

- Local anaesthetics belong to two classes, amino-amide or amino-ester (Figure 5.6), and are structurally related to cocaine, with the suffix "-caine". Their rate of action and potency is proportional to lipid solubility, and duration of action is proportional to protein binding.
- Amide group – from fast- to slow-acting:
  - Lignocaine/Lidocaine (Xylocaine®)
  - Prilocaine (Citanest®)
  - Ropivacaine (Naropin®)
  - Bupivacaine (Marcaine®)
- Ester group:
  - Procaine
  - Cocaine
  - Tetracaine/Amethocaine
- Local anaesthetics are weak bases, usually prepared as a hydrochloride salt to render them water-soluble. All act at neuronal cell membranes to inhibit sodium transfer, and reversibly decrease the rate of membrane depolarization and repolarization. Amino-amides are metabolized in the liver, while most amino-esters are metabolized by pseudocholinesterase.

Lignocaine/lidocaine

- Lignocaine is the most commonly used anaesthetic in venous practice. When used by injection, it typically acts within four

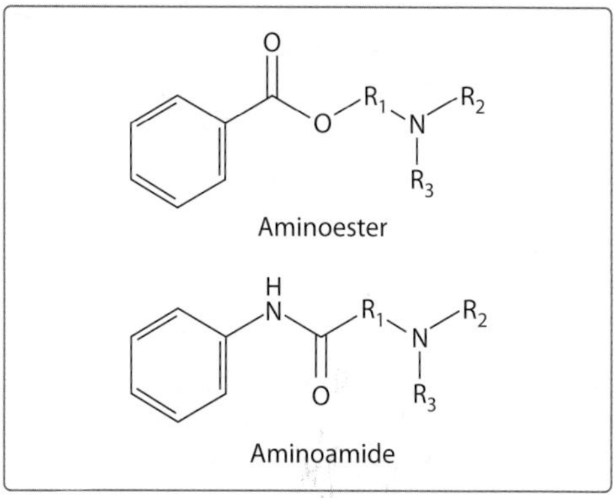

Figure 5.6 Local anaesthetic agent groups.

minutes and lasts for one-half to three hours. Lignocaine is 70% plasma protein-bound. The elimination half-life is about 90–120 minutes in most patients, prolonged in patients with hepatic impairment or congestive heart failure, and it is mostly metabolized in the liver by the enzyme CYP3A4. Its metabolism is decreased in patients taking cimetidine, β-blockers, phenytoin or procainamide. Lignocaine is excreted in the urine, mostly as metabolites. Small amounts cross the placenta or into breast milk. Maximum quoted safe doses are 3 mg/kg for lignocaine, 2.5 mg/kg for ropivicaine and 2 mg/kg for bupivacaine.

- The action is prolonged by adding 1:100,000 adrenaline, which causes vasoconstriction. Added adrenaline reduces bruising but not haematoma or pigmentation. The maximum safe dose is considerably increased if adrenaline is added, and plasma levels then peak at about 12 hours. The manufacturer's quoted safe limit of 3 mg/kg for lignocaine is equivalent to 20 mL of 1% (200 mL of 0.1%) for a 67 kg person of plain lignocaine, and 7 mg/kg or 50 mL 1% (500 mL of 0.1%) of lignocaine with adrenaline. However, higher levels are used in practice. Experience in liposuction has shown that doses up to 35 mg/kg are safe, but it is not clear whether this also applies to perivenous tumescence.
- Plain lignocaine has a pH of 5–7 and adrenaline has a pH of 3–5 so that sodium bicarbonate may be used to buffer the anaesthetic to neutralize the pH and minimize injection pain, and to reduce the time of onset of anaesthetic effect. Although bupivacaine has a longer duration of action than lignocaine, it is much more cardiotoxic when given intravenously.

Allergy

- Local anaesthetic molecules are too small to be antigens but can be a hapten on plasma proteins. A true immunologic reaction to a local anesthetic is rare and most reported reactions are vasovagal or psychogenic. Allergic reactions attributed to local anaesthetics can be caused by preservatives in the solution such as methylparaben and metabisulfite included to prevent bacterial growth, or antioxidants added to prevent oxidation of vasopressors in adrenaline-containing vials. Intradermal skin testing for local anesthetics and additives should be performed in patients whose history suggests a possible allergic reaction, and if future local anesthesia is necessary. If a patient has a history of lignocaine allergy, prilocaine or bupivacaine without vasopressors is often safe.

Toxicity

- Local anaesthetic systemic toxicity is least with fast-acting and more frequent with long-acting agents. It usually presents with progressing neurological symptoms including perioral and tongue paraesthesia, a metallic taste and dizziness, then slurred speech, diplopia, tinnitus, restlessness, anxiety or drowsiness, muscle twitching and finally convulsions and coma, followed by cardiovascular collapse. Occasionally, patients progress to seizures without prior neurological symptoms, and rarely present with cardiac arrest. Cardiovascular toxicity can be heralded by bradycardia with long PR-interval and widened QRS complexes, conduction block, multifocal ectopic beats, arrhythmias, tachycardia or ventricular fibrillation. Treatment is with 100 mL 20% intralipid over one minute, then 15 mls/minute until stable, with a maximum of 500 mL. Fortunately, toxicity should be short-lived using lignocaine due to its brief half-life.

Sedatives

Penthrane

- Penthrane (methoxyfluorane) gas is a fluorinated hydrocarbon and was developed as a volatile analgesic. Its effects begin after about eight breaths and persist for several minutes after it is ceased. Small amounts remain in the fat reservoir for several days, some 20% is recovered unchanged in exhalation and about 30% is excreted as urinary metabolites.

It lost favour in anaesthesia due to nephrotoxicity, but continues to be used in small doses by paramedics. It is contraindicated if there is impaired renal, cardiac or respiratory function, malignant hyperthermia or known allergy, and drug interactions increase risk of nephrotoxicity with tetracycline, or hypotension with β-blockers. Side-effects include laryngospasm, hypotension and unpredictable behaviour. It is recommended not to drive or operate heavy machinery for 24 hours after treatment.

Benzodiazepines

- Oral diazepam or temazepam or intravenous midazolam can be given to anxious patients for premedication or during procedures. Side effects include hypotension.

Propofol

- This short-acting general anaesthetic has excellent procedural sedation qualities. Its onset is within two minutes and duration about five minutes if not repeated. Side-effects include transient apnoea and hypotension. Patients are usually able to wake up and walk away within a few minutes after a procedure. It wears off more quickly than intravenous midazolam.

Veno-active drugs

- Veno-active drugs are widely prescribed in some countries but are not available in others. There is reasonable evidence that they reduce oedema, relieve symptoms and help ulcer healing, with minimal risk of side-effects or complications.[9] However, they have no demonstrated effect on prevention or progression of varicose veins.
- A Cochrane review concluded that: 'Moderate-quality evidence shows that phlebotonics may have beneficial effects on oedema and on some signs and symptoms related to chronic venous insufficiency such as trophic disorders, cramps, restless legs, swelling and paraesthesia when compared with placebo but can produce more adverse effects. Phlebotonics showed no differences compared with placebo in ulcer healing. Additional, high-quality randomized clinical trials focused on clinically important outcomes are needed to improve the evidence base'.[10]
- The following groups of veno-active agents are used in clinical practice.
  - Rutosides.
  - Flavonoids.
  - Procyanidins.
  - Alpha-benzopyrones.
  - Saponins.
  - Quinones.
  - All are plant extracts, apart from quinones, which are synthetic.
- Veno-active drugs act to:
  - increase venous tone by inhibiting noradrenaline breakdown by catechol-O-methyltransferase to prolong noradrenergic activity
  - protect microvascular permeability by inhibiting adhesion and migration of leukocytes, release of inflammatory mediators and expression of leukocyte (L-selectin) and endothelial (ICAM-1, VCAM-1) mediators
  - increase lymphatic drainage by improved lymphatic peristalsis
  - decrease capillary permeability and lymph flow to decrease the risk of oedema
  - inhibit leukocyte adhesion to endothelial cells and migration into the vein wall
  - limit red cell aggregation to decrease blood viscosity and increase red cell velocity
  - facilitate fibrinolysis
- Plant extracts and synthetic quinones increase venous tone through the noradrenaline pathway. Sulodexide has anti-inflammatory effects on the venous wall and can restore venous endothelial function.
- Gastrointestinal or autonomic side-effects occur in approximately 5% of patients. Veno-active drugs should not be prescribed for more than three months unless symptoms recur after treatment is discontinued. It is not appropriate to combine several veno-active drugs in the same prescription.

Rutosides – Paroven

- Paroven (hydroxyethylrutosides) acts to reduce capillary permeability and restore the veno-arteriolar reflex to lessen oedema and improve venous symptoms. Peak plasma levels after oral administration occur within eight hours, but it is distributed to tissues and particularly vessel endothelium of vessels to be then slowly released back into the circulation so that its action persists for longer. It is eliminated through the liver and by renal excretion. Trans-placental passage is minimal, but is best avoided in pregnancy.
- Recommended dosage for Paroven forte is 500 mg twice daily pending symptom relief at about two weeks, then once daily. It is not recommended for oedema due to heart, kidney or liver disease. Adverse effects include gastro-intestinal disturbance, tiredness and skin rashes.

Flavinoids – Daflon

- Daflon or micronized purified flavonoid fraction (MPFF – 90% diosmine and 10% other flavonoids expressed as hesperidin) is indicated for symptom relief and may also have possible benefit for healing ulcers. It acts to decrease leukocyte activation by inhibiting expression of endothelial intercellular adhesion molecule 1 (ICAM-1) and vascular cell adhesion molecule (VCAM), as well as surface expression of some leucocyte adhesion molecules. It affects platelet function, inhibits noradrenaline degradation and enhances lymphatic peristalsis to increase lymph flow.
- It is prescribed as 500 mg twice daily. It has few known side-effects, and interactions with other drugs have not been reported.

Procyanids – Pycnogenol

- Pycnogenol is a patented formulation of French Maritime Pine Bark extract which is standardized to 65%–75% procyanidin compounds. Procyanidins are chain-like structures consisted of catechins similar to some found in green tea. Most of Pycnogenol's

benefits appear related to nitric oxide being increased thereby improving blood flow and also blood glucose control.

Other medications

Anticoagulant, anti-platelet and thrombolytic drugs are discussed in Chapter 21.

Pentoxifylline

- Pentoxifylline (Trental) is used to improve blood flow with arterial disease, but has also been shown to enhance ulcer healing. A Cochrane review concluded that: 'Pentoxifylline is an effective adjunct to compression bandaging for treating venous ulcers and may be effective in the absence of compression'.[11]
- It reduces blood viscosity, inhibits platelet aggregation, decreases fibrinogen levels and activates leukocytes to increase blood circulation and tissue oxygenation.
- It is prescribed as 400 mg three times daily, and may take several weeks to show benefits. It is not recommended if there is a bleeding tendency or marked impairment of liver or kidney function. It can increase the effect of anticoagulants such as warfarin. Most side-effects are gastrointestinal, and it should be taken with meals. Concurrent caffeine intake should be minimized.

Prostaglandin E-1

- Prostaglandin E-1 (PGE-1) is available for parenteral, oral or topical use. It improves blood flow to assist ulcer healing, and has several other uses. It is a constituent of membrane phospholipids, and acts on membrane receptors of intercellular adenyl-cyclase to increase cyclic adenosine monophosphate levels. This results in reduced platelet adhesiveness and aggregation, inhibition of smooth muscle cell proliferation in the media, reduced blood viscosity, enhanced fibrinolysis and activation of white blood cells. This leads to reduced endothelial permeability and inhibition of vasoconstrictive effects of thromboxane A2, serotonin, leukotrenes and endothelin, and stimulates formation and growth of a collateral circulation.

Sulodexide

- Sulodexine is a pro-fibrinolytic agent consisting of 80% low molecular weight heparin and 20% dermatan sulfate. Its actions resemble that of heparin, but it has less anticoagulant effect and better oral absorption. It simultaneously potentiates antiprotease activities of both antithrombin III and heparin cofactor II. Sulodexide may enhance healing of venous ulcers. It is not clear whether it has adverse effects.

Vasodilators

- Vasodilators are mostly used to treat heart disease and hypertension, but are also prescribed for peripheral vascular disorders. They act to relax smooth muscle in arterial resistance and venous capacitance vessels, and reduce cardiac inotropy and chronotropy. Vasodilators should be discouraged for use in patients with veno-lymphatic diseases unless prescribed for other cardiovascular conditions.
- *Alpha-adrenergic antagonists* are competitive antagonists to binding of noradrenaline at alpha-adrenoceptors ($\alpha1$ and $\alpha2$) on vascular smooth muscle synapses.
- *Beta-adrenergic blocking agents* act by preventing adrenaline and noradrenaline from binding to receptors.
- *Calcium-channel blockers* restrict calcium inflow required for smooth muscle cell contraction. They frequently cause leg oedema.
- *Angiotensin converting enzyme (ACE) inhibitors* act in both circulating plasma and in the heart and kidneys to restrict angiotensin II formation. They also block breakdown of bradykinin, which is a vasodilator.
- *Angiotensin II receptor antagonists* block angiotensin II receptors on blood vessels and in the heart.
- *Potassium-channel openers* such as diazoxide reduce intracellular calcium causing smooth muscle relaxation.

Stanozolol

- Stanozalol has been proposed to improve ulcer healing. It is a synthetic anabolic steroid derived from dihydrotestosterone. Unlike most injectable anabolic steroids, stanozolol is not esterified and is manufactured as an aqueous suspension or as oral tablets, as C17 α-alkylation allows the hormone to survive first-pass liver metabolism when ingested. In humans, it has been demonstrated to be successful in treating anaemia and hereditary angioedema.

Corticosteroids

- These have an anti-inflammatory action via multiple effects, especially leukocyte adhesion and phospholipase A2 production of prostaglandins and leukotrienes. They have not been shown to be helpful for venous disease except associated dermatitis, and they may exacerbate oedema.

Fish oil

- Fish oils contain the omega-3 fatty acids eicosapentaenoic acid (EPA) and docosahexaenoic acid (DHA), precursors of certain eicosanoids that are known to reduce inflammation in the body. There is reasonably good evidence for benefit for hypertriglyceridemia, hypertension and cardiovascular disease, and is commonly being taken by patients with venous disease, but higher doses increase the risk of bleeding and may cause matting after treatment of surface veins.

Magnesium

- Magnesium supplements may reduce the frequency and severity of muscle cramps, perhaps by an effect on neuro-transmitters.

Foetal exposure to drugs

- The placenta and foetus can be regarded as a foreign allograft which must evade attack by the mother's immune system. The placenta secretes neurokinin B-containing phosphocholine molecules to avoid detection by the host immune system. The foetus produces lymphocytic suppressor cells that inhibit maternal cytotoxic T cells by inhibiting response to interleukin 2. Many other placental transporters are now being revealed, and trans-placental passage of drugs can no longer be predicted simply from their physical and chemical properties. In general, lipid-soluble drugs cross the placental barrier while highly ionized and polar molecules do not.

Categories for prescribing medicines in pregnancy – Australian Department of Health

A summary of categories for effects of drugs in pregnant women and women of child-bearing age are:[12]

Category A

- Drugs taken by a large number of women without any proven increase in direct or indirect harmful effects on the foetus.

Category B

- Drugs taken by a limited number of women without an increase in direct or indirect harmful effects on the human foetus having been observed.

  B1 – Studies in animals have not shown evidence of an increased occurrence of foetal damage.
  B2 – Studies in animals are inadequate or lacking, but available data show no evidence of an increased occurrence of foetal damage.
  B3 – Studies in animals have shown an increased occurrence of foetal damage, the significance of which is considered uncertain in humans.

Category C

- Drugs which have caused or may be suspected of causing harmful effects on the human foetus or neonate without causing malformations.

Category D

- Drugs which have caused or may be expected to cause an increased incidence of human foetal malformations.

Category X

- Drugs which have such a high risk of causing permanent damage to the foetus that they should not be used in pregnancy or when there is a possibility of pregnancy.

History

- The ancient Incas in Peru used the leaves of the coca plant as a local anaesthetic from which cocaine was isolated and first used for local anaesthesia in 1884.
- Lignocaine, the first amino amide-type local anaesthetic, was synthesized under the name 'xylocaine' by Swedish chemist Nils Löfgren in 1943 and tested by his colleague Bengt Lundqvist, who performed the first injection anaesthesia experiments on himself.

References

1. Cooley-Andrade O, Connor DE, Ma DD, Weisel JW, Parsi K. Morphological changes in vascular and circulating blood cells following exposure to detergent sclerosants. *Phlebology* 2016;31:177–91. http://www.ncbi.nlm.nih.gov/pubmed/25694419
2. Connor DE, Cooley-Andrade O, Goh WX, Ma DD, Parsi K. Detergent sclerosants are deactivated and consumed by circulating blood cells. *Eur J Vasc Endovasc Surg* 2015;49:426–31. http://www.ncbi.nlm.nih.gov/pubmed/25686663
3. Cooley-Andrade O, Jothidas A, Goh WX, Connor DE, Parsi K. Low-concentration detergent sclerosants stimulate white blood cells and release proinflammatory and proangiogenic cytokines *in vitro*. *J Vasc Surg Venous Lymphat Disord*. 2014;2:433–40. http://www.ncbi.nlm.nih.gov/pubmed/26993550
4. Parsi K. Interaction of detergent sclerosants with cell membranes. *Phlebology* 2015;30:306–15. http://www.ncbi.nlm.nih.gov/pubmed/24827732
5. Parsi K, Exner T, Connor DE, Herbert A, Ma DD, Joseph JE. The lytic effects of detergent sclerosants on erythrocytes, platelets, endothelial cells and microparticles are attenuated by albumin and other plasma components *in vitro*. *Eur J Vasc Endovasc*

Surg 2008;36:216–23. http://www.ncbi.nlm.nih.gov/pubmed/18396426

6. Tessari L, Cavezzi A, Frullini A. Preliminary experience with a new sclerosing foam in the treatment of varicose veins. *Dermatol Surg* 2001;27:58–60. http://www.ncbi.nlm.nih.gov/pubmed/11231246

7. Pollak JS, White RJ. The use of cyanoacrylate adhesives in peripheral embolization. *J Vasc Interv Radiol* 2001;12:907–13. http://www.afinitica.com/arnews/sites/default/files/techdocs/nBCA%20in%20Med%20Rev.pdf

8. Rosen RJ, Contractor S. The use of cyanoacrylate adhesives in the management of congenital vascular malformations. *Semin Intervent Radiol* 2004;21:59–66. https://www.ncbi.nlm.nih.gov/pmc/articles/PMC3036205/

9. Nicolaides AN. Venoactive medications and the place of Daflon 500 mg in recent guidelines on the management of chronic venous disease. *Phlebolymphology* 2009;16:340. http://www.phlebolymphology.org/wp-content/uploads/2014/09/Phlebolymphology65.pdf

10. Martinez-Zapata M, Vernooij RWM, Uriona Tuma S, Stein AT, Moreno RM, Vargas E, Capellà D, Bonfill Cosp X. Phlebotonics for venous insufficiency. *Cochrane Database System Rev* 2016;(4):Art. No.: CD003229. http://www.cochrane.org/CD003229/PVD_drugs-improve-blood-flow-people-who-have-poor-blood-circulation-veins-their-legs

11. Jull AB, Arroll B, Parag V, Waters J. Pentoxifylline for treating venous leg ulcers. *Cochrane Database System Rev* 2012;12:Art. No.: CD001733. http://onlinelibrary.wiley.com/doi/10.1002/14651858.CD001733.pub3/abstract?systemMessage=Wiley+Online+Library+will+be+unavailable+on+Saturday+17th+December+2016+at+09:00+GMT/+04:00+EST/+17:00+SGT+for+4hrs+due+to+essential+maintenance

12. Australian categorisation system for prescribing medicines in pregnancy. 2011. https://www.tga.gov.au/australian-categorisation-system-prescribing-medicines-pregnancy

6 Clinical presentations for chronic venous diseases

Definitions

This chapter includes recommendations from the European Society for Vascular Surgery, Society for Vascular Surgery, American Venous Forum and the Australian and New Zealand Clinical Practice Guidelines for Prevention and Management of Venous Leg Ulcers.[1-5]

- There is ambiguity regarding terms commonly used that refer to venous diseases.
- *Chronic venous disease* literally should include the wide range of cosmetic and symptomatic venous disorders at any site in the body that have a gradual onset and natural history. However, the term is commonly incorrectly limited to lower limb venous disease associated with visible superficial veins.
- *Chronic venous insufficiency* is sometimes used as an alternative to chronic venous disease but is more often loosely reserved for chronic venous disease in the lower limbs associated with skin complications. It is difficult to understand what is 'insufficient'.
- *Superficial venous disease* refers to visible veins at any site and has the following manifestations, either alone or in combination, arbitrarily defined as:
  - *Telangiectases* (flares) – dilated intradermal veins 0.1–1 mm diameter.
  - *Reticular veins* – dilated subdermal veins 1–3 mm diameter.
  - *Varicose veins* – subcutaneous dilated veins ≥3 mm diameter measured in the upright position.
- *Varicose disease* more precisely refers to visible varicose veins with reflux in deeper superficial veins, with or without reflux or obstruction in deep veins. This is usually *lower limb varicose disease* affecting lower limb tributaries and saphenous or other superficial veins, but varicose veins can occur elsewhere.

CEAP classification

- The CEAP classification was developed in 1994.[4] The aim was to classify chronic venous disease of the lower limbs for:
  - C – clinical class based upon objective signs
  - E – etiology in relation to whether disease was congenital or acquired
  - A – anatomical distribution of reflux and obstruction in the superficial, deep and perforating veins
  - P – pathophysiology whether due to reflux or obstruction
- *Basic CEAP* was refined to a more comprehensive *advanced CEAP* in 2004 to include a descriptor for no venous abnormality (n), the date of classification and the nature of clinical investigation performed.[5]

6.1 CEAP classification

C – Clinical classification:

- C0 – no visible or palpable signs of venous disease
- C1 – telangiectases or reticular veins
- C2 –varicose veins
- C3 – oedema
- C4 – skin changes ascribed to venous disease:
  a. pigmentation or eczema
  b. lipodermatosclerosis or atrophy blanche.
- C5 – skin changes with healed ulcer
- C6 – skin changes with active ulcer.

E – Etiologic classification:

- Ec – congenital problems apparent at birth or recognized later
- Ep – primary problems that are not congenital with no identifiable cause
- Es – secondary problems that are acquired with known pathology such as post-thrombotic or post-traumatic.

A – Anatomic classification

- As – superficial veins:
  1. telangiectases and reticular veins
  2. great saphenous vein above knee
  3. great saphenous vein below knee
  4. small saphenous vein
  5. non-saphenous veins.
- Ad – deep veins:
  6. interior vena cava
  7. common iliac vein
  8. internal iliac vein
  9. external iliac vein
  10. pelvic – gonadal, broad ligament
  11. common femoral vein
  12. deep femoral vein
  13. femoral vein
  14. popliteal vein
  15. crural veins – anterior tibial veins, posteriorly tibial veins, peroneal veins
  16. muscular veins – gastrocnemial, soleal, other.
- Ap – perforator veins:
  17. thigh
  18. calf.

P – Pathophysiologic classification:

- Pr – reflux
- Po – obstruction
- Pro – both
- Pn – none.

Examples

- Typical great saphenous vein reflux using the extended classification – C2EpA123Pr 2/6/2015 Level 2 (DUS).
- Great saphenous vein reflux but no visible varices and asymptomatic – C0EpA23Pr.
- Post-thrombotic syndrome with lipodermatosclerosis – C4EdA11-15Pro.
- Asymptomatic telangiectasia with incidental great saphenous vein reflux – C1EpA123Pr.

Telangiectasia and reticular veins

- Telangiectases seen in clinical practice are dilations of capillaries or small venules at 200–300 μ deep to the epidermis, although some can be arterio-venous anastomoses.
- The most common locations are the lateral thigh and upper one-third of calf. Most receive backflow from feeder reticular veins or directly from incompetent venous tributaries. Their colour reflects their degree of oxygenation with more red veins closer to afferent arterioles and more purple veins closer to draining venules. Small red and blue telangiectases are sub-epidermal, larger violet telangiectases, termed venulectases are intradermal while blue reticular veins are sub-dermal.
- Reticular veins are larger and lie deeper than telangiectases mostly situated on

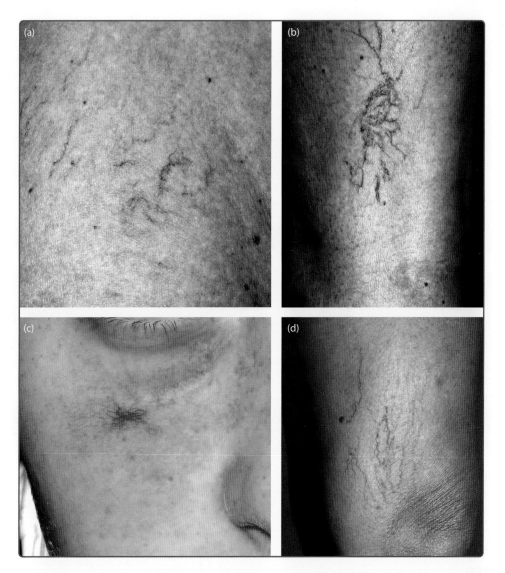

Figure 6.1 Types of common telangiectases. (a) Simple – not associated with a feeder vein. (b) Arborised (dendritic, candelabra) – fed by superficial reticular veins. (c) Spider – fed by a small central perforating arteriole. (d) Papular – circumscribed and no visible feeder.

the inner and posterior thighs, back of the legs, ankles and occasionally on the face (Figure 6.2). Reticular veins can feed into telangiectases, and these feeder veins need to be controlled to successfully treat the smaller veins. Reticular veins are usually of a blue or purple colour and may form clusters. They can be associated with pain or discomfort.

- The Edinburgh Vein Study made the following observations relating to telangiectasia:[6]
  - Telangiectases alone or in combination with varicose veins were found in 79% of men and 88% of women.

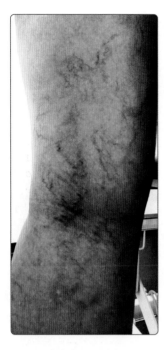

Figure 6.2 Reticular veins.

- There was a significant association between the grade of telangiectasia and severity of varicose veins.
- Telangiectasia was not responsible for leg symptoms.
- The Bonn Vein study found telangiectases or reticular veins alone in 58.4% of men and 59.5% of women.[7]

Uncomplicated varicose disease

- The Edinburgh Vein Study made the following findings relating to varicose veins:[8]
  - The incidence was similar in men and women and increased with age.
  - Body mass index had a significant correlation with prevalence even after correction for age.
  - Nearly one-half deteriorated over 13 years.
  - Almost one-third developed skin changes and a risk of ulceration.
  - Age, family history of varicose veins, history of deep venous thrombosis and being overweight influenced the risk of progression to skin changes.

- The Bonn Vein study found that the prevalence of varicose disease was 31% (27% men, 34% women) consisting of C2: 14.3% (12% men, 16% women), C3: 13.4% (12% men, 15% women), C4: 2.9% (3% men, 3% women), C5: 0.6% and C6: 0.1%. Approximately one-half reported venous symptoms (49% men, 62% women).[7]

Sites of reflux

- Refluxing connections between deep and saphenous veins demonstrated by ultrasound are as follows:[9]

Great saphenous vein

	Females	Males
Sapheno-femoral junction	65%	80%
Low pelvic/abdominal veins	35%	10%
Perforators	3%	3%
Unknown	7%	7%

Small saphenous vein

Sapheno-popliteal junction	65%
Great saphenous tributaries	15%
Thigh extension	15%
Popliteal perforator	5%

Thigh extension

Posterior circumflex thigh vein to great saphenous vein (vein of Giacomini)	70%
Abdominal or pelvic veins	15%
Femoral vein	10%
Deep veins in buttock	5%

- Flow in the thigh extension and vein of Giacomini can be in either direction, making it difficult to define which constitutes reflux.
  - Downward flow from the great saphenous vein, pelvic veins or deep veins to the small saphenous vein.
  - Provoked upward flow from the small saphenous to the great saphenous vein.

Recurrent varicose veins

- Patterns of reflux for recurrent varicose veins are more complex than for untreated disease. Appreciable numbers of patients develop recurrent varicose veins after any form of treatment due to:
  - residual veins in the treated territory that were not eliminated at the time.
  - true recurrence in the venous territory of veins that were previously treated.
  - new varicose veins in a territory other than that previously treated.
- Recurrence after treatment for great saphenous reflux affects the great saphenous territory in two-thirds, or new disease with small saphenous or perforator reflux in one-third. Frequently, there are multiple deep-to-superficial connections. Ultrasound demonstrates the following refluxing connections to the great saphenous vein for recurrent varicose veins.[9]

Sapheno-femoral junction	25%
Low pelvic/abdominal veins	50%
Perforators	15%
Unknown	10%

- Similar considerations apply to the saphenopopliteal junction after small saphenous vein treatment, where veins from the popliteal fossa connect to the small saphenous vein or calf tributaries.

Complicated varicose disease

- Complications can result from superficial or deep reflux alone or both combined. Complications include venous eczema, lipodermatosclerosis and venous ulceration, active or healed. Superficial vein thrombosis and bleeding from varices can also occur. The prevalence of active or healed ulcers is approximately 1%, rising to 4% over 65 years of age, and the prognosis is poor in that only 50% heal at four months, 20% remain open at two years and 8% remain open at five years.[3] Venous leg ulcers are the most common clinical wound problem seen in general practice, and community nurses spend some 50% of their time treating leg ulcers.

Venous eczema and pigmentation

- Venous eczema presents in the leg as itchy red weeping crusted plaques or dry fissured scaly plaques (Figure 6.3). Colonization with *Pseudomonas* is common. Secondary infection can occur with *Staphylococcus aureus*, resulting in yellowish crusts. Cellulitis due to infection with *Streptococcus pyogenes* occasionally occurs, with pain and fever, redness, swelling, a red streak up the leg and swollen inguinal lymph nodes. Secondary eczema can spread to other areas on the body. It needs to be distinguished from contact dermatitis due to an allergic reaction to ointments or creams used for treatment, which is usually more diffuse.
- Pigmentation with brownish skin discoloration results from haemosiderin staining secondary to extravasation of iron-containing red blood cells into the subcutaneous tissues compounded by secondary melanin deposition (Figure 6.4). Colour reversal is

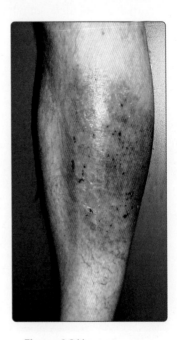

Figure 6.3 Venous eczema.

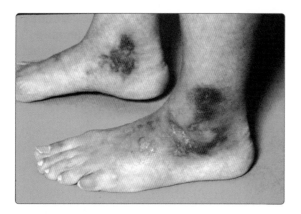

Figure 6.4 Venous pigmentation.

slow and incomplete over the years, even after correcting underlying venous hypertension. Attempts to lighten discolouration with skin bleaching and lasers are generally unsuccessful.

Atrophie blanche

- Atrophie blanche appears as localized whitish atrophic areas of skin surrounded by dilated capillaries with variable hyperpigmentation (Figure 6.5) and is not to be confused with a healed ulcer scar. It results

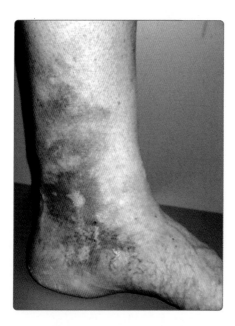

Figure 6.5 Atrophie blanche.

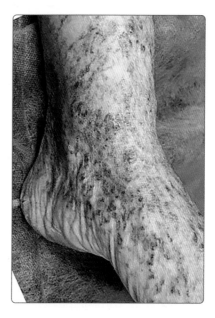

Figure 6.6 Corona phlebectatica.

from obstruction of dermal arterioles causing multiple tiny patches of infarction and is usually a consequence of venous hypertension, but can be due to vasculitis or livedoid vasculopathy.

Corona phlebectatica

- Corona phlebectatica is a fan-shaped pattern of numerous small intradermal veins on the medial or lateral aspects of the ankle and foot (Figure 6.6) and is associated with underlying venous reflux.

Lipodermatosclerosis (LDS)

- Progression towards LDS heralds the onset of irreversible skin changes that put the patient at risk for leg ulcers.
- Acute LDS results from painful inflammation of subcutaneous fat in the ankle region (Figure 6.7). It commonly affects patients who are obese. It is often mistaken for cellulitis, but it does not require antimicrobial therapy.
- Chronic LDS appears as skin induration, increased pigmentation and swelling (Figure 6.8). Eventually this leads to scarring with the *inverted champagne bottle* appearance of the ankle (Figure 6.9).

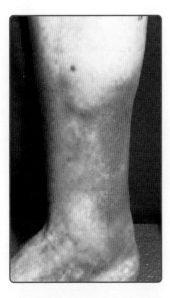

Figure 6.7 Acute lipodermatosclerosis.

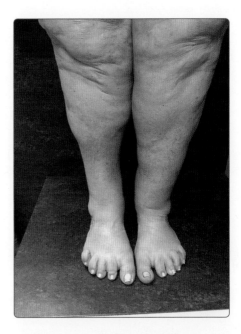

Figure 6.9 Champagne-bottle deformity of the right leg.

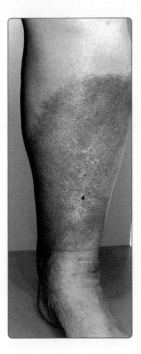

Figure 6.8 Chronic lipodermatosclerosis.

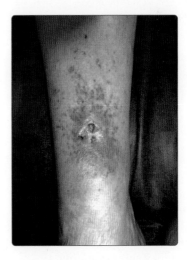

Figure 6.10 Venous ulcer.

Ulceration

- Venous ulcers result from advanced chronic venous hypertension. They are invariably associated with other features such as varicose dermatitis, haemosiderin staining and LDS (Figure 6.10).[10] Venous ulcers must initially be differentiated from arterial ulcers and malignancy, usually a squamous cell carcinoma known as a Marjolin's ulcer.*

- The most common causes for leg ulcers which often overlap are:[11]

---

* Jean-Nicolas Marjolin (1780–1850), French surgeon and pathologist working at the Hôtel-Dieu in Paris.

Table 6.1 Unusual causes of leg ulcers

Vasculitis	Rheumatoid arthritis
	Systemic lupus erythematosus
	Allergy
	Pyoderma gangrenosum
	Wegener's granulomatosis
	Scleroderma
Metabolic	Diabetes mellitus
	Gout
	Calciphylaxis of renal failure
Haematological	Polycythaemia rubra vera
	Leukaemia
	Sickle cell anaemia
	Thalassaemia
	Spherocytosis
Infectious	Bacterial
	Mycobacterial
	Fungal
	Tropical ulcer
Miscellaneous	Drug induced for example, hydroxyurea
	Self-inflicted
	Post-irradiation
	Burns, frostbite
	Insect bites
	Sarcoidosis

- venous 45%–80%
- arterial 5%–20%
- diabetic (arterial and neuropathic components) 15%–25%
- squamous cell carcinoma
- infections
- other causes (see Table 6.1)

Other telangiectatic conditions

Essential telangiectasia

- This benign condition usually affects females from puberty to about 40 years.[11–13] Although asymptomatic, cosmetic

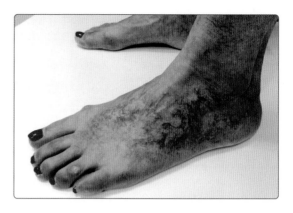

Figure 6.11 Essential telangiectasia.

disturbance can be profound. It has a lace-work pattern of red or pink dilated capillaries usually less than 0.2 mm in diameter (Figure 6.11). Pressure causes temporary blanching. It is not associated with any underlying systemic disorder.

- *Peripheral essential telangiectasia* occurs only on the lower limbs. *Generalized essential telangiectasia* is less common and can progressively involve the torso and upper limbs and eventually the whole body (Figure 6.12).
- Treatment is by vascular lasers targeting haemoglobin or intense pulsed light with a 560 nm filter, with sclerotherapy if required.

Benign hereditary telangiectasia

- This inherited autosomal dominant condition is likely to affect multiple family members. Lesions usually appear between ages two and 12 years, but rarely at birth, become more prominent during pregnancy and are asymptomatic and cause only mild cosmetic concern. Telangiectases are present on light-exposed sites and appear as macular, reticulated, punctate or mottled lesions.

Poikiloderma of Civatte

- This common benign condition typically affects women and occurs in sun-exposed areas of the neck with sparing under the chin. It refers to thinning of the skin (poikiloderma) with increased pigmentation and telangiectasia, red-brown lesions and prominent hair

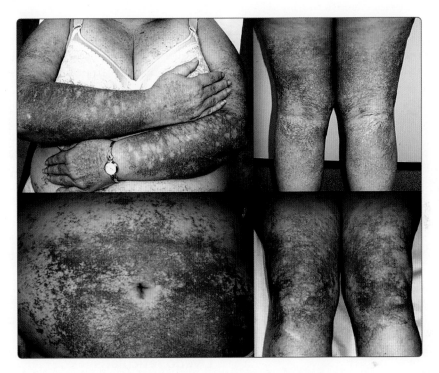

Figure 6.12 Generalized essential telangiectasia.

follicles (Figure 6.13). Contributing factors are fair skin, sun exposure, photosensitizing components of cosmetics and toiletries and hormonal factors.

Spider naevi

- These are common on the face and upper chest (Figure 6.14). They have a central red arteriole and radiating capillaries that quickly fill after blanching. They may be seen

in children or adults, but are more numerous in the presence of extra oestrogen, for example in pregnancy or with impaired liver function. Spider naevi in children normally resolve spontaneously and do not require treatment. Spider naevi are best treated with

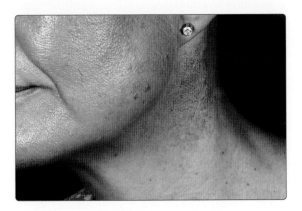

Figure 6.13 Poikiloderma of Civatte.

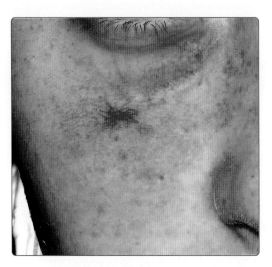

Figure 6.14 Spider naevus.

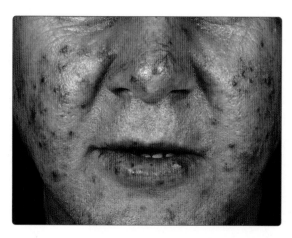

Figure 6.15 Hereditary haemorrhagic telangiectasia.

vascular lasers which carries a lower risk of ulceration than sclerotherapy.

Hereditary haemorrhagic telangiectasia (Osler–Weber–Rendu disease)

- This rare autosomal dominant inherited disorder results from mutations in the receptor-like kinase genes found on chromosomes 9 and 12. It affects both sexes, and features usually do not develop until puberty or adulthood. Lesions appear as small red to purplish spots or dark red lacy lines involving the skin and mucous membranes (Figure 6.15), with a tendency to cause recurrent epistaxis or more serious gastro-intestinal, central nervous or pulmonary bleeds.

Ataxia telangiectasia

- This rare autosomal recessive inherited disease presents in childhood in either sex and is characterized by cerebellar ataxia, growth and mental retardation and telangiectases around the eyes spreading to the ears and cheeks. Compromised immunity results in increased risk of infections and malignancies.

Patterned telangiectatic disorders

- These congenital or acquired conditions consists of patches of superficial telangiectases in a unilateral linear or serpiginous distribution becoming apparent either early in life or in states of relative oestrogen excess such as in pregnancy or chronic liver disease.

Other conditions

- Telangiectasia can be associated with other inherited syndromes, liver disease, Cushing's syndrome and connective tissue disorders such as *systemic sclerosis* and its more limited form the *CREST syndrome.*
- Telangiectasia can complicate scarring due to trauma, irradiation or heat exposure (erythema ab igne), skin tumours such as basal cell carcinoma and medications including corticosteroids and oestrogen.

Disorders of vascular perfusion

Livedo reticularis

- This represents various vasospastic disorders that appear as a reticular network of violet mottling in unbroken circles on the skin that can be blanched.[11–13] The conditions affect dermal perfusion of the hexagonal angiosome, a cone-shaped area with a 1–4 cm base supplied by a central arteriole (Figure 6.16). Arteriolar spasm or occlusion causes sluggish flow, central blanching, ischaemia or infarction. Partial involvement of several angiosomes causes a segmental branched pattern termed *livido racemosa.*
- Primary livedo reticularis (cutis marmorata) is a benign physiological condition due to vasospasm induced by cold, smoking or emotional stress. It usually occurs in the lower limbs affecting younger women. However, it may herald subsequent antiphospholipid syndrome or Sneddon syndrome (see below). Treatment involves avoiding precipitating factors, while a calcium channel-blocker such as nifedipine may help improve appearance.
- Secondary livedo reticularis is a pathologic variant associated with autoimmune diseases, or is veno-oclusive from

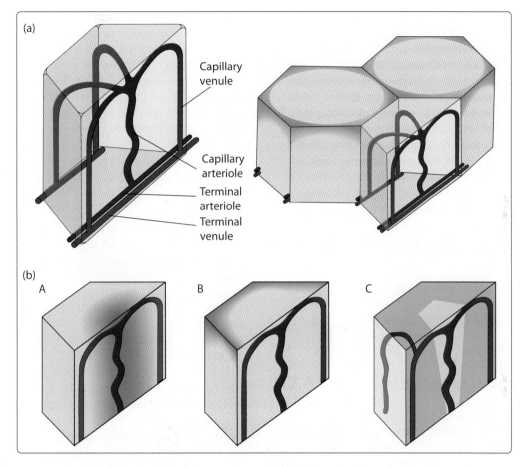

Figure 6.16 (a) Hexagonal arteriolar unit of an angiosome. (b) A – Arteriolar occlusion causing a central dermal infarct. B – Venocongestion such as with livido reticularis. If occluded with inflammation, it could appear as purpura. C – Central dermal infarct from arteriolar atrophy causing atrophie blanche.

hyperviscosity, cryoglobulins, drugs such as amantadine or infection such as hepatitis C or mycoplasma. It usually spreads beyond the legs to the buttocks and torso. It is necessary to differentiate the usually painless, symmetrical, unbroken vessel network of primary livedo reticularis from the frequently painful, irregular, asymmetrical and broken pattern observed in the secondary condition often associated with livedo racemosa.

- Investigation for the secondary form includes antiphospholipid antibody levels, while a skin biopsy may be necessary when serologic findings are indeterminate. The differential diagnosis includes erythema ab igne, livedoid vasculopathy and acrocyanosis.

- Treatment is for the underling condition, but long-term anticoagulation is required if secondary to the antiphospholipid syndrome or Sneddon syndrome.

Livedoid vasculopathy

- Livedoid vasculopathy is a non-inflammatory thrombotic condition associated with abnormal coagulation factors.[14] Histology shows segmental hyalinizing changes at the subintimal region of small dermal vessels with thrombotic occlusions. Strictly speaking, it is not a vasculitis as there are no neutrophilic inflammatory changes.

- Typically, it occurs in the lower limbs of middle-aged women and is remitting and relapsing over many years. It has been associated with prothrombotic mutations and the antiphospholipid syndrome.

- It appears as recurrent livedo reticularis and painful skin ulcers, particularly around the ankle and back of the feet, that heal to produce atrophie blanche, although this is separate to atrophie blanche complicating lower limb varicose disease. There may be associated acrocyanosis or Raynaud's phenomenon.
- Treatment includes aspirin, dipyridamole, low molecular weight heparin, pentoxifylline, nifedipine or intravenous immunoglobulins.

Sneddon syndrome

- This refers to the coexistence of cerebrovascular events with livedoid vasculopathy, usually with a racemosa rash and hypertension. Treatment options include enoxaparin, pentoxifylline, aspirin, dipyridamole and steroids.

Thermal disorders (Figure 6.17)

Raynaud's phenomenon*

- Raynaud phenomenon consists of episodic attacks brought on by cold or emotional stress resulting in a triphasic colour change of the digits from white to blue to red. Vasoconstriction results from abnormalities of small blood vessels and their sympathetic nervous control and intravascular factors, including platelet activation. As arteriolar vasoconstriction subsides, stasis leads to deoxygenation of blood and cyanosis, and rewarming then leads to vasodilation and hyperaemia.
- Primary Raynaud's disease is benign and is common in young women, particularly in cool climates. It does not progress to tissue necrosis.
- Secondary Raynaud's phenomenon can result from haematologic disorders, autoimmune diseases, occupational hazards, endocrine

diseases and occlusive arterial disease. These can progress to digital tissue necrosis which may lead to calcinosis.

- Non-pharmacologic treatment requires lifestyle changes to avoid cold and keep warm. A vasodilating calcium channel-blocker such as nifedipine can reduce attacks and severity of symptoms. Iloprost, a synthetic analogue of prostacyclin can be used. Pain control with opioids, chemical or surgical sympathectomy and spinal cord stimulation may be necessary in severe cases.

Erythromelalgia

- This uncommon disorder results when heat exposure causes peripheral vessels in the hands and feet to vasodilate leading to hyperaemia and intense burning pain. It affects children, adolescents or younger to middle-aged women. It appears to be associated with small nerve fibre neuropathy and microvascular functional changes.
- An autosomal dominant familial form that most often begins in childhood is due to sodium-channel abnormalities from mutation of the gene SCN9A. Secondary forms can be a manifestation of myeloproliferative disorders, drugs such as calcium channel-blockers, auto-immune diseases and neuropathic or neoplastic conditions.
- The soles of the feet are more often affected than the hands. Symptoms are generally bilateral and paroxysmal. An attack may last for several minutes or hours to days and is generally aggravated by dependency, alcohol, warm rooms, summer heat, exercise or simply wearing shoes and socks or gloves. Ulceration or even gangrene can occur in secondary forms.
- The differential diagnosis includes complex regional pain syndrome, cellulitis, peripheral neuropathy, Raynaud syndrome and acrocyanosis.
- Treatment is through avoiding aggravating conditions and learning to cool the involved areas. Topical lignocaine, aspirin or non-steroidal anti-inflammatory drugs, vasoconstrictors, anti-migraine drugs and even sympathectomy may be required.

---

* Auguste Gabriel Maurice Raynaud (1834–1881), Parisian physician, one of a select few to achieve eponymous fame with a doctoral dissertation, 'De l'asphyxie locale et de la gangrène symétrique des extrémités'.

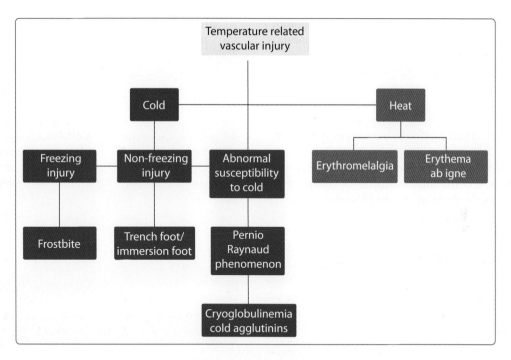

Figure 6.17 Summary of thermal disorders.

Acrocyanosis

- Acrocyanosis manifests as symmetrical cyanotic discoloration affecting the hands, feet or both. The extremities are usually cold despite normal pulses and are sometimes swollen, the palms and soles are typically sweaty, and cyanosis worsens with cooling and improves with warming. Unlike Raynaud's syndrome, cyanosis is persistent and there is no pain, ischaemia or ulceration. It results from precapillary vasoconstriction with hypoxic dilatation of post-capillary venules.
- Primary acrocyanosis is a benign condition seen most often in young women. It may be more common in cooler climates and a familial predisposition has been reported. It can be precipitated by vasoconstrictors and tricyclics. The condition is benign and treatment is usually not required, although a trial of an α-adrenergic blocking agent may be considered.
- Acrocyanosis can be secondary to haematologic conditions, malignancies or autoimmune diseases, and treatment is for the underlying cause.

Erythema ab igne

- Erythema ab igne is a hyperpigmented skin condition due to repeated or chronic exposure to a heating source that is not hot enough to burn the skin. Patients have no symptoms beyond slight burning or itching. Skin discoloration is reticular, erythematous or brownish hyperpigmentation, and ulceration and bullous lesions can occur in chronic cases, while dysplastic changes can predispose to actinic keratosis and squamous cell carcinoma. Aside from eliminating the cause, treatment for the skin discolouration includes topical tretinoin or hydroquinone.

Frostbite and chilblains

- Frostbite represents cold-induced skin necrosis of the digits or ears, nose and cheeks. Tissue injury results from extra- and intracellular ice crystal formation and intracellular dehydration causing ischaemia. Frostnip is superficial cooling of tissues without cellular destruction.

- Chilblains (pernio) occur in susceptible individuals with exposure to cold. Acute chilblains are characterized by symmetrical intense itching, numbness or burning of the toes and fingers and less commonly of the nose, ears and cheeks shortly after exposure to cold or damp conditions, that disappears within a few weeks. There are single or multiple erythematous, brownish or purple–blue skin lesions that may progress to blisters or ulcers.
- Chronic chilblains develop each year during the cold months after repeated cold exposure and results in cyanotic papules, macules or nodules.
- Keeping warm and wearing insulated gloves are paramount. Pharmacologic treatment includes topical steroids for the inflammatory symptoms, while some may benefit from a calcium channel-blocker such as nifedipine, orally or as a topical gel.

Bier spots: angioplastic macules

- This is an uncommon idiopathic benign physiologic vascular anomaly, usually affecting the limbs of young women. There is a pattern of vascular mottling forming a pattern of irregular-shaped white macular areas against an erythematous or blue cyanotic background that blanches with pressure. They require no treatment apart from counselling.

Disorders with pigment alteration

Pigmented purpuric dermatoses

- These are characterized by an appearance of orange–brown speckled discolouration caused by red blood cell extravasation and marked haemosiderin pigmentation of the skin (Figure 6.18). They can be caused by venous hypertension as well as by contact dermatitis and drug sensitivities. When large and brown, they are easily confused with lipodermatosclerosis when they do not have the patchy cayenne pepper spots. Pigmented purpuric dermatoses have several variants: when patchy it is referred to as Schamberg disease, and when scaly with overlying

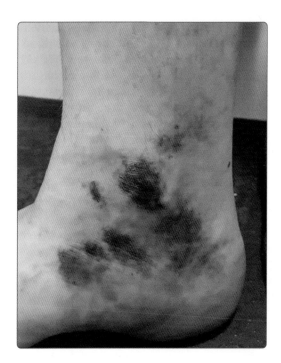

Figure 6.18 Pigmented purpuric dermatosis.

varices, it is known as *lichen aureus*. More than 50% are associated with venous hypertension. Differential diagnosis includes leukocytoclastic vasculitis and cutaneous T-cell lymphoma (mycosis fungoides).

Other causes of pigment alteration

- Other causes include haemosiderin deposition following trauma, poikiloderma of Civatte or post-inflammatory hyper-pigmentation. From time to time, phlebologists may encounter iatrognenic causes of hyperpigmentation such as minocycline staining of the skin, staining from intramuscular iron injections in the buttocks or intravenous extravasation of iron infusions in the cubital fossa.

Petechiae, purpura and ecchymosis

- These common but non-specific medical signs result from red blood cell extravasation, particularly in dependent areas. Petechiae are <2 mm, purpura 0.2–1 cm and

Table 6.2 Causes of petechiae and purpura

Platelet disorders – thrombocytopenic purpura
• Primary
• Secondary
• Post-transfusion
Vascular disorders – non-thrombocytopenic purpura
• Microvascular injury – senile purpura
• Hypertensive
• Vasculitis
Coagulation disorders
• Disseminated intravascular coagulation
• Scurvy
Infections
• Meningococcemia and Ricketsia
Acute radiation poisoning
Psychogenic

ecchymoses >1 cm diameter. If not palpable, they usually signify a non-inflammatory condition, and if palpable signify an inflammatory disease. Underlying mechanisms are shown in Table 6.2.

Vasculitis

- Inflammatory leukocytes can damage vessel walls causing bleeding and distal ischaemia. There is often malaise and multisystem involvement, including renal, gastro-intestinal and lungs. It is categorized by blood vessel size and type (Figure 6.19).
  - *Small-vessel vasculitis* causes palpable purpura and includes the more common and usually benign leukocytoclastic vasculitis, Henoch–Schönlein purpura, cryoglobulinemic vasculitis and vasculitis secondary to auto-immune disease, viral infections or serum sickness.
  - *Medium-vessel vasculitis* includes polyarteritis nodosa, which can cause nodules and purpura, blancheable livedo racemosa and ulcerations.
  - *Large-vessel vasculitis* such as temporal arteritis.

- *Systemic lupus erythematosus* is a multi-system collagen disease often seen in young women. Besides vasculitis, it causes a malar erythema or 'butterfly rash' with telangiectases and discoid lupus lesions seen as scaly plaques, often on the head and face.
- *Rheumatoid disease* can cause leg ulcers, digital infarcts and a purpuric vasculitis.

Exercise-induced vasculitis

- This is a harmless form of cutaneous small vessel vasculitis, also called golfer's vasculitis.[11] It is a neutrophilic inflammatory disorder involving small to medium-sized vessels of the skin and subcutaneous tissue. It affects one or both lower limbs with single or multiple episodes of an urticarial rash and purpuric spots, oedema and intense itching. Lesions resolve over 3–4 weeks, but a purplish-brown mark may persist for longer. It most often affects middle-aged women who are otherwise healthy.

Other vascular entities

- *Venous lakes* are dark blue phlebectasias that are compressible. They occur on sun-exposed skin such as the lips in older patients (Figure 6.20). They can be treated with sclerotherapy or lasers.
- *Cherry angiomas or* Campbell de Morgan spots occur anywhere on the body – although predominantly the torso – and increase in number with age. They can be red, purple or black. They respond well to surface laser.
- *Angiokeratomas* are vascular ectasias from vessels in the papillary dermis with overlying hyperkeratosis. Various forms are described, but the localized and scrotal variants are the most commonly encountered.

Panniculitis

- Panniculitis is a term used to describe inflammation of subcutaneous fat that can result from multiple causes. The affected areas appear as raised nodules or lumps under the skin or as a plaque or large flat area of thickened skin, the overlying skin may be reddened or show darker brownish

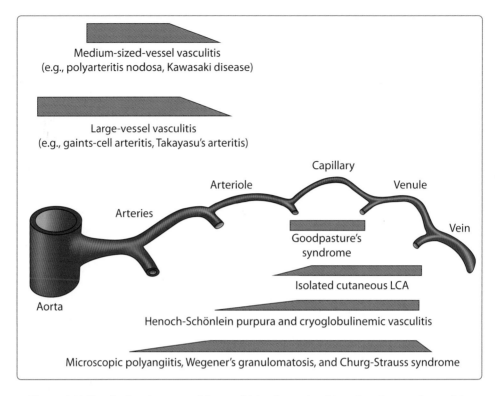

Figure 6.19 Sites for involvement of the small blood vessels with various forms of vasculitis.

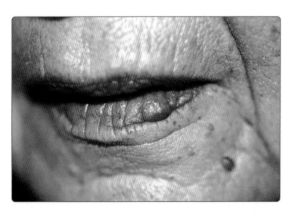

Figure 6.20 Venous lake of the lip.

pigmentation, and the area is often tender. When inflammation has settled and with chronicity, the affected skin becomes fibrotic and firm forming lipodermatosclerosis. The acute red hot painful inflammatory phase is frequently misdiagnosed as cellulitis and treated unnecessarily with antibiotics.

- Panniculitis without systemic disease can be due to trauma or cold. Panniculitis with systemic disease can be caused by autoimmune disorders such as lupus erythematosus or scleroderma, lymphoproliferative disease such as lymphoma or histiocytosis, sarcoidosis with cutaneous involvement, or pancreatitis or pancreatic cancer. Superficial thrombophlebitis is also classified as a subset of panniculitis where inflammation of the affected veins 'spill over' into the adjacent subcutaneous tissue resulting in clinical and histological panniculitis.

References

1. Wittens C, Davies AH, Bækgaard N, Broholm R, Cavezzi A, Chastanet S, de Wolf M et al. Management of chronic venous disease. Clinical practice guidelines of the European Society for vascular surgery. *Eur J Vasc Endovasc Surg* 2015;49:678–737. https://www.researchgate.net/publication/280483468_Editor's_Choice_-_Management_of_Chronic_Venous_Disease

_Clinical_Practice_Guidelines_of_the_European_Society_for_Vascular_Surgery_ESVS

2. Gloviczki P, Comerota AJ, Dalsing MC, Eklof BG, Gillespie DL, Gloviczki ML, Lohr JM et al. The care of patients with varicose veins and associated chronic venous diseases: Clinical practice guidelines of the Society for Vascular Surgery and the American Venous Forum. *J Vasc Surg* 2011;53:2S–48S. https://www.ncbi.nlm.nih.gov/pubmed/21536172

3. Australian and New Zealand Clinical Practice Guideline for Prevention and Management of Venous Leg Ulcers. 2011. http://www.awma.com.au/publications/2011_awma_vlug.pdf

4. Beebe HG, Bergan JJ, Bergqvist D, Eklof B, Eriksson I, Goldman MP, Greenfield LJ et al. Classification and grading of chronic venous disease in the lower limbs. A consensus statement. *Eur J Vasc Endovasc Surg* 1996;12:487–91. http://www.ncbi.nlm.nih.gov/pubmed/8980442

5. Eklöf B, Rutherford RB, Bergan JJ, Carpentier PH, Gloviczki P, Kistner RL, Meissner MH et al. American Venous Forum International Ad Hoc Committee for Revision of the CEAP Classification. Revision of the CEAP Classification for chronic venous disorders: Consensus statement. *J Vasc Surg* 2004;40:1248–52. http://www.ncbi.nlm.nih.gov/pubmed/15622385

6. Ruckley CV, Evans CJ, Allan PL, Lee AJ, Fowkes FGR. Telangiectasia in the Edinburgh Vein Study: Epidemiology and association with trunk varices and symptoms. *Eur J Vasc Endovasc Surg* 2008;36:719–24. http://www.ejves.com/article/S1078-5884(08)00460-7/abstract

7. Rabe E, Pannier F. What have we learned from the Bonn Vein Study? *Phlebolymphology* 2006;13:188–94. http://www.phlebolymphology.org/what-have-we-learned-from-the-bonn-vein-study/

8. Robertson L, Lee AJ, Evans CJ, Boghossian S, Allan PL, Ruckley CV, Fowkes FG. Incidence of chronic venous disease in the Edinburgh Vein Study. *J Vasc Surg Venous Lymphat Disord* 2013;1:59–67. https://www.ncbi.nlm.nih.gov/pubmed/26993896

9. Myers KA and Clough A. *Practical Vascular Ultrasound. An Illustrated Guide.* 2014; CRC Press. https://www.crcpress.com/Practical-Vascular-Ultrasound-An-Illustrated-Guide/Myers-Clough/p/book/9781444181180

10. Mosti G, De Maeseneer M, Cavezzi A, Parsi K, Morrison N, Nelzen O, Rabe F et al. Society for Vascular Surgery and American Venous Forum Guidelines on the management of venous leg ulcers: The point of view of the International Union of Phlebology. *Int Angiol.* 2015;34:202–18. https://www.researchgate.net/publication/309670926_Evidence-based_S3_guidelines_for_diagnostics_and_treatment_of_venous_leg_ulcers

11. DermNet New Zealand. http://www.dermnetnz.org/topics/

12. Parsi K. Dermatological manifestations of venous disease. Part I. *Aust NZ J Phlebol* 2007;10:11–9. http://www.sydneyskinandvein.com.au/PDF_Uploads/39_DermManPart1.pdf

13. Parsi K. Dermatological manifestations of venous disease. Part II. *Aust NZ J Phlebol* 2008;11:11–42. http://www.sydneyskinandvein.com.au/PDF_Uploads/42_DermManPart2.pdf

14. Alavi A, Hafner J, Dutz JP, Mayer D, Sibbald RG, Criado PR, Senet P, Callen JP, Phillips TJ, Romanelli M, Kirsner RS. Livedoid vasculopathy: An in-depth analysis using a modified Delphi approach. *J Am Acad Dermatol* 2013;69:1033–42. https://www.ncbi.nlm.nih.gov/pubmed/24028907

Pathogenesis of varicose disease

The chapter includes opinions relating to venous leg ulcers from an Australian and New Zealand Clinical Practice Group.[1]

Work is still in progress to define the multiple influences that result in superficial veins becoming varicose and to determine why skin complications may subsequently develop.

Pathology of varicose veins

- Varicose veins are characterized by patchy damage to all layers of the vein wall which allow the weakened vein to dilate.[2] Veins have hypertrophic segments with smooth muscle cell disruption and increased extracellular matrix, and atrophic segments with decreased smooth muscle and extracellular matrix. Inflammatory cells infiltrate all layers.
- The *intima* shows damaged endothelial cells, patches of sub-endothelial fibrosis and a disrupted elastic lamina. The *media* has disrupted smooth muscle cell bundles and fibrosis from increased collagen and elastin. Smooth muscle cells accumulate and, in part, change from a contractile to synthetic lipid-rich phase, then migrate to the sub-intima. There is a decrease in the normal rate of smooth muscle cell apoptosis, which can interfere with normal tissue integrity. Fibroblasts become slow-growing and senescent.
- There is more *collagen* in varicosities than in normal veins, and increased collagen synthesis in smooth muscle cell cultures from varicose veins compared to controls. Cell cultures show an increase in type I and decrease in type III collagen from both varicose veins and dermal fibroblasts of patients with varicose disease, indicating a systemic alteration for collagen synthesis.
- There is decreased *elastin* synthesis with age, shown by reduced components such as tropoelastin and lysyl oxidase-like 1 (LOXL-1), and there is an even greater decrease in LOXL-1 in patients with varicosities than in age-matched controls. Thickened and fragmented elastic fibres are seen both in varicose vein segments and in the skin of patients with varicose veins, providing further evidence for a systemic influence with varicose disease. Fibrillin-1 is a major component of elastic fibres and is increased in both varicose vein tissue and the skin of patients with varicose disease.
- Changes in the *extracellular matrix* include increased levels of laminin, which is involved in vein wall remodelling. Transforming growth factor-beta (TGF-β) is increased, particularly in tortuous segments of varicose veins.
- Gradual thickening of *valves* with age may also inhibit their normal function. Increase in elastic tissue and sub-endothelial collagen deposition starts at the valve cusp base, and the number of competent valves gradually decreases by some 20% at 60 years.[3]

Development of varicose disease

- The venous system is permanently subjected to high pressures, particularly in lower limb veins due to standing. There is still debate as to whether varicose veins result from high pressures from above due to gravity distending essentially normal veins (the descending theory) or whether normal pressures from above distend abnormal veins (the ascending theory). Accordingly, whether disease is mostly acquired or at least in part due to intrinsic and hereditary processes is still to be determined. Either way, all manifestations result from the effects of venous congestion and hypertension.

- The descending or 'veins down' hypothesis has been part of the traditional teaching, as it has been attractive to attribute disease to the erect human posture. Congenital absence of proximal guarding valves has been implicated.
- The ascending or 'veins up' hypothesis is supported by anatomical studies that show that vein dilations are on the caudal side of venous valves,[4] and by ultrasound studies that show predominant distal disease in young subjects gradually progressing to more proximal levels with ageing.[5,6]

- A hypothesis is that weakening of the vein wall, loss of collagen and smooth muscle at the valve ring and thinning of valve cusps are primary mechanisms.[7] This may result from local hypoxic damage due to vortices that form in the valve sinus as the valve opens, causing damage to the adjacent vein wall. Normal haemodynamic stresses associated with hydrostatic pressure then potentiate these changes.

Mediators of varicose disease

- The effects on all tissues in the vein wall are mediated through chemical agents and blood cells (Figure 7.1).

Endothelial injury, blood cells and inflammation

- Venous hypertension results in vein wall distension and loss of normal fluid shear stress.[2] Endothelial cells respond by releasing the vascular cell adhesion molecule (VCAM), intercellular adhesion molecule (ICAM), and E-selectin. These are activated

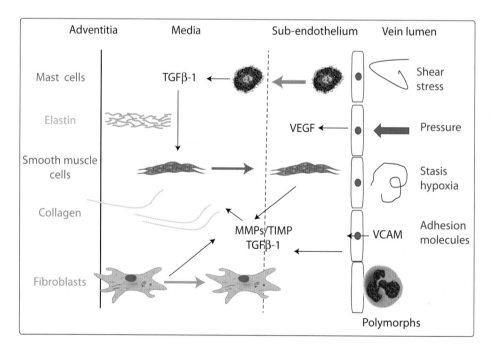

Figure 7.1 Mechanisms for changes in the venous wall with varicose veins. TGFβ-1: transforming growth factor β-1; MMPs: metalloproteinases; TIMP: tissue inhibitor metalloproteinase (deficient); VEGF: vascular endoothelial growth factor; VCAM: vascular cell adhesion molecule.

by tumour necrosis factor-alpha (TNF-α) and interleukin-1 (IL-1)) to recruit blood cells and mediate their adhesion to endothelial cells, and are involved in the inflammatory and immune responses.

- Injured endothelial cells release inflammatory cytokines and growth factors, with increased production of vasodilators such as nitric oxide and prostacyclin and impaired effect of vaso-constrictors such as noradrenaline.

- Leukocytes attach to the endothelium, and activated neutrophils and macrophages migrate into the vein wall and venous valves. These can produce inflammatory agents that destroy elastin and collagen to weaken the vein wall. This initiates a cascade reaction with further recruitment of macrophages and lymphocytes, stimulation of cytokines and growth factors and progressive damage to endothelial cells and the vein wall.

Matrix metalloproteinases

- Increased levels of tissue and plasma matrix metalloproteinases (MMPs) and tissue inhibitors of metalloproteineses (TIMP) occur in both varicose vein tissue and the skin of patients affected with varicose disease, indicating a systemic influence.[8] MMP-1, MMP-2, MMP-3, MMP-9, TIMP-1 and TIMP-3 activity is increased in the endothelium and diffusely in smooth muscle cells and fibroblasts throughout the media.

- MMPs are proteases that degrade collagen and elastin in the vein wall. This causes an increased collagen:elastin ratio in varicose veins and in adjacent segments of unaf-fected saphenous veins when compared to veins in subjects without varicose disease. The MMP/TIMP interaction is complex, with variations in the action of different enzymes on each component tissue in the vein wall.

Cytokines and growth factors

- Cytokines mediate the effects of inflamma-tion.[9] Chemokines, interleukins, lympho-kines and tumour necrosis factor are involved in varicose disease. They are synthesized by endothelial cells, smooth muscle cells and macrophages, and they attract monocytes, macrophages, mast cells and neutrophils, which contribute to inflammation and oedema in the vein wall.

- Varicose veins have elevated levels of the vascular growth factors VEGF-121 and VEGF-165 and their receptors VEGFR1-flt-1 and VEGFR2, as well as platelet-derived growth factor (PDGF) and fibroblast growth fac-tor (FGF). Their interactions may determine how veins adapt to various stimuli such as changes in wall shear stress.

- Transforming growth factor (TGF-β1) is involved in vascular remodelling, recruits macrophages and fibroblasts, and inhibits MMP-1 to restrict collagenase synthesis and increase TIMP activity. TGF-β1 levels are par-ticularly increased in the tortuous segments of varicose veins.

Pathogenesis of complications

- It is not fully understood how venous hyper-tension causes the inflammation and fibrosis seen with complications of varicose disease, leading to lipodermatosclerosis and even-tual ulceration.[10,11] A sequence of events is postulated.

Inflammation

- Venous hypertension causes extravasation of red blood cells and increased capillary per-meability to macromolecules. Red blood cell degradation products and interstitial proteins attract cytokines, growth factors and other chemical agents to initiate an inflammatory reaction in the dermis. Leukocytes collect around capillaries and post-capillary venules, and extracellular matrix and collagen form vascular cuffs. Adhesion molecules are activated which cause macrophages, lympho-cytes and mast cells to move into the dermis.

- T-lymphocytes and macrophages accumu-late in the dermis in areas of lipodermato-sclerosis and adjacent to ulcers, but not in normal skin. Neutrophils are not seen in the dermis but are trapped in the microcircula-tion. Endothelial monocytes become inter-stitial macrophages which release growth factors, and these cells have an ability to metabolize the amino acid arginine to either a 'killer' molecule (nitric oxide) or a 'repair' molecule (ornithine). Growth factors including platelet-derived growth factor (PDGF) and vascular endothelial growth factor (VEGF) are also produced and these recruit leukocytes.

Skin damage and ulceration

- Monocytes and mast cells travel to the site and produce TGF-β1 and other chemicals. This interferes with dermal fibroblast and endothelial cell function leading to decreased fibroblast proliferation and function and impaired collagen synthesis. Impaired fibroblast proliferation increases the longer the damage persists. Metalloproteinase activity is altered.
- The extracellular matrix normally provides a good substrate for keratinocytes to migrate in a wound, and this activity is impaired. Exudate in an ulcer base has a high collagenase activity, which also inhibits fibroblast proliferation and function.

Infection

- The stages of wound infection including those for venous ulcers have been well defined.[12]
- *Contamination.* Virtually all open wounds are contaminated with endogenous and exogenous microbes. Host defences respond to destroy bacteria by phagocytosis unless compromised.
- *Colonization.* Colonization occurs if these microbes undergo limited proliferation within the wound without evoking a host reaction, but wound healing is not impaired.
- *Local infection.* Wound infection occurs when bacteria or other microbes move deeper into wound tissues and proliferate sufficient to invoke a local host response. Wound culture does not distinguish colonization from infection.
- *Spreading infection.* Surrounding tissues are invaded by spreading infection causing symptoms and signs beyond the ulcer.
- Microbes progressively join and incorporate secreted extracellular substances to form a biofilm which acts as a barrier against the host immune response and allows microbes to proliferate. Host defence responses to eradicate the biofilm lead to inappropriate over-recruitment of neutrophils, cytokines and proteases, which causes tissue destruction that in turn provides nutrition for the biofilm. Wound management includes attempts to remove this biofilm by cleansing and debridement.

Ulcer healing

- Ulcer healing requires control of venous hypertension to allow the extracellular matrix to be rebuilt by fibroblasts with a normal balance between collagen I and III, and for epithelial regrowth to occur.
- Healing occurs through four overlapping stages:
  - Haemostasis
  - Inflammation
  - Tissue proliferation
  - Tissue maturation
- The inflammatory phase over the first few days is partially triggered by platelets and fibrin and starts with intrinsic debridement of damaged tissues by white cell phagocytosis. Macrophages are activated and release cytokines and growth factors to initiate inflammation with angiogenesis and granulation tissue formation.
- Tissue proliferation involves fibroblasts that lay down collagen and extracellular matrix, and epithelial cells grow in from the margins to cover the area. Keratinocytes secrete collagenases and proteases such as MMPs that break down the overlying scab or eschar. They also produce growth factors that are stimulated by integrins and MMPs to cause cells to proliferate at the wound edges.
- Myofibroblasts contract the wound, remodelling of fibrous tissue occurs to strengthen repair, and excessive unwanted cells undergo apoptosis. Collagen develops approximately 20% of its normal tensile strength by three weeks, increasing to a maximum 80% by 12 weeks.
- The growth factors involved include epidermal growth factor (EGF), transforming growth factor-α (TGF-α), vascular

endothelial growth factor (VEGF), platelet derived growth factor (PDGF), fibroblast growth factors 1 and 2 (FGF-1, FGF–2) and keratinocyte growth factor (KGF). The predominant cytokines are interleukin-1 (IL-1) and tumour necrosis factor (TNF). TGF-β facilitates polymorph migration from surrounding blood vessels. FGF, TGF-β and TGF-α, PDGF and plasma-activated complements C3a and C5a are released by macrophages into the wound and overlying scab or eschar. Macrophages also release factors that promote multiplication of endothelial cells and fibroblasts including TGF, TNF and PDGF and IL-1.

- Wound healing is delayed by local factors such as ischaemia, oedema, infection, over- or under-hydration and excessive movement, and by systemic factors such as diabetes, smoking and alcohol consumption, immuno-suppression, systemic disease, older age and malnutrition, with low albumin, vitamins C, B complex and E deficiency and zinc and selenium deficiency.

7.1 Postulated mechanisms for development of complications with varicose disease

- Venous hypertension causes extravasation of red blood cells and fibrinogen (Figure 7.2).
- Degradation products initiate an inflammatory reaction in the dermis. Growth factors are produced and recruit leukocytes.
- Activated adhesion molecules facilitate movement of macrophages, lymphocytes and mast cells into the dermis.
- T-lymphocytes and macrophages accumulate in the dermis in areas of skin damage but are not seen in normal skin.
- Neutrophils are trapped in the microcirculation.
- Monocytes and mast cells travel to the site and produce transforming growth factor and other chemicals that interfere with dermal fibroblast and endothelial cell function.
- A high collagenase activity in ulcer exudate inhibits fibroblast proliferation and function.

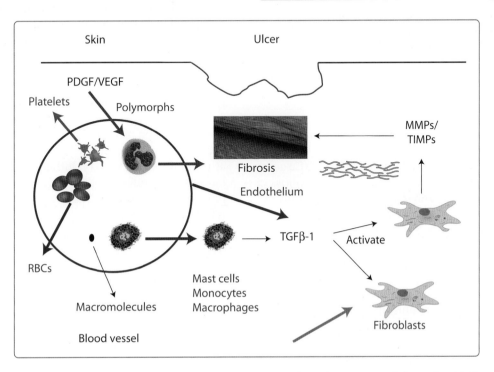

Figure 7.2 Mechanisms for venous ulcer formation. TGFβ-1: transforming growth factor β-1; MMPs: metalloproteinases; TIMP: tissue inhibitor metalloproteinase (deficient).

Heredity

- Epidemiological studies support a genetic basis for varicose disease.[13] About 80% of patients with varicose veins have a positive family history compared to 20% without the disease, and there is a 75% risk for developing varicose veins in monozygotic twins compared to a 50% risk for dizygotic twins. Different ethnic groups show marked differences in prevalence. However, despite demonstrating familial aggregation and clustering of the varicose vein phenotype, single-centre studies have displayed widespread disparity, with no accurate estimate of inheritance in the general population. The magnitude of genetic contribution has yet to be clarified.
- Genes that mediate the inflammatory reaction are more active and those responsible for collagen production are less active in patients with varicose veins. Several genes have been implicated which influence angiogenesis through vascular endothelial growth factors, venous wall integrity relating to different forms of collagen, and MMPs that cause extracellular matrix degradation. There are 46 chromosomes in humans and each chromosome has about 900 genes, so there are likely to be genes involved that have not yet been identified.

Genes linked to varicose veins

- It is possible that mutation of the FOXC2 gene is involved in inheritance of varicose veins. FOXC2 is a member of the forkhead family of transcription factors that bind to DNA and is located on the 16th chromosome. It is at that position that transfer RNase lays down a family of micro-filamentous proteins termed *actin* which provide a scaffold for soft tissue structures including venous valves and vein walls, as well as controlling smooth muscle function. It is postulated that FOXC2 mutation impairs transfer RNse instructions to cause a weakened actin to be laid down which in turn causes the vein wall to dilate and venous valves to fail.

- FOXC2 gene mutation was first identified as being a cause of the rare inherited condition of lymphoedema distichiasis, but has since been linked to varicose veins in the general population. Mutation occurs in 25%–30% of the adult population, it is autosomal dominant, is not sex-linked and has variable penetration, so that gene mutation could cause varicose veins to appear in one or both legs, in different veins or in one sibling but not in another. Studies in twins show a strong familial concordance for FOXC2 gene mutation with varicose veins and haemorrhoids, particularly for dizygotic twins.
- Ehlers–Danlos syndrome comprises multiple connective tissue disorders with abnormal collagen synthesis, and patients with this syndrome frequently have varicose veins. It is associated with the COL (collagen alpha chain) gene. However, the similar condition of Marfan syndrome is not associated with an increased prevalence of varicose veins, and the genetic differences that account for this have still to be determined.
- Matrix Gla-protein (MGP) is significantly increased in varicose compared to normal veins, contributing to altered extracellular matrix, and this may be due to gene mutation.
- Connexins form a family of gap junction proteins; at least three members are required for normal vein development, and gene mutations have been proposed as interfering with vein function.
- Thrombomodulin is an endothelial cell surface glycoprotein receptor that binds thrombin, and the thrombomodulin gene has been related to endothelial injury predisposing to varicose veins.
- Plasminogen activator inhibitor (PAI) regulates the fibrinolytic system, and PAI-1 4G/5G gene polymorphism has been association with varicose disease.
- A correlation between hyperhomo-cysteinemia and varicose disease has been demonstrated, and genetic mutation for methylene tetrahydrafolate reductase (MTHFR) has been linked to this association.

Genes linked to complications of varicose disease

- HFE C282Y hemochromatosis gene mutation is present in about 15% of patients with varicose veins, and can cause iron overload in the area of skin changes. The C282Y allele is no more prevalent in patients with varicose veins without ulcer disease than in normal subjects, so that it is only relevant to ulcer formation.
- Low-factor XIII activity has been demonstrated in the blood of patients with venous ulceration, and topical factor XIII treatment may improve venous ulcer healing. The factor XIII-34L gene variant is associated with a shorter healing time after surgery for venous ulcer surgery suggesting that it has a role in tissue regeneration.
- The oestrogen receptor-B gene is more likely to be present, and oestrogen has been shown to improve the rate of wound healing.
- TNF-A polymorphism is associated with inflammatory conditions. There is a two-fold increase in the risk of ulceration in carriers of the TNFA-308A allele, and leg ulcer wound fluid levels of TNF-A decrease as ulcers start to heal.

Progression of varicose disease

- Once veins are damaged, several factors then promote development and progression of varicose veins.

Ageing

- Disease will inevitably progressively worsen with age. Venous valves are progressively lost with age. Disease progressively advances up the limb to eventually render the terminal saphenous valves incompetent.

Pregnancy

- Although the prevalence of varicose veins is approximately equal between men and women and in women who have never been pregnant, they frequently either present or rapidly worsen during pregnancy. This mostly occurs in the first trimester, well before the uterus is sufficiently enlarged to cause mechanical iliac vein obstruction, and the process is considered to result from venous wall relaxation due to progesterone. Oral hormone replacement and contraceptives do not increase the risk of developing varicose veins.

Obesity

- The population is becoming increasingly obese. Obesity is significantly more frequent in patients with advanced varicose disease, though less frequent in those with telangiectasia.[14] Fat tissue in obese subjects usually contains plasminogen activator inhibitor (PAI)-1, interleukin-6 and the adhesion molecule P-selectin, which all contribute to vein damage. Increased intra-abdominal pressure results in increased ilio-femoral venous pressure and reduced flow from lower limb veins.
- Obese patients with lower limb venous disease are more likely to be symptomatic. Diagnosis is more difficult and treatment less effective in obese patients. Bariatric surgery usually improves chronic venous disease.

Increased intra-abdominal pressure

- A study of almost 10,000 Danish workers showed that the risk of requiring treatment for varicose veins was almost doubled for those standing or walking at least 75% of their working hours, for both men and women, independent of body mass index or of the number of children for women.[15]

History

- Hippocrates (460–370BC) introduced the term 'varicose' from the Greek word 'grapelike'. Galen (131–201AD) also provided a description of varicose veins. A Byzantine physician, Oribasius of Pergamum (325–405), devoted three chapters of text to varicose veins.
- Al-Zahrawi or Albucasis (936–1013) lived and worked in Cordoba and was considered the greatest medieval surgeon. His major contribution was the Kitab at-Tasrif, a 30-volume encyclopedia of medical practice that included descriptions of varicose veins

and their treatment by surgical techniques not much different to current practice.

- Ambroise Paré (1510–1590) working in Paris described a relation between varicose veins and pregnancy in 1545. Hieronymus Fabricius ab Acquapendente of Padua (1537–1619) appears to have been the first to relate varicose veins to valvular incompetence. Richard Lower (1631–1691), an English physician, described the relation between varicose veins and weakening of the vein wall in 1670.
- Rudolf Virchow (1821–1902), Professor of Pathology in Berlin, was probably the first to describe a hereditary tendency to varicose veins, in 1846.

References

1. Australian and New Zealand Clinical Practice Guideline for Prevention and Management of Venous Leg Ulcers 2011. http://www.awma.com.au/publications/2011_awma_vlug.pdf
2. Pocock ES, Alsaigh T, Mazor R, Schmid-Schönbein GW. Cellular and molecular basis of venous insufficiency. *Vasc Cell* 2014;6:24. https://www.ncbi.nlm.nih.gov/pmc/articles/PMC4268799/
3. Caggiati A. The venous valves of the lower limbs. *Phlebolymphology* 2013;20:87–95. http://www.phlebolymphology.org/the-venous-valves-of-the-lower-limbs/
4. King ESJ. The genesis of varicose veins. *Aust NZ J Surg* 1950;20:126–133. Text available from editor on request.
5. Boisseau MR. Recent findings in the pathogenesis of venous wall degradation. *Phlebolymphology* 2007; 14:59–68. http://www.phlebolymphology.org/recent-findings-in-the-pathogenesis-of-venous-wall-degradation/
6. Caggiati A, Rosi C, Heyn R, Franceschini M, Acconcia MC. Age-related variations of varicose veins anatomy. *J Vasc Surg* 2006;44:1291–5. http://www.ncbi.nlm.nih.gov/pubmed/17145433
7. Corcos L, De Anna D, Dini M, Macchi C, Ferrari PA, Dini S. Histopathology of great saphenous vein valves in primary venous insufficiency. *Phlebolymphology* 2004;47:304–311.

http://www.phlebolymphology.org/histopathology-of-great-saphenous-vein-valves-in-primary-venous-insufficiency/
8. Raffetto JD, Khalil RA. Mechanisms of varicose vein formation: Valve dysfunction and wall dilation. *Phlebology* 2008;23:85–98. https://www.ncbi.nlm.nih.gov/pubmed/18453484
9. Del Rio Solá L, Aceves M, Dueñas AI, González-Fajardo JA, Vaquero C, Sanchez Crespo M, García-Rodríguez C. Varicose veins show enhanced chemokine expression. *Eur J Vasc Endovasc Surg* 2009;38:635–641. http://www.sciencedirect.com/science/article/pii/S1078588409004006?np=y&npKey=21190bc07de2b7f1ec97c4975621323f1837a8503340ac3226c1bf1051f46c5b
10. Simka M. Cellular and molecular mechanisms of venous leg ulcers development – the 'puzzle' theory. *Int Angiol* 2010;29:1–19. http://www.ncbi.nlm.nih.gov/pubmed/20224526
11. Lim CS, Davies AH. Pathogenesis of primary varicose veins. *Br J Surg* 2009;96:1231–1242. https://www.ncbi.nlm.nih.gov/pubmed/19847861
12. Swanson T, Angel D, Sussman G, Cooper R, Haesler E, Ousey K, Carville K et al. *International Wound Infection Institute. Wound infection in clinical practice. International Consensus Update.* 2016. https://www.bbraun.com/content/dam/b-braun/global/website/products-and-therapies/wound-management/Docs/askina-calgitrol-ag-scientific-evidence/IWII%20Consensus_Final%20web.pdf.bb-.03454072/IWII%20Consensus_Final%20web.pdf
13. Krysa J, Jones GT, van Rij AM. Evidence for a genetic role in varicose veins and chronic venous insufficiency. *Phlebology* 2012;27:329–335. https://www.ncbi.nlm.nih.gov/pubmed/22308533
14. Seidel AC, Belczak CE, Campos MB, Campos RB, Harada DS. The impact of obesity on venous insufficiency. *Phlebology* 2015;30:475–80. https://www.ncbi.nlm.nih.gov/pubmed/25193821
15. Tuchsen F, Hannerz H, Burr H, Krause N. Prolonged standing at work and hospitalisation due to varicose veins: A 12 year prospective study of the Danish population. *Occup Environ Med* 2005;62:847–850. https://www.ncbi.nlm.nih.gov/pmc/articles/PMC1740939/pdf/v062p00847.pdf

8 | Selecting treatment for superficial venous disease

Treatment options

> This chapter includes recommendations from the European Society for Vascular Surgery, Cochrane Database, NICE Guidelines, Society for Vascular Surgery and American Venous Forum.[1–5]

- These include:
  - conservative management
  - superficial cosmetic procedures
  - direct-vision sclerotherapy
  - ultrasound-guided sclerotherapy (UGS)
  - catheter-directed sclerotherapy
  - mechanical occlusion chemically assisted (MOCA)
  - endovenous laser ablation (EVLA)
  - radio-frequency ablation (RF)
  - steam ablation
  - cyanoacrylate closure (CAC)
  - surgery
- Sclerotherapy techniques can be collectively referred to as chemical ablation and are performed using either liquid or foamed sclerosant. EVLA, RF and steam ablation are collectively termed endovenous thermal ablation (ETA).

Opinions from consensus statements

Representative organizations have offered recommendations for optimal treatment based on evidence from the literature, summarized below. These usually need to be updated by their time of publication.

European Society for Vascular Surgery

Classes of recommendation

I. Evidence and/or general agreement that management is beneficial, useful, effective.[1]
II. Conflicting evidence and/or divergence of opinion about the usefulness/efficacy of management.
  IIa. Weight of evidence/opinion is in favour of usefulness/efficacy.
  IIb. Usefulness/efficacy is less well-established from evidence/opinion.
III. Evidence or general agreement that management is not useful/effective and in some cases can be harmful.

Levels of evidence

A. Data derived from multiple randomized clinical trials or meta-analyses.
B. Data derived from a single randomized clinical trial or large non-randomized studies.
C. Consensus of opinions of experts and/or small studies, retrospective studies or registries.

Recommendations

- Liquid or foam sclerotherapy is not recommended as first-choice treatment for chronic venous disease C2–6 due to saphenous reflux and should only be used as primary treatment in selected cases – Class IIIA.

- Foam sclerotherapy is recommended as second-choice treatment for varicose veins and more advanced stages of chronic venous disease that are not eligible for surgery or endovenous ablation – Class IA.
- Foam sclerotherapy should be considered as primary treatment in patients with recurrent varicose veins, and in elderly and frail patients with venous ulcers – Class IIaB.
- Endovenous thermal ablation is recommended in preference to surgery or foam sclerotherapy for the treatment of great saphenous reflux for chronic venous disease – Class IA.
- Endovenous thermal ablation techniques should be considered for the treatment of small saphenous reflux with chronic venous disease, and access to the small saphenous vein should be gained no lower than mid-calf – Class IIaB.

Cochrane database

- They evaluated ETA and foam UGS versus open surgery by high ligation and stripping from 13 trials with over 3000 patients and reached the following conclusions.[2]
- The quality of the studies was acceptable but none tried to conceal the treatment type from participants, researchers or clinicians who measured outcomes. The available evidence is limited; there were large differences between the way studies reported outcomes and more randomized controlled trials are required.
- For foam UGS compared with surgery, there was no difference between treatment groups for recurrence rates and technical failure.
- Comparing EVLA and surgery, there was no difference between recurrence or recanalization rates, but early technical failure and later neovascularization were both higher for surgery than for EVLA.
- Comparing RF and surgery, there were no differences between treatment groups for recurrence, recanalization, neovascularization or technical failure rates.
- Quality of life generally increased similarly in all treatment groups and complication rates were low, especially major

complications. Pain was similar between treatment groups.
- New techniques may result in less pain after the procedure, fewer complications and a quicker return to work and normal activities with improved patient quality of life, as well as avoiding the need for a general anaesthetic. Evidence supports foam UGS, EVLA and RF as being no worse than open surgery.

The National Institute for Health and Care Excellence (NICE)

- Do not offer compression hosiery as a stand-alone treatment for varicose veins unless interventional treatment is not suitable – based on low- and very low-quality evidence.[3,4]
- If intervention is recommended:
  - Offer ETA by RF or EVLA.
  - If ETA is unsuitable, offer foam UGS.
  - If foam UGS is unsuitable, offer truncal vein stripping surgery.
  - This was based on low- and very low-quality evidence from direct comparisons in randomized controlled trials.
  - Cost-effectiveness analysis showed no significant benefit for UGS compared to ETA when studied long-term.[6]
- They identified a need for clinical research to address clinical and cost-effectiveness for:
  - Compression stockings versus no compression for the management of symptomatic varicose veins.
  - Concurrent phlebectomies or foam sclerotherapy for varicose tributaries with truncal ETA compared to tributary ablation some weeks later.
  - Optimal treatment by compression, ETA, foam UGS or surgery for varicose disease at each of the CEAP stages comparing clinical C2–3, C4 and C5–6.

Society for Vascular Surgery and American Venous Forum

- Recommendations were strong (Grade 1) if benefits clearly outweigh the risks, burden and costs, or weak (Grade 2) if benefits are closely balanced with risks and burden. The level of available evidence to support the evaluation was high (A), medium (B) or low or very low (C) quality.[5] Recommendations were:

- Treatment by compression for patients with symptomatic varicose veins (Grade 2C) but not as primary treatment if the patient is a candidate for saphenous vein ablation (Grade 1B).
- Compression as primary treatment to aid healing of venous ulceration (Grade 1B) and ablation of incompetent superficial veins in addition to compression to decrease risk of ulcer recurrence (Grade 1A).
- For great saphenous reflux:
  - ETA rather than high ligation and inversion stripping of the saphenous vein to the level of the knee (Grade 1B).
  - Phlebectomy or sclerotherapy to treat varicose tributaries (Grade 1B),
  - Foam UGS as an option (Grade 2C).
- Avoid selective treatment of perforating vein reflux in patients with uncomplicated varicose veins (Grade 1B), but treat pathologic perforating veins located underneath healed or active ulcers (Grade 2B).

Randomized clinical trials

- Details of trials addressing various options have been summarized.[7,8]

Rasmussen and colleagues

- Their European trial compared treatment of 500 patients with varicose veins and great saphenous reflux randomized to EVLA, RF, foam UGS or surgical stripping with tumescent anaesthesia.[9] Tributaries were treated by phlebectomy. The patients were examined with ultrasound before and at three days, one month and one year after treatment.
  - At one year, technical ultrasound success rates were 94.2% for EVLA, 95.2% for RF, 83.7% for foam UGS and 95.2% for surgery.
  - Both RF and foam UGS were associated with a faster recovery and less post-operative pain than EVLA or stripping.

Brittenden and colleagues

- Their multicentre study in the United Kingdom of 798 patients treated by EVLA, foam UGS or surgery measured technical success, disease-specific and generic quality of life, clinical success and complications.[10]
  - Successful ablation of saphenous trunks was less common with foam UGS than for surgery.
  - Disease-specific quality of life was slightly worse after foam UGS than after surgery, but was similar for EVLA and surgery. There were no significant differences between the foam, laser or surgery groups for generic quality of life. Measures of clinical success were similar for all groups.
  - The frequency of procedural complications was lower for EVLA than for foam UGS or surgery, although the small risk of serious adverse events was similar for all groups.
  - In a later study, they found that cost-effectiveness analysis showed no significant benefit for UGS compared to ETA when studied long-term.[11]

Venous ulcers
The ESCHAR study

- This followed 500 patients with open or recently-healed leg ulcers and superficial venous reflux randomized to compression alone or compression plus saphenous surgery.[12] There was an advantage for surgery, although methodologic problems with the conclusions include concern as to compliance with compression and a relatively large number of patients randomized to surgery who refused operation.
- Ulcer healing rates at three years were 89% for the compression group and 93% for compression plus surgery, and rates of ulcer recurrence at four years were 56% for the compression group and 31% for the compression plus surgery. Recurrence rates in relation to superficial and deep venous disease were:

- isolated superficial reflux – 51% for compression and 27% for compression plus surgery (five years).
- superficial with segmental deep reflux – 52% for compression and 24% for compression plus surgery (three years).
- superficial and total deep reflux – 46% for compression and 32% for compression plus surgery (three years).

Authors opinions

- EVLA and RF are used to ablate saphenous veins and incompetent perforators, while EVLA is also used for relatively straight tributaries and arteriovenous malformations. Steam ablation promises to allow both saphenous veins and tributaries to be controlled. Cyanoacrylate embolisation (CE) avoids the need for tumescent anaesthesia.
- ETA shows faster recovery and return to work and normal activities, higher patient satisfaction, less pain and better short-term quality of life than traditional surgery, with comparable efficacy for eliminating venous reflux and relieving symptoms for both.
- ETA and surgery show better long-term success than UGS. EVLA and RF probably have a similar outcome.
- There is less perioperative pain for procedures that do not require tumescent anaesthesia such as MOCA and CE.
- Cost-effectiveness analysis shows no significant benefit for UGS compared to ETA when studied long-term.[6,10] Similarly, ETA is as cost-effective as surgery, taking all associated costs into account, including time away from work and other societal costs.[13]
- Many consider it necessary to treat both the saphenous veins and tributaries in an affected part of the limb although management of perforators is more controversial. However, other practitioners have developed techniques to preserve the saphenous veins, limiting treatment to tributaries (see Chapter 14). Ultrasound surveillance after primary intervention frequently shows residual refluxing saphenous veins in the distal segment of a saphenous vein where the proximal segment

has been treated by surgery or endovenous techniques, and this is a frequent cause for unresolved symptoms, persistent varicosities and early recurrence unless treated.
- In the past when surgery was the only option to treat a venous ulcer, intervention was usually deferred until healing was advanced and bacterial contamination was minimal to avoid infection in surgical wounds. With the advent of endovascular procedures, intervention can now be safely performed much earlier.

History

- The Egyptian Ebers Papyrus of herbal knowledge dating to about 1550 BC which is now held in the library of the University of Leipzig warned against intervention for varicose veins: 'If thou examine a swollen blood vessel under the skin of a limb and its aspect increases, becomes sinuous and serpentine, like something swollen with air, then thou will say concerning it, it is a swollen blood vessel – Thou shall not touch something like this'.[14]
- Hippocrates (460–370BC) was somewhat opposed to surgery for varicose veins and at most recommended making tiny incisions to remove them supplemented by compression, with emphasis that this could lead to ulcers.
- Plutarch reported on varicose vein surgery for the Roman general Gaius Marius: 'Refusing to be bound, he presented to him one leg, and then without a motion or a groan but with a steadfast countenance and in silence, endured incredible pain under the knife. When, however, the physician was proceeding to treat the other leg, Marius would suffer him no further declaring that he saw the cure to be not worth the pain.'[15]

References

1. Wittens C, Davies AH, Bækgaard N, Broholm R, Cavezzi A, Chastanet S, de Wolf M et al. Management of chronic venous disease. Clinical practice guidelines of the European Society for Vascular Surgery. *Eur J Vasc Endovasc Surg* 2015;49:678–737. https://www.

researchgate.net/publication/280483468_Editor's_ Choice_Management_of_Chronic_Venous_Disease_ Clinical_Practice_Guidelines_of_the_European_ Society_for_Vascular_Surgery_ESVS

2. Nesbitt C, Bedenis R, Bhattacharya V, Stansby G. Endovenous ablation (radiofrequency and laser) and foam sclerotherapy versus open surgery for great saphenous vein varices. *Cochrane Database System Rev* 2014;7:CD005624. http://onlinelibrary.wiley.com/ doi/10.1002/14651858.CD005624.pub3/pdf

3. NICE guidelines. Varicose veins: diagnosis and management. [CG168] July 2013. https://www.nice.org.uk/ guidance/cg168

4. Marsden G, Perry M, Kelley K, Davies AH. Diagnosis and management of varicose veins in the legs: Summary of NICE guidance. *BMJ* 2013;347:f4279. http://www.bmj. com/content/347/bmj.f4279

5. Gloviczki P, Comerota AJ, Dalsing MC, Eklof BG, Gillespie DL, Gloviczki ML, Lohr JM et al. The care of patients with varicose veins and associated chronic venous diseases: Clinical practice guidelines of the Society for Vascular Surgery and the American Venous Forum. *J Vasc Surg* 2011;53:2S–48S. https://www.ncbi.nlm.nih. gov/pubmed/21536172

6. Marsden G, Perry M, Bradbury A, Hickey N, Kelley K, Trender H, Wonderling D, Davies AH. A Cost-effectiveness analysis of surgery, endothermal ablation, ultrasound-guided foam sclerotherapy and compression stockings for symptomatic varicose veins. *Euro J Vasc Endovasc Surg* 2015;50:794–801. https://www. researchgate.net/publication/280696295_A_Cost-effectiveness_Analysis_of_Surgery_Endodermal_ Ablation_Ultrasound-guided_Foam_Sclerotherapy_ and_Compression_Stockings_for_Symptomatic_ Varicose_Veins

7. Eklof B, Perrin M. Randomized controlled trial in treatment of varicose veins (1). *Phlebolymphology* 2011;18:196–207. http://www.phlebolymphology.org/ randomized-controlled-trials-in-the-treatments-of-varicose-veins/

8. Perrin M, Eklof B. Randomized controlled trials in the treatment of varicose veins (2). *Phlebolymphology* 2012;19:91. http://www.phlebolymphology.org/ randomized-controlled-trials-in-the-treatment-of-varicose-veins-2/

9. Rasmussen L, Lawaetz M, Serup J, Bjoern L, Vennits B, Blemings A, Eklof B. Randomized clinical trial comparing endovenous laser ablation, radiofrequency ablation, foam sclerotherapy, and surgical stripping for great saphenous varicose veins with 3-year follow-up. *J Vasc Surg Ven Lymph Dis* 2013;1:349–56. http://www. jvsvenous.org/article/S2213-333X(13)00096-6/abstract

10. Brittenden J, Cotton SC, Elders A, Ramsay CR, Norrie J, Burr J, Campbell B et al. A randomized trial comparing treatments for varicose veins. *N Engl J Med* 2014;371:1218–1227. https://www.ncbi.nlm.nih.gov/ pubmed/25251616

11. Brittenden J, Cotton SC, Elders A, Tassie E, Scotland G, Ramsay CR, Norrie J et al. Clinical effectiveness and cost-effectiveness of foam sclerotherapy, endovenous laser ablation and surgery for varicose veins: results from the Comparison of Laser, Surgery and foam Sclerotherapy (CLASS) randomised controlled trial. *Health Technol Assess.* 2015;19:1–342. https://www.ncbi. nlm.nih.gov/pubmed/25858333

12. Gohel MS, Barwell JR, Taylor M, Chant T, Foy C, Earnshaw JJ, Heather BP et al. Long term results of compression therapy alone versus compression plus surgery in chronic venous ulceration (ESCHAR): randomised controlled trial. *BMJ* 2007;335:83. https:// www.ncbi.nlm.nih.gov/pmc/articles/PMC1914523/

13. Gohel MS, Epstein DM, Davies AH. Cost-effectiveness of traditional and endovenous treatments for varicose veins. *Br J Surg* 2010;97:1815–1823. http:// www.flebologiaitaliana.it/articoli/costo-efficacia%20 del%20trattamento%20tradizionale%20o%20 endovenoso%20per%20varici.pdf

14. Perrin M. History of venous surgery (1). *Phlebolymphology* 2011;18:123–9. http://www.phlebolymphology.org/ history-of-venous-surgery-1/

15. The Parallel Lives by Plutarch. Vol. IX, Loeb Classical Library edition, 1920. http://penelope.uchicago.edu/Thayer/E/ Roman/Texts/Plutarch/Lives/Marius*.html#nnn

9 Preparing for treatment of superficial venous disease

Patient selection

- Whether or not to advise intervention depends on the reason for a patient's presentation.
  - Patients with impending or actual complications are encouraged to undergo intervention unless there is an overriding contraindication.
  - Patients with appreciable cosmetic disturbance or symptoms will frequently request treatment which is usually offered unless there are significant contraindications.
  - Some patients present to explore whether it is best to treat their disease early before it gets too bad or if it is acceptable to wait. Progression of disease is virtually certain, but the rate is unpredictable, and many will never develop complications or even symptoms. It is up to the patient to decide, and no pressure should be brought to bear, for this is prone to an unhappy outcome.
  - Many patients present simply because they, their families or their treating doctors feel that they should be evaluated, and these should be treated with caution, as the results of treatment may not be appreciated.
  - It is equally important to guide patients as to priorities for treatment, both to meet their expectations and to indicate when these are not realistic. An example is the patient with impending skin complications who insists upon limited cosmetic treatment only.

Conservative management

- It is usually appropriate to advise conservative management if the patient is old or in poor health, unless compelled to intervene because of complications. Conservative management may be necessary due to absolute or relative contraindications to intervention.

Intervention

- The patient's concerns should determine whether there is a need for further investigation and determine also the most appropriate advice for treatment. Failure to address these concerns is likely to lead to an unsatisfactory outcome.
- The choice of best treatment is based in part on factors that concern the treating doctor.
  - What is the likelihood of durable technical success?
  - Does the anatomy allow access without risk of damage to important adjacent nerves and arteries?
  - Which procedure involves the least pain and risk of complications?
  - Which is the most cost-effective?

9.1 Contraindications to intervention for superficial venous disease

Absolute

- Acute deep vein thrombosis and/or pulmonary embolism.[1]
- Deep venous obstruction.
- Severe peripheral arterial occlusive disease.
- Local infection.
- Severe generalized infection or illness.
- Long-lasting immobility and confinement to bed.

Relative

- Pregnancy.
- Breast feeding – interruption for two to three days.
- Poor general health.
- Limited mobility.
- Morbid obesity.
- High thrombo-embolic risk.
- Acute superficial venous thrombosis.
- Recent surgery.
- Recent long-haul travel.
- Diabetes – wound healing.
- Intolerance to compression.

NB. Treatment for superficial venous disease is contraindicated if there is deep vein obstruction, but can be effective in reducing venous load if there is deep venous reflux. Current treatment with anticoagulant drugs is not a contraindication to endovenous treatment.

9.2 Specific contraindications to chemical ablation

- Known allergy to the sclerosant or strong predisposition to allergies.[1]
- Known symptomatic right-to-left shunt, such as a patent foramen ovale, if using foam.
- Neurological disturbances following previous sclerotherapy.
- Severe needle phobia.
- Severe migraines or asthma.

- The decision is also based in part on factors that concern the patient.
  - What is the most effective method to relieve symptoms and improve appearance?
  - Which is the safest?
  - Which involves the least peri- and post-operative pain?
  - Which will cause the least inconvenience during recovery and the most rapid return to normal activities, with minimal time lost for the procedure and recovery?
  - Will compression be necessary and for how long?
  - Which is the least expensive?
- Patients must be warned that they should not expect all veins to disappear and that there would be no more than improvement in appearance, that further they should anticipate not only the need for multiple treatment sessions but also that lasting success requires long-term review.

Selection

- Arrange for pre-treatment ultrasound scanning to map refluxing saphenous veins and tributaries in most patients who are being considered for intervention. Ideally, this should include patients with smaller cosmetic veins to ensure that there is no unrecognized reflux in saphenous or other veins, but cost of ultrasound scanning frequently prohibits its use, for example in a young asymptomatic woman with a few thigh telangiectases.
- If intervention is warranted, then the technique recommended largely depends on ultrasound findings.
  - Clinical telangiectases and reticular veins without clinical or ultrasound evidence of saphenous or major contributory reflux can be treated by direct-vision sclerotherapy or other cosmetic techniques.
  - There is a dilemma for clinical cosmetic veins and ultrasound finding of incidental saphenous or major tributary reflux, for conventional belief is that the underlying reflux should be treated first to ensure good results from subsequent sclerotherapy,

although this opinion has yet to be tested. This will usually involve more extensive treatment than was anticipated by the patient.

- Appreciable varicose veins without ultrasound evidence of saphenous reflux are best managed by ultrasound-guided sclerotherapy (UGS) or by ambulatory phlebectomy.
- Appreciable varicose veins with ultrasound evidence of associated saphenous reflux are now best treated by endovenous techniques.
- Appreciable varicose veins with ultrasound evidence of sapheno-femoral incompetence but no great saphenous reflux is a situation where high saphenous ligation and phlebectomy can be considered.
- Endovenous interventions are preferred for recurrent varicose veins, and redo varicose vein surgery is no longer recommended, as results are poor and risk of wound and other complications, such as nerve and lymphatic damage, is high.

The first consultation

The history

- Start by asking about the reasons for presentation.
  - Concern about appearance or worsening chronic symptoms.
  - Complications such as eczema or ulceration, variceal bleeding or superficial vein thrombosis.
  - Advice regarding future medical implications.
  - A recommendation from a family member or referring doctor.
- Symptoms tend to be more severe in the early stages of disease, and the presence and severity of symptoms do not correlate well with the size and extent of varicose veins or development of complications. Not all patients are aware that their symptoms had been due to venous disease until after treatment. Conversely, many symptoms are due to conditions other than varicose veins.

- Symptoms have been assessed in detail by a consensus group.[2]
  - Pain, aching, throbbing, tightness, heavy legs.
  - Fatigue, cramps, restless legs.
  - Swelling of the ankles and feet.
  - Itching, bleeding.
- Pain associated with larger varicose veins is usually a dull ache. Symptoms are usually worse as the day progresses and precipitated by prolonged standing or activities involving straining. Symptoms usually worsen with menstruation.
- Pain is frequently described as being:
  - made worse by prolonged standing
  - worse by the end of the day
  - partly relieved by exercise
  - eased by compression stockings
- Take a history to include features relevant to venous disease and treatment.
  - Date of onset.
  - Family history of varicose veins or thrombo-embolism.
  - History of miscarriages and pregnancies.
  - Past venous complications such as skin changes or ulceration.
  - Past venous thrombo-embolism.
  - Past treatment for venous disease.
  - Migraine headaches.
  - Asthma.
  - Allergies.
  - Medications.
  - Smoking habits.
- Ask whether a female patient is or could become pregnant. It is essential to ensure that no medications that could harm the foetus be administered. Categories for harmful effects from agents are given in Chapter 5.
- Take a general history.
  - Occupation.
  - Smoking habits, alcohol intake and other substances.
  - Associated general and local diseases – hypertension, diabetes, cardiovascular disease, cerebrovascular disease or intermittent claudication.
  - HIV and hepatitis status.
  - Past medical and surgical history.
  - Attitude to needles, history of syncope.

Thrombo-embolism

- Enquire as to a history of past thrombo-embolic events, family history of thrombosis, or multiple late miscarriages or complications during pregnancy, for these might lead to suspicion of underlying thrombophilia. However, most patients proceed to treatment regardless of the outcome of testing for thrombophilia, so that usual practice now is to move away from testing and to simply manage patients with prophylactic anticoagulation if there is a strong suspicion.

Medications

- Advise that current medications be continued, with the following reservations.
    - Ask female patients if they are taking an oral contraceptive or undergoing hormone replacement therapy. Sodium tetradecyl sulphate manufacturers state that sclerotherapy should not be performed whilst on the oral contraceptive due to risk of thrombosis, while polidocanol manufacturers recommend that sclerotherapy should be avoided if there are 'multiple prothrombotic risk factors'. However, there is no scientific evidence to support this, and many experienced practitioners argue that the risks of an unwanted pregnancy outweigh the risk of remaining on the oral contraceptive. There should be individual discussion as to whether or not taking hormones should be suspended. The oral contraceptive and fish oil may increase the risk of matting, but further studies are required for this to be verified.
    - Ask whether medications that reduce blood clotting such as aspirin, fish oil or warfarin are being taken, to warn that these could increase post-treatment bruising. They do not need to be stopped as they do not reduce the likelihood of a successful outcome.
    - Enquire as to whether minocycline or iron supplements have been prescribed as this could increase the risk of pigmentation after treatment with sclerosants. If so, advise that either supplement should be discontinued four weeks before intervention.
- Enquire as to calcium-channel blockers which may be a cause of peripheral oedema in addition to or instead of venous disease.

Venous ulceration

- Ask about specific features.[3]
    - Is it the first time or is there a recurrence, and if a recurrence then how many previous times and when?
    - Are there medical conditions causing lack of mobility that might impair the calf muscle pump?
    - Is there evidence of systemic disease?
    - Attempt to distinguish a venous ulcer from ulceration due to occlusive arterial disease, vasculitis or a neoplasm. Nocturnal pain is usually not severe with a venous ulcer and very severe with an arterial ulcer. Ask about trophic changes such as hair and skin changes seen with arterial and neuropathic disease.
    - Enquire as to the duration of the current ulcer, previous ulcers and the time they have taken to heal, time spent free of venous ulcers and strategies used to manage previous venous ulcers. Consider using a pain scale.
    - Ask about food and fluid intake.

Examination

- Stand the patient for a few minutes to fill the veins.
- Inspect both lower limbs and the perineum, pubic region and abdominal wall. Look for the nature, size and distribution of veins. Visible distended superficial veins in the leg and thigh are usually diseased, but normal veins are prominent in athletes, translucent skin may allow normal veins to be visible, and normal veins are typically distended and visible at the ankle and in the foot.
- Inspect for telangiectases, prominent varicose veins, skin changes and scars from prior surgery. Photograph any findings as patients often forget the original appearance and may insist that pre-existing lesions were instead caused by treatment.

- Lightly palpate for dilated veins that may not yet be visible. Feel for thrombosed superficial veins and for fascial defects at the site of perforating veins, although these are difficult to distinguish from fat atrophy at the site of varicosities. Request a forced cough which may produce a palpable thrill or sudden expansion in a varicose vein if reflux is present.
- Traditional Trendelenburg's and Perthe's tests using tourniquets have proven to be unreliable. A European consensus considers that they no longer have a place in mapping the distribution of venous disease as they have been replaced by ultrasound scanning.[4]
- Note discoloured skin near the affected veins and in the lower leg, corona phlebectatica, atrophie blanche, lipodermatosclerosis, scarring from a healed ulcer or active ulceration.

Venous ulceration

- Examine the limb to attempt to distinguish a venous ulcer from ulceration due to occlusive arterial disease, vasculitis or a neoplasm. The appearance of the pigmented surrounding skin usually points to a venous cause. Palpate for arterial pulses.
- Make note of the anatomical distribution of an ulcer in relation to the skin draining regions of the great and small saphenous veins. Ulcers relating to great saphenous reflux are usually on the medial aspect, whereas those from small saphenous reflux may be on either side.

9.3 Comparison of venous and arterial ulcers

Venous ulcers	Arterial ulcers
• Medial gaiter area	• Lateral or over malleoli, metatarsal heads, toes
• Ulcer shallow with irregular sloping edges	• Ulcer punched out, dry and scabbed
• Varicose veins, oedema and pigmentation	• Skin pale, cold, shiny and hairless
• Some pain	• More painful

- Measure the ulcer length, width and depth, and consider tracing the ulcer margins and using planimetry. Note the amount and type of exudate, appearance of the ulcer bed, condition of the ulcer edges and signs of clinical infection.
- Measure the ankle and calf circumferences to assess oedema.
- Attempt to assess the gait, strength of calf muscle contraction and range of ankle movements to evaluate the calf muscle pump.
- Investigate all patients with a duplex ultrasound scan.

Advice to patients before treatment

- Defer treatment if there is impending long-distance travel. The risk of thrombo-embolism begins to rise for any form of travel of more than about five hours' duration,[5] and although evidence is lacking, it is reasonable to assume that this risk might be further increased if intervention were to be performed within a short time before or after travel. It is best to avoid possible accusation that travel-related thrombosis was due to treatment. Changes predisposing to venous thrombo-embolism persist for up to several weeks after travel. Accordingly, it is prudent to advise that treatment be avoided within an arbitrary four weeks of impending long-distance travel or two weeks after return. If travel is essential near the time of treatment, then cover the trip with prophylactic anticoagulation and stockings.
- Antibiotic prophylaxis to reduce the risk of bacterial endocarditis with heart valve disease is not generally required. The American Heart Association recommends that patients with high-risk heart conditions, prosthetic heart valves and prosthetic joints should receive an anti-staphylococcal agent such as cephalothin prior to a procedure, but there are no guidelines for venous procedures.
- Wear slacks or loose trousers and sandals or loose shoes to allow for the thickness of bandages and stockings.

Advice to patients after treatment

- Advise the patient to walk for 15 minutes immediately after treatment and then at least once daily. However, there is no evidence that this improves results or lessens post-operative problems.
- Maintain normal daytime activities and avoid standing still for long periods. Resume normal exercise activities within 24–36 hours.
- A check ultrasound scan may be arranged shortly after treatment to ensure that the treated vein is occluded, determine whether any further veins require treatment and exclude the small risk of deep vein thrombosis.
- Maintain compression stockings through the day. Early evidence suggested benefit from several days of post-treatment compression, but this has not been proven, and there is no consensus as to what compression regime should be used.[6,7] Most practitioners in Australasia use 20–40 mm Hg compression stockings for one to two weeks, continuous for the first one to three days, in the belief that this will provide comfort and will reduce trapped blood, but there is a trend towards less compression. A French study that compared compression stockings against no compression after UGS found no difference in occlusion rates on ultrasound, symptoms and side effects, patient satisfaction, quality of life or rate of mobilization, and this has resulted in a marked decrease in post-treatment compression by French phlebologists.[8,9]
- The NICE guidelines suggest 'If offering compression bandaging or hosiery for use after interventional treatment, do not use for more than seven days'.[10] However, they indicate that this is based on low- and very low-quality evidence. They identified a need for studies to compare compression bandaging or stockings after interventional treatment with no compression, and if there is benefit then the optimal duration for compression.

Consent

- Signed informed consent should include the following:
  - An indication that all treatment options have been explained.
  - What the proposed treatment involves, its risks, complications and costs.
  - Acknowledgement that risks for continuing medications such as hormones have been accepted.
  - What mechanisms are available for a complaints process.
- The patient should have received a detailed printout of what to expect, before, during and after treatment.

References

1. Rabe E, Breu FX, Cavezzi A, Coleridge Smith P, Frullini A, Gillet JL, Guex JJ et al. Guideline Group. European guidelines for sclerotherapy in chronic venous disorders. *Phlebology*. 2014;29:338–54. http://journals.sagepub.com/doi/pdf/10.1177/0268355513483280

2. Perrin M, Eklof B, Van Rij A, Labropoulos N, Vasquez M, Nicolaides A, Blattler W et al. Venous symptoms: The SYM Vein Consensus statement developed under the auspices of the European Venous Forum. *Int Angiol* 2016;35:374–98. https://www.ncbi.nlm.nih.gov/pubmed/27081866

3. Kunimoto BT. Assessment of venous leg ulcers: an in-depth discussion of a literature guided approach. *Ostomy/Wound Mgmt* 2001;47:38–53. https://www.ncbi.nlm.nih.gov/pubmed/11889721

4. Wittens C, Davies AH, Bækgaard N, Broholm R, Cavezzi A, Chastanet S, de Wolf M et al. Management of Chronic Venous Disease. Clinical Practice Guidelines of the European Society for Vascular Surgery. *Eur J Vasc Endovasc Surg* 2015;49:678–737. https://www.researchgate.net/publication/280483468_Editor's_Choice_-_Management_of_Chronic_Venous_Disease_Clinical_Practice_Guidelines_of_the_European_Society_for_Vascular_Surgery_ESVS

5. Johnston RV, Hudson MF, on behalf of the Aerospace Medical Association Air Transport Medicine Committee. Travelers' thrombosis. *Aviat Space Environ Med* 2014;85:191–4. https://www.asma.org/asma/media/asma/Travel-Publications/Medical%20Guidelines/Travelers-Thrombosis.pdf

6. Bootun R, Onida S, Lane TR, Davies AH. To compress or not to compress: The eternal question of the place of compression after endovenous procedures.

Phlebology 2016;31:529–31. https://www.ncbi.nlm.nih.gov/pubmed/26447136

7. El-Sheikha J, Carradice D, Nandhra S, Leung C, Smith GE, Wallace T, Campbell B, Chetter IC. A systematic review of the compression regimes used in randomised clinical trials following endovenous ablation. *Phlebology* 2017;32:256–71. https://www.ncbi.nlm.nih.gov/pubmed/27178404

8. Hamel-Desnos CM, Guias BJ, Desnos PR, Mesgard A. Foam sclerotherapy of the saphenous veins: randomised controlled trial with or without compression. *Eur J Vasc Endovasc Surg* 2010;39:500–7. https://www.ncbi.nlm.nih.gov/pubmed/20097585

9. Tripey V, Monsallier JM, Morello R, Hamel-Desnos C. French sclerotherapy and compression: Practice patterns. *Phlebology* 2015;30:632–40. https://www.ncbi.nlm.nih.gov/pubmed/?term=hamel-desnos+tripey

10. NICE guidelines. Varicose veins: diagnosis and management. [CG168] July 2013. https://www.nice.org.uk/guidance/cg168

10 Investigations for chronic venous diseases

This chapter incorporates recommendations from a consensus group representing the Union Internationale de Phlebologie.[1,2]

Non-invasive investigations have largely replaced invasive techniques. Ultrasound examination is now routinely requested for most patients.[1-4] Investigations for pressure and volume changes have clinical value in selected patients and are used for research.[5]

Indications for ultrasound

- The purpose is to detect reflux in veins that are not visible to clinical inspection. Ultrasound is particularly valuable for patients with complications from primary varicose disease or with recurrent varicose veins where disease patterns can be complex. Some patients present with leg oedema or leg pains without obvious varicose veins where the investigation can either detect occult venous disease or exclude a venous cause. Ultrasound is used to help plan for endovenous or surgical treatment, guide the procedure and perform surveillance after intervention.
- There are differences in techniques for ultrasound scans for chronic venous disease described in this chapter and those for deep vein thrombosis described in Chapter 15. Chronic venous scans involve testing for vein morphology and normal flow or reflux due to gravity in deep, superficial and perforator veins, mostly with the patient erect. In contrast, venous thrombosis scans concentrate on patency or occlusion of superficial and deep veins, mostly with the patient supine.
- Superficial venous disease has come to be defined by reflux in superficial veins shown by ultrasound, but symptoms or complications seen in real life are due to venous pooling and venous hypertension. Other investigations such as air plethysmography can provide a broader picture, but are not routinely performed in most practices.

Ultrasound techniques

Plan the scan and prepare the patient

- Reflux is more likely to develop later in the day. Scan in a warm room as cold surroundings can cause veins to constrict and apparently become competent in patients with borderline reflux. Allow more time for scanning if the patient is elderly, large or incapacitated.
- Explain what is going to be done, such as the Valsalva manoeuvre. Ask about past deep vein thrombosis and venous interventions.
- Examine the leg in a bright light for the site of varicosities to help predict venous patterns. Look for surgical scars which may be the only evidence for past vein treatment.
- Check for skin changes from eczema, lipodermatosclerosis or ulceration, and look to

see where to avoid placing the hand for distal compression. Cover open areas for mutual protection.

- Warn patients to sit down quickly if they feel faint, as fainting may occur after standing for some time for the examination. Consider turning off sound, as the noise from reflux with spectral Doppler can increase anxiety and a tendency to faint.

Set up the machine

Transducers

- Use a medium- to high-frequency (10–18 Mhz) linear-array transducer for most studies.
- Change to a lower-frequency (2–5 MHz) curved-array transducer for an obese or oedematous limb, for deep veins in the thigh, such as the femoral vein at the adductor hiatus, or for peroneal veins.
- Change to a low-frequency curved- or phased-array transducer to scan the inferior vena cava or iliac, pelvic or ovarian veins.

B-Mode

- Use low gain and power to prevent over-saturation of surrounding tissues or artefact within veins.
- Use a high contrast setting to highlight vein walls and to show the lumen as a black background when testing for reflux, and a low contrast setting to show detail in surrounding tissue.

Colour Doppler

- Set colour to blue for flow towards the heart and red away from the heart.
- Set a low colour velocity range of +10 to −10 cm/s or even lower for very small veins, but increase the range if this produces unacceptable high colour artefact or reduced frame rate.
- Select an even colour hue across the frequency range as velocity information and aliasing are not used to test for venous disease.
- Optimize colour gain and priority settings to allow good colour filling without 'bleeding'.

Spectral Doppler

- Orientate the probe for an augmentation signal to appear below and a reflux signal to show above the baseline.
- Set the velocity range to 40–50 cm/s when testing for reflux and reduce the range for low-flow states. Set the wall filter to a minimum so that low-flow traces are not filtered out. Open the sample volume to obtain as much information from the veins as possible. Set the Doppler display sweep to the slowest speed to easily identify flow patterns.

Detect venous reflux

- There is transient reflux for ≤0.5 sec as normal valves close. The accepted definition of reflux is reverse flow for >0.5 sec for saphenous veins, lower leg veins and perforators, and >1 sec for femoro-popliteal veins.
- Induce reflux in proximal veins by the Valsalva manoeuvre.* Alternatively, use manual compression to squeeze then release the thigh, calf or foot depending on the level being examined. Other techniques include pneumatic calf cuff deflation, eliciting flow by active foot dorsiflexion and relaxation, or manual compression of varicose vein clusters. The 'Paraná' manoeuvre† is to push the patient gently to induce a calf contraction and is particularly useful if the leg is oedematous or too painful to squeeze.

Make measurements

- Measure representative vein diameters. The most reproducible point to measure saphenous vein diameter a few cm distal to its junction with the deep vein, although the most representative level is still debated.
- Record the level of landmarks such as the position of the sapheno-popliteal junction, other deep to superficial connections and perforating veins in relation to surface

---

* Antonio Maria Valsalva (1666–1723), Italian anatomist.
† Described by Claude Franceschi at a CHIVA congress in 1998 in the town of Paraná, Argentina.

landmarks such as the knee and groin creases, and the medial and lateral malleoli.

- Perforators pass through the deep fascia which is a distinct hyperechoic band on B-mode, and this is the most representative site to measure perforator vein diameter.

10.1 Limitations of venous ultrasound

- It can be difficult to obtain the best angle for insonation and Doppler sampling.
- Scarring can cause increased beam attenuation.
- The colour display is in two dimensions whereas flow is three-dimensional.
- The small sample size for spectral Doppler provides information only for a small segment in a larger field of view.

Scan the patient

- Scan with the patient standing or tilted on a table in reverse Trendelenburg to >60°. Face the patient towards the sonographer with the leg being examined rotated outwards and weight taken on the opposite leg. Use light transducer pressure to ensure that superficial veins are not compressed making it difficult for them to be seen.
- Initially ignore varicosities and scan for sites of reflux to these veins, and only if this fails should varices be traced back to the saphenous veins.
- To mark veins prior to endovenous ablation or surgery, place the patient supine with the limb in the operation position, as shifting from standing to supine changes the relation between veins and surface landmarks and causes up to 25% decrease in the saphenous vein diameter.[6]
- Identify each vein with B-mode in transverse, change to colour Doppler to test for reflux in longitudinal, then use spectral Doppler to measure duration of reverse flow. Experienced sonographers tend to rely on colour Doppler to make a visual diagnosis as to whether reflux is present. Follow each vein along its full length with B-mode,

and periodically test for reflux with colour Doppler. Identify perforators passing through the deep fascia.

Veins above and at the knee

- Scan for the great saphenous vein (GSV), anterior accessory saphenous vein (AASV), sapheno-femoral junction (SFJ), common femoral, deep femoral and femoral veins, thigh perforators and tributaries.

Position the patient and select windows

- Examine veins in the groin through the femoral triangle. Scan the GSV through a medial window and the AASV through an anterior window. Examine deep veins in the thigh from an antero-medial approach.
- Image quality may deteriorate as the deep vein passes through the adductor hiatus. Straighten the leg and use an anterior approach through the vastus medialis muscle to view the vein – it is further from the transducer but the image is better. Alternatively, scan from antero-medial while pushing with the other hand from behind.

Scan the GSV and AASV above the knee

- Commence in the groin in transverse to show the SFJ and common femoral vein as the 'Mickey Mouse sign' (Figure 10.1). If the junction is not present due to ligation of the GSV then 'Mickey's' medial ear is missing.
- The GSV and AASV lie in the subcutaneous tissue within a compartment which is delineated by the muscular fascia below and the saphenous fascia above seen on ultrasound as the *saphenous eye* (see Figure 2.16). Tributaries and non-saphenous veins are in the subcutaneous tissue and they do not lie in any compartment.
- If present, determine connections for reflux by colour or spectral Doppler, that is, from incompetence at the SFJ, veins from the low abdomen or pelvis, thigh or calf perforators or the vein of Giacomini.
- In transverse, determine whether the destination for reflux is into the GSV or major thigh tributaries. Measure the level of inflow of reflux to the GSV if it is distal to the SFJ.

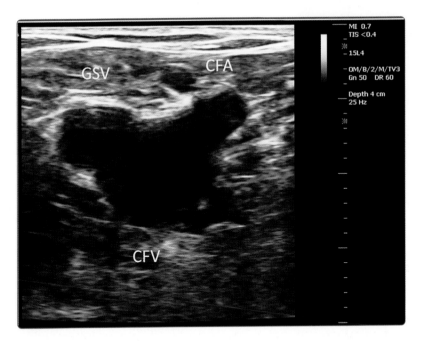

Figure 10.1 The 'Mickey Mouse' sign in the left lower limb. The 'head' is the common femoral vein and the two 'ears' are the common femoral artery on the lateral side and the great saphenous vein on the medial side.

- Scan for saphenous reflux distal to communication with a significant tributary. Suspect a connection for reflux if there is a sudden increase in GSV diameter. Follow the full length of the GSV and tributaries to the knee. Test at intervals for compressibility and reflux.
- Measure diameters at the SFJ and at intervals along the GSV and AASV if there is reflux.

The alignment sign

- The GSV and AASV can be distinguished by ultrasound from their relation to the femoral artery and vein; the AASV lies superficial to the femoral artery and vein whereas the GSV is more medial (Figure 10.2).

Tibio-gastrocnemius angle sign

- The tibio-gastrocnemius angle sign is useful to detect the GSV if it is present just below the knee. It lies in the triangle formed by the tibia, medial gastrocnemius muscle and fascial sheath (Figure 10.3). The GSV is absent or hypoplastic in the lower thigh, knee area

and upper leg in many subjects (see Figure 2.17).

Scan the common femoral and femoral veins

- Test the common femoral vein in longitudinal with spectral Doppler for phasicity with normal respiration, cessation of flow with deep inspiration and reflux with the Valsalva manoeuvre. Lack of phasicity may indicate proximal obstruction and the test should be extended later to show the iliac veins and inferior vena cava.
- Test the femoral confluence for reflux or thrombosis. Follow the full length of femoral vein to the popliteal vein testing for reflux or thrombosis. Slow outflow during distal compression suggests obstruction between the test and augmentation sites.

Scan thigh perforators

- Use colour Doppler to test for outward flow in perforators by thigh muscle contraction. Use spectral Doppler if flow direction and duration are ambiguous.

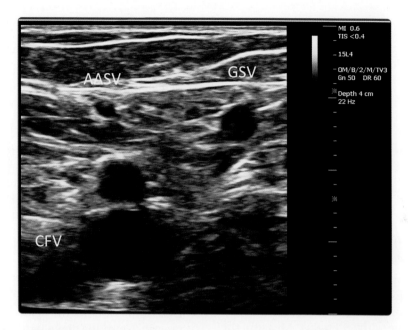

Figure 10.2 Alignment sign in the right lower limb. The anterior accessory saphenous vein lies superficial to the femoral artery and vein, while the great saphenous vein is more medial.

- Look for perforators on the medial thigh as the full length of GSV and deep veins are examined. Look for lateral, posterior and anterior thigh perforators if clinical assessment shows varices in these regions. Measure the levels of refluxing perforators from the inguinal ligament or skin crease behind the knee, and measure their diameters with B-mode. Insonate the fascia at 90° to ensure maximum specular reflection to help identify perforators passing through the fascia.

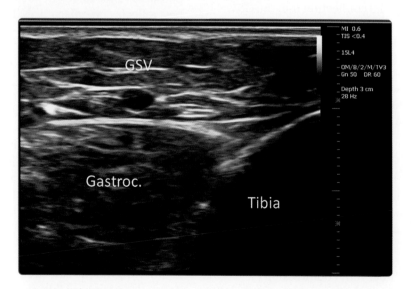

Figure 10.3 Tibio-gastrocnemius angle sign in the left lower limb. The great saphenous vein lies superficial to the angle of the gastrocnemius just beside the tibia if it is present at the knee.

Posterior veins of the thigh and calf

- Scan for the small saphenous vein (SSV), thigh extension, sapheno-popliteal junction (SPJ), vein of Giacomini, popliteal vein, gastrocnemius veins, soleal sinuses and perforators.

Position the patient and select windows

- Turn the patient to face away to use posterior windows.

Scan the SSV, thigh extension and vein of Giacomini

- Start at the back of knee. Determine whether the SPJ is present. If so, show the junction in longitudinal. Determine if there is SPJ incompetence with SSV reflux. Measure the level of the SPJ in relation to the skin crease behind the knee.
- Look for alternative connections for reflux including communication with popliteal fossa perforators, GSV tributaries, pelvic veins traced to the buttock or perineum, thigh extension or vein of Giacomini.
- Examine the thigh extension and vein of Giacomini. Determine the distal SSV connection and proximal connection into the GSV, deep or pelvic veins.
- If there is reflux, measure diameters at the SPJ and along the SSV, thigh extension and vein of Giacomini.
- Note the presence and position of the sciatic, tibial, common peroneal and sural nerves, and look for a saphenous artery.

Scan the popliteal and medial gastrocnemius veins

- Test the popliteal vein for reflux or thrombosis proximal and distal to the SPJ. Test the medial gastrocnemius veins for reflux or thrombosis. Examine the popliteal vein after extending the knee to provoke possible popliteal vein compression (see Chapter 16).

Veins below knee

Position the patient and select windows

- Consider sitting the patient on the side of the bed facing the sonographer with the foot on the knee to allow calf muscles to drop away to better fill the veins.
- Image the GSV from a medial approach and scan from the medial or postero-medial aspect for the posterior tibial and peroneal veins. Peroneal veins can also be seen through a posterior or antero-lateral window. Many sonographers show the peroneal veins from a medial approach, in the same image but deep to the posterior tibial veins and in front of the fibula.

GSV below knee

- Determine whether the below-knee GSV is present. Continue down its length as for the above-knee GSV. Examine for reflux and thrombosis. Measure diameters in B-mode if reflux is present.

Calf veins

- With experience, all tibial veins can be identified. Examine for reflux or thrombosis throughout the posterior tibial veins and peroneal veins. Reflux in posterior tibial veins best reflects clinical features. It is optional to scan the anterior tibial veins.

Calf perforators

- Test for outward flow by colour Doppler after a calf muscle squeeze, isometric calf muscle contraction or foot squeeze. Wait for >15 seconds to allow calf muscles to refill before repeating the squeeze. Use spectral Doppler if flow direction and duration is ambiguous with colour Doppler. Definitions of what constitutes abnormal outward flow constituting 'reflux' or 'incompetence' is uncertain and debated but flow of >0.5 s in a perforator with diameter >3.5 mm measured at the deep fascia is considered abnormal. Look for perforators around the calf circumference, and if they show outward flow then measure their level from the medial or lateral malleolus and use B-mode to measure their diameters at the deep fascia.

Recurrent varicose veins

- These are the most difficult studies. Patterns of reflux are frequently different to primary varicose veins, so be aware of the many possible sites.
- If there has been previous surgery to the GSV, examine the medial and posterior thigh for recurrence of a refluxing GSV and connections for reflux from the common femoral vein, pelvic, round ligament, gluteal, abdominal, ovarian or pudendal tributaries or thigh perforators.
- After past treatment to the SSV, examine the popliteal fossa for connections at the SPJ, from popliteal or posterior calf perforators or from the thigh extension or vein of Giacomini.
- Examine the leg for recurrence through calf perforators.

Continuous–wave Doppler

- The hand-held continuous-wave (CW) Doppler unit is still used by some to assess each GSV, SSV and deep veins. However, duplex ultrasound has largely replaced this technique; the European Society for Vascular Surgery consensus statement holds that CW Doppler is not recommended for the diagnostic work-up of chronic venous disease.[7]
- Most probes need to be held at 30°–45° to the surface to obtain the best signal, and there is no signal if held at 90°.

Great saphenous vein

- Stand the patient with the knee slightly bent, heel on the ground and weight taken on the opposite leg. Listen in the groin for the common femoral artery pulse, move the probe medially to listen for reflux in the common femoral vein after squeezing the calf, then move the probe a little more medial and down to be over the GSV and listen for reflux

after squeezing the calf. If there is reflux, then repeat and use a finger of the free hand to occlude the GSV below the probe to determine whether this stops reflux.
- Repeat listening over a distal varicosity to determine whether there is reflux and whether this can be stopped by pressure over the GSV. To detect whether a varicosity and the GSV are connected, tap on one while listening over the other with the CW transducer to hear if there is a signal.

Small saphenous vein

- Stand the patient on a step facing away with the knee slightly bent, heel on the step and weight on the opposite leg. Listen for the popliteal artery signal, move the probe to the SSV just lateral to the artery, squeeze the calf and listen for reflux after releasing the squeeze.
- If there is reflux, repeat and use a finger of the free hand after releasing the squeeze to occlude the SSV above the probe to determine whether this stops reflux.

Venography

- Invasive venography has been largely replaced by non-invasive contrast computed tomography and contrast magnetic resonance imaging.

Ascending venography

- This can be used to assess deep veins. Inject contrast into a dorsal foot vein with an ankle tourniquet applied to direct flow into deep veins. Contrast flow is slowed by a second thigh cuff with the patient semi-erect on a tilt table. Deep veins are well seen up to the level of the common femoral vein.

Descending venography

- Inject contrast through a catheter in the ipsilateral or contralateral femoral or popliteal vein. This demonstrates superficial or deep reflux as well as information relating to the site and function of venous valves after a Valsalva manoeuvre. The procedure has potential complications.

Varicography

- Inject contrast directly into a superficial vein as a roadmap to show sites of connections in patients with recurrent varicose veins, or to show the best sites for incisions to ligate connections.

Other non-invasive investigations

Air plethysmography

- Volume changes in the lower limb can be measured using air plethysmography (APG). The technique employs a cuff that extends from knee to ankle and senses pressure changes in response to changes in volume.
- The initial test is performed with the subject supine to measure the capacity of the lower limb venous system for both the degree and rate of swelling after inflating a thigh venous tourniquet, and the rate of outflow after the tourniquet is released (Figure 10.4). This helps to identify venous outflow obstruction and the extent of collateral formation.
- Normally, the limb increases its volume by some 70–100 mL before approaching a steady state (Vc-mL). After, the tourniquet is then suddenly released, the volume ejected in

one second (V1-mL) is measured and allows calculation of a one-second outflow fraction equal to V1/Vc. This fraction is >40% in normal limbs with no outflow obstruction and <30% in limbs with severe outflow obstruction.

- The limb is then elevated to empty the veins, the tourniquet is removed and the subject stands (Figure 10.5).
  - The rate and amount of venous filling termed the functional venous volume (VV-mL) is noted. VV is 80–150 mL in normal limbs and up to 400 mL in limbs with varicose disease.
  - The 90%VV is more reproducible and allows calculation of a 90% filling time (VFT90).
  - The venous filling index (VFI) = VV/time to fill (mL/sec). VFI is <2 ml/sec in normal limbs in which the veins fill slowly from the arterial side and may increase up to 30 ml/sec in limbs with severe venous reflux.
- Measurements are then taken after one tip-toe to induce calf muscle pumping.
  - The volume expelled is the ejection volume (EV-mL). The normal EV is 65–130 mL.
  - The ejection fraction (EF) = EV/VV × 100%. The normal EF is >60%, 30%–70% in limbs with primary varicose

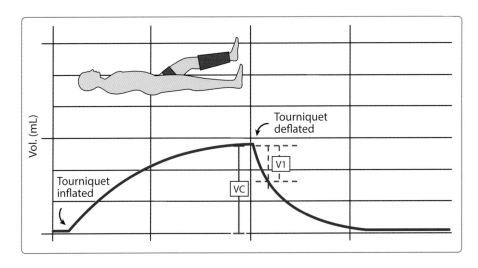

Figure 10.4 Volume changes in a lower limb determined by air plethysmography with a subject lying at rest after inflating a thigh venous tourniquet to measure maximum volume, then at one second after deflation to calculate a one second venous outflow fraction.

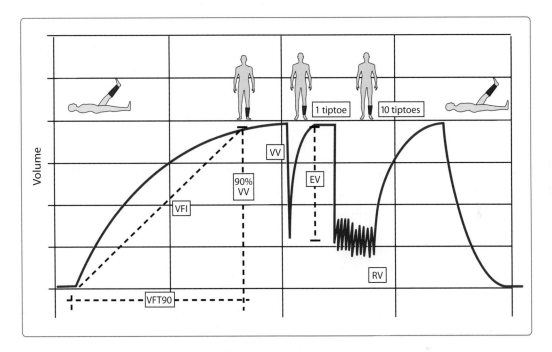

Figure 10.5 Volume changes in a lower limb determined by air plethysmography with a subject standing, then performing one tip-toe and 10 tip-toe exercises.

disease and as low as 10% in limbs with deep venous disease.

- This is followed by 10 tip-toes to assess the combined effect of venous reflux, obstruction and ejection capacity. The residual volume (RV-mL) and residual volume fraction (RVF) = RV/VV × 100% are measured. The RVF is 5%–35% in normal limbs, 20%–70% in limbs with primary varicose veins, and up to 100% with deep venous disease.

Photoplethysmography

- The technique measures light reflection from the skin on the dorsum of the foot or behind the medial malleolus. Reflection from red blood cells in the dermis relates to local blood volume. Light absorption decreases as veins empty and venous pressure falls with exercise. Only the post-exercise recovery time is reproducible and it is normally >20 s.

Strain gauge plethysmography

- A strain gauge can measure calf volume before and after exercise to calculate

expelled volume and refilling time to distinguish between superficial and deep reflux.
- Strain gauge plethysmography can be used to assess the 'reflux burden' before and after treatment, and correlates with ulcer risk.

Foot volumetry

- The foot is placed in an open water bath, and volume in the bath is measured with a sensor. Blood volume refilling after exercise without and with a tourniquet can help distinguish between superficial and deep venous reflux and quantify its degree.

Other invasive investigations

Ambulatory venous pressure

- Venous pressure is measured through a needle in a dorsal foot vein connected to a pressure transducer, amplifier and recorder (Figure 10.6). At rest, intravenous pressure corresponds to the hydrostatic pressure and pressures are identical in superficial and deep veins at the same level. Moving from

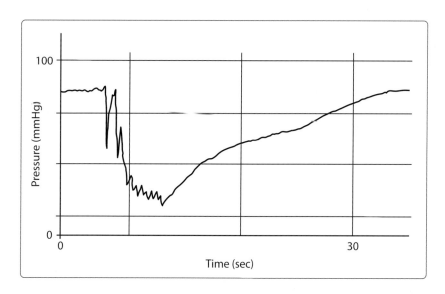

Figure 10.6 Ambulatory venous pressure measurements from a dorsal foot vein at rest standing, then after 10 tip-toe exercises with recovery after ceasing exercise, in a normal subject.

the horizontal to standing position causes hydrostatic pressure to increase equally in both arteries and veins of the foot, by some 80–90 mmHg. Capillary flow is not affected because the arteriovenous pressure gradient remains constant.

- A subject performs 10 tip-toes then stands still while pressure recovers to baseline. The exercise is then repeated after inflating a narrow pneumatic cuff at the ankle. Measurements are the pressure at rest (P0-mmHg), mean pressure toward the end of the 10 tip-toes (P10-mmHg), the difference between the two pressures and the recovery time (RT-sec) best measured at 50% or 90% RT.
- In normal limbs, the pressure falls rapidly to less than 30 mmHg and recovery through capillary inflow is slow, typically 20–40 seconds. In limbs with varicose disease, reflux occurs between contractions, P10 remains high in the range 25–70 mmHg while RT90 is fast in the range 10–20 seconds. In limbs with deep venous disease, P10 remains high and may even increase above resting levels, usually in the range 55–85 mmHg, and RT90 is typically <15 seconds.

Femoral venous pressure

- Record pressure from a needle in the common femoral vein at rest and after exercise to detect inadequate recanalization or collateral formation due to an ilio-caval occlusion. The pressure is compared to central venous pressure or pressure in a hand vein.

References

1. Coleridge-Smith P, Labropoulos N, Partsch H, Myers K, Nicolaides A, Cavezzi A. Duplex ultrasound investigation of the veins in chronic venous disease of the lower limbs--UIP consensus document. Part I. Basic principles. *Eur J Vasc Endovasc Surg.* 2006;31:83–92. http://www.ncbi.nlm.nih.gov/pubmed/16226898
2. Cavezzi A, Labropoulos N, Partsch H, Ricci S, Caggiati A, Myers K, Nicolaides A, Smith PC. Duplex ultrasound investigation of the veins in chronic venous disease of the lower limbs--UIP consensus document. Part II. Anatomy. *Eur J Vasc Endovasc Surg.* 2006;31:288–99. http://www.ncbi.nlm.nih.gov/pubmed/16230038
3. Myers KA and Clough A. *Practical Vascular Ultrasound. An Illustrated Guide.* 2014; CRC Press. https://www.crcpress.com/Practical-Vascular-Ultrasound-An-Illustrated-Guide/Myers-Clough/p/book/9781444181180

4. Zygmunt J, Pichot O, Dauplaise T. *Practical Phlebology: Venous Ultrasound*. 2013; CRC Press. https://www.crcpress.com/Practical-Phlebology-Venous-Ultrasound/Zygmunt-Pichot-Dauplaise/p/book/9781853159480

5. Nicolaides AN. Investigation of chronic venous insufficiency. *Circulation* 2000;14(102):E126–163. http://circ.ahajournals.org/content/102/20/e126

6. Van der Velden SK, De Maeseneer MG, Pichot O, Nijsten T, van den Bos RR. Postural diameter change of the saphenous trunk in chronic venous disease. *Eur J Vasc Endovasc Surg*. 2016;51:831–7. http://www.ncbi.nlm.nih.gov/pubmed/27090741

7. Wittens C, Davies AH, Bækgaard N, Broholm R, Cavezzi A, Chastanet S, de Wolf M et al. Management of chronic venous disease. Clinical practice guidelines of the European Society for Vascular Surgery. *Eur J Vasc Endovasc Surg* 2015;49:678–37. https://www.researchgate.net/publication/280483468_Editor's_Choice_-_Management_of_Chronic_Venous_Disease_Clinical_Practice_Guidelines_of_the_European_Society_for_Vascular_Surgery_ESVS

11 Conservative treatment

This chapter includes recommendations from the International Wound Infection Institute, European Society for Vascular Surgery, Society for Vascular Surgery, American Venous Forum, NICE and Australian and New Zealand Clinical Practice for Prevention and Management of Venous Leg Ulcers.[1–7]

Conservative treatment consists of general advice, compression, local wound care and pharmacological agents. It may be the only treatment advised or may supplement intervention.

Compression

- Compression aims to improve venous haemodynamics by applying a pressure high enough to overcome intravenous pressure, adjusted to the body position. An ideal compression device exerts a low resting pressure in the supine position that is well tolerated at night, causes a pressure increase when the patient stands, and provides a pressure sufficient to reduce venous reflux while walking to promote venous return to the heart.
- Compression can be achieved using bandages, stockings, velcro-devices or intermittent pneumatic compression.[8–12] Compression may be used for chronic venous disease, following intervention to treat venous disease, for acute superficial and deep vein thrombosis, and for lymphoedema.
- A lack of evidence from randomized controlled trials is offset by ample lower-quality evidence based on observational studies and clinical experience to show improved symptoms and quality of life after treatment for chronic venous disease.
- Compression as primary treatment acts to:
  - narrow superficial and deep veins
  - increase venous blood velocity
  - reduce or abolish venous reflux and hypertension
  - improve the microcirculation
  - reduce oedema
- Compression after definitive treatment for venous disease acts to:
  - increase deep venous flow
  - reduce the risk of deep vein thrombosis
  - reduce post-treatment inflammatory oedema and trapped blood
  - improve superficial venous occlusion rates when combined with pressure pads
  - reduce matting and pigmentation
- Compliance with wearing stockings or using bandages can be poor due to:
  - difficulty applying and removing them, particularly for the elderly
  - itching causing scratching and skin damage
  - discomfort in the hot weather
  - unattractive appearance
  - high cost of stockings and bandages
  - poor education and skills to understand the importance of compression and how to apply bandages
- Ensure that the patient is not taking medications that cause oedema, including some calcium channel-blockers, anti-hypertensive drugs, non-steroidal anti-inflammatory drugs, endocrine agents or anti-psychotic drugs.

Definitions

- The *compression pressure* exerted due to the elastic properties of stockings or bandages is defined by the force they exert on the body surface.[8] One Pascal (Pa) is the force of one Newton per square metre. Expressed in mmHg, 1 mmHg = 133.3 Pa. The Laplace equation: $P = \Upsilon/r$, where Υ is the wall tension and r is the radius, indicates that compression pressure is directly proportional to the tension of a textile but inversely proportional to the radius of the curvature to which it is applied. It is zero over a completely flat surface, low over the flat thigh, greater over the curved tibia and high over sharp edges. The pressure developed beneath a bandage is also governed by the width and number of layers applied. The pressure measured under static conditions is the *resting pressure* while that measured during movement is the *working pressure*.
- *Stiffness* is the increase of compression per centimetre increase in limb circumference. Stiffness increases with multilayer bandages or if two compression stockings are worn one over the other, thus causing more friction between the layers.
- A technique has been developed to calculate a *static stiffness index* (SSI) to allow for complexities resulting from different textiles and multiple layers. A pressure sensor is fixed to the medial leg about 12 cm above the ankle where the calf muscle and tendon interaction causes variance with position, and SSI is the difference between the interface pressure in the standing and lying positions (mmHg). Pressure amplitudes and peaks during walking are also parameters for stiffness and correlate well with SSI, but they are difficult to measure.
- Elastic *hysteresis* is the pattern of recoil from a stretch, where the recoil force is less than the stretch force, resulting in weaker tension and generation of heat during the recoil phase. A stocking or bandage has high hysteresis if it is unable to keep up with the circumferential changes of the leg during normal walking and low hysteresis if it maintains its strength.

Stiffness corresponds to the slope of a hysteresis curve.

Stockings

- As opposed to dress or athletic stockings and socks, compression stockings are manufactured using elastic rubber fibres to exert extra pressure. They can be made as knee-high, thigh-high, waist-high, pantihose or maternity stockings. Stockings can be made to incorporate silver textile fibres which may provide anti-microbial protection. Stockings used for treatment are selected for pressure according to the condition and severity of disease.
- Pressure under a stocking is determined by its manufacture and is presented as various *classes*, which unfortunately vary between countries. Attempts are being made to introduce international standards to describe pressures and stiffness of stockings both at rest and during ambulation.[8]

	mmHg	mmHg	mmHg	mmHg
	Class 1	Class 2	Class 3	Class 4
British standard	14–17	18–24	25–35	N/A
German standard	18–21	23–32	34–46	>49
French standard	10–15	15–20	20–36	>36
European standard	15–21	23–32	34–46	>49
USA Standard	15–20	20–30	30–40	N/A

- It has been proposed to classify stockings with a pressure on the distal lower leg of less than 20 mmHg as mild, 20–40 mmHg as moderate, 40–60 mmHg as strong and >60 mmHg as very strong.
- No two patients have the same body size and shape, so that it is necessary to be aware of the available sizes and to measure limbs to achieve the best fit. Some patients will require custom-made stockings. To remain effective,

they should be replaced every three to four months with constant use.

- Stockings are manufactured to exert *graduated compression*, usually from ankle to thigh, to create a smooth pressure gradient for flow. However, manufacture to exert maximum pressure over the calf to compress the large calf veins may be the most crucial component for compression.

11.1 Advice if compliance is poor

- Try below-knee class 1 stockings.
- Use two class 1 stockings one over the other on the same limb as these are easier to apply than a class 2 stocking and compression is additive.
- Leave compression off at night.
- Consider low-stretch bandages or Velcro devices instead.

Bandages

- The pressure exerted by a bandage depends on its composition and the tension with which it is applied. An *elastic* or *long-stretch* bandage can stretch by more than 100% and an *inelastic* or *short-stretch* bandage by less than 100%. The haemodynamic efficacy depends on the interface pressure. Compression by more than 50 mmHg in the upright position is desirable to reduce ambulatory venous hypertension. However, the pressure with an inelastic bandage should be lower in the resting position to be tolerated and not cause restricted arterial supply.
- Inelastic short-stretch three-layer bandages with cohesive surfaces do not give way when calf muscles contract during walking, thus causing high peaks of interface pressure. They can be applied at a tolerable pressure at rest so that pressure during walking will produce a peak with every muscle systole to cause intermittent narrowing of veins. An elastic bandage would need to be applied at an intolerable high pressure at rest to achieve the same high standing working pressure.

However, inelastic bandages give higher pressure than elastic stockings at calf level during walking. Perhaps this intermittent pumping is more effective for fluid drainage than constant pressure.

- The skill of the person applying the bandages is the most important factor in determining their efficacy. Even experienced staff frequently apply them too loosely. Inelastic and multicomponent bandages lose pressure very quickly due to rapid oedema reduction so that they may need to be re-applied frequently. Compression is most effective when combined with walking exercises.

Selection of compression

- Stockings or bandages reduce oedema and inflammation even when applied with low pressure, and stronger compression may be poorly tolerated. However, stronger compression materials that exert higher pressures more effectively reduce reflux and increase venous pumping function in the upright position.
- Compression stockings that exert 10–20 mmHg pressure are sufficient to prevent leg swelling after prolonged sitting. So-called thrombo-prophylactic stockings accelerate venous blood flow velocity in the supine but not in the upright position, and are only of use in sedentary in-hospital patients, for example after surgery.
- The compression pressure must be higher than the intravenous pressure to narrow superficial and deep leg veins. The pressures required depend on the body position; about 20 mmHg in the supine and 50–70 mmHg in the upright position at lower leg level.
- High compression pressures of 50–70 mmHg can be achieved with multiple compression stockings or strongly-applied compression bandages. Ideally these high values should be exerted only during standing and walking and should fall immediately when the patient lies down. With the same resting pressure, inelastic compression material reduces venous reflux more effectively than elastic bandages due to their higher 'working pressure.'

- Stiff material can cause intermittent occlusion of leg veins with each muscle contraction during walking. For a short time, the sub-bandage pressure peaks during muscle systole to overcome the intravenous pressure and occlude the vein, acting like an artificial valve that suppresses reflux during each muscle systole. At the same time, muscle contractions pump blood out during walking.
- Sustained external compression should never exceed the intra-arterial pressure which is reduced in limbs with peripheral arterial disease. However, intermittent compression with peak pressures above arterial systolic pressure followed by long intervals without pressure can improve arterial blood flow. Stiff bandages applied with care at low resting pressure produce intermittent pressure peaks in a similar way when the patient is walking or moving the ankles. The resulting massage effect of inelastic compression can reduce oedema and increase arterial blood flow.

Measuring for lower limb stockings

- Circumferences are measured for the ankle at its narrowest point, calf at its widest point, and upper thigh 5 cm below the buttock crease (Figure 11.1). Lengths are measured for below-knee or thigh-high stockings.

Uncomplicated disease

- It may be decided to choose expectant treatment to relieve symptoms using compression and pharmacologic agents (also see Chapter 5). Patients with severe symptoms, oedema, and impending skin complications particularly benefit from these conservative measures. Compression is the most important element of management. Other measures include weight reduction, leg elevation avoiding knee hyperextension that could cause popliteal vein compression, moving about rather than standing and active exercise.

Venous ulcer management

- Compression and local treatment is an integral part of management for venous ulcers, usually prior to intervention to correct venous

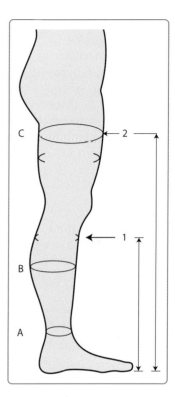

Figure 11.1 Measurements for stocking sizes. Circumference: A – narrowest level at ankle; B – widest level of calf; C – high-thigh. Length: 1 – floor to 1–2 cm below knee-crease: 2 – thigh-high.

hypertension, but sometimes as sole treatment if there is a contraindication to intervention. Endovenous intervention is now preferred to surgery.

Compression

Ulcer healing

- Compression bandages improve ulcer healing rates compared with standard care without compression. An alternative to traditional bandaging is non-elastic compression with the Unna boot, a compression dressing impregnated with zinc oxide paste.
- An inelastic bandage produces a much higher working pressure during muscle systole than an equivalent elastic bandage, and it is this stronger haemodynamic effect that is the reason for them being used to treat venous ulcers.

- A three- or four-layer bandage technique incorporating both elastic and inelastic bandages has been found to provide more effective compression than lower grades of compression with a single-layer inelastic bandage. A multi-layered bandage becomes progressively less elastic with each layer.
- Intermittent pneumatic compression improves venous flow and promotes healing of venous ulcers in combination with elastic stockings and possibly as sole treatment. However, the effect is not great, as it does not fully replicate physiological foot and calf pump compression with walking.
- A venous ulcer is unlikely to heal as long as oedema persists, so patients should wear the highest level of compression that is tolerable. A wound that has copious exudate almost certainly has had inadequate compression rather than inappropriate dressings.

Ulcer recurrence

- Compression by stockings should be maintained after ulcer healing to reduce the risk of recurrence, particularly in patients with deep vein occlusion or gross incompetence not amenable to intervention. Compression bandages are usually replaced by elastic stockings, and patients should wear the highest level of compression that is comfortable, although less compression is required at night, especially if the arterial circulation is compromised.

Dressings

- After cleansing an ulcer to remove devitalized tissue and exudate, apply a suitable dressing to protect the region and promote moist wound healing.[7] Measure wound healing by planimetry of the surface area or by time to complete healing. In addition, assess progress by changes in the wound bed for the phases of healing, the haemostatic phase then the inflammatory phase, granulation phase and epithelialization. Simple venous ulcers should heal in 8–12 weeks with best care, and if not, then a review for an alternative diagnosis is required.

- There is no convincing evidence that any one dressing is better than others, no dressing is suitable for all ulcers and an ulcer needs regular assessment to select a dressing for each stage of healing.

Dressing types

- It is important to choose an absorbent local dressing to provide the best moist environment for healing. Polyurethane dressing with an incorporated adhesive layer (PolyMem®) is moist, highly absorbent and protective and can be left on for up to seven days. Foam dressings (Biatain®) and cellulose fibre dressings (Aquacel®) are also highly absorbant.
- Calcium alginate polysaccharide from seaweed (Kaltostat®) forms a gel on the ulcer which provides a moist environment. It reduces pain, can pack cavities, is absorbent for exudative wounds, promotes haemostasis and is low-allergenic. It may require a secondary dressing.
- Polyurethane film coated with adhesive hydrocolloid (Duoderm®) retains moisture and is easily removed, but is not suitable for high-exudate ulcers. It can be left on for up to seven days.
- Semi-permeable transparent polyurethrane film (OpSite®, Tegaderm®) allows some moisture evaporation, acts as a barrier to external contamination and enables inspection, but it can cause exudate to pool and be traumatic to remove.
- Non-adherent gauze impregnated with paraffin (Tulle Gras®) or an antiseptic or antibiotic (Jelonet®, Sofra-Tulle®) reduces wound adhesion and provides a moist environment, but it does not absorb exudate, requires a secondary dressing and may induce allergy.
- Non-adherent dry thin perforated plastic film coating attached to an absorbent pad (Melolin®, Tricose®) has low wound adherence and can absorb light exudates, but is not suitable if there is high exudate, can dry out and stick to the wound and may require a secondary dressing.
- Porous polyester fabric with adhesive backing (Hypafix) is used to cover other

dressings. It conforms to body contours, provides good pain relief and helps control oedema. It remains permeable, allowing exudate to escape and be washed and dried off so that dressing changes can be left for several days.

Selection of dressing

- The aim is to remove slough, control infection and reduce exudate so as to promote a granulating base with epithelium growing in from the edges.
  - Dry necrotic ulcer – semi-permeable hydrocolloid for moisture retention left for 3–4 days.
  - Slough covered ulcer – hydrocolloid or alginate for moisture retention and fluid absorption left for 3–4 days.
  - Infected ulcer – avoid semi-occlusive dressings and consider alginate or hydrocolloid if high exudate, and leave for 1–2 days.
  - Other chronic ulcers – hydrocolloid, alginate or foam left for 5 days.

Dermatitis under adhesive dressings

- Most skin reactions related to adhesive tape are mechanical irritant dermatitis rather than true contact dermatitis, though the latter must be considered when topical medications are being applied. A scaly erythema under an adherent dressing requires removal of the dressing, simple moisturisers and rarely a cortisone cream.

Topical agents

- These may be useful if there is clear evidence of infection rather than simple contamination, but they cause toxic effects on fibroblasts and macrophages *in vitro*. A combination of a surfactant betaine and antimicrobial polyhexanide (Prontosan) is a very good antiseptic to wash down limbs and, in gel form also makes a good dressing.
- Cadexomer iodine products made as ointments, powders and impregnated dressings (Iodosorb) are able to absorb exudate, have broad-spectrum antimicrobial properties and promote autolytic debridement of the wound bed. They are usually not associated with significant adverse events, but should not be used in patients with known thyroid disease. However, povidone iodine can actually delay wound healing and should not be used.
- Topical silver creams or silver-impregnated dressings are held to promote healing through a broad-spectrum antimicrobial effect if the ulcer is infected, but there is no strong evidence that they are effective.
- Topical honey such as Manuka honey found in Australia and New Zealand is a super-saturated sugar solution and has long been used to treat wounds. Honey is thought to aid wound healing through an osmotic effect that draws fluid from the wound to the surface, through promotion of a moist healing environment and by lowering wound pH, all of which promote autolysis, and it may have antibacterial properties. However, there is no strong evidence that it is effective, and it causes pain and increased exudate.
- Recommendations from a consensus statement from the European Society for Vascular Surgery[2] include:
  - Alginate, foam, hydrocolloid and silver donating dressings do not increase venous ulcer healing rates and more research is needed before recommending them.
  - Topical cadexomer iodine is more effective than standard care in achieving complete healing when added to compression therapy.
  - Zinc oxide impregnated paste bandages achieve better ulcer healing than alginate dressings but further research is needed to investigate their role.
  - Local allergic side effects might limit the use of topical antimicrobial dressings.

Other measures

- Systemic antibiotics have a minimal role in venous ulcer treatment, but can be prescribed if a wound shows features of infection such as spreading erythema and fever. A wound swab should be taken to guide appropriate choice of antibiotic if it is prescribed, but does not help to distinguish between contamination and infection. Culture of a biopsy is even more specific.

- Physiotherapy and self-exercising to improve joint mobility and activate the calf muscle pump is beneficial. Massage to improve lymphatic drainage and reduce oedema promotes healing.
- Leg elevation removes hydrostatic pressure, but prolonged bed rest negates the benefits of calf muscle pumping from exercise. Rest with leg elevation is advised if compression cannot be tolerated due to acute inflammation. Although bed rest in hospital is still occasionally recommended, patient compliance to remain in hospital is poor and ulcer recurrence is very common.
- Vacuum assisted closure (VAC) uses negative pressure in the range of 75–125 mmHg to improve blood flow, decrease local tissue oedema, and remove excessive fluid from the ulcer bed, assisting formation of healthy granulation tissue. A Cochrane-based review on the efficacy of VAC therapy in chronic wounds found evidence for a positive effect.[13]
- Other modalities such as hyperbaric oxygen therapy and dressings that incorporate growth factors are still being evaluated. Oral pentoxifylline is believed to increase ulcer healing in patients receiving compression, and oral flavonoids and sulodexide may also be effective. It is not known whether therapeutic ultrasound, oral aspirin, rutosides, thromboxane alpha2 antagonists, zinc, debriding agents or intravenous prostaglandin E1 are beneficial. Peri-ulcer injections of granulocyte–macrophage colony-stimulating factor may enhance healing. It is usual to advise weight loss, good diet and giving up smoking. Larval therapy has been used for debridement.

Definitive treatment

- Debridement is necessary with local dressings to soften eschar, autologous or enzymatic dressings to help separation and surgical excision of necrotic tissue if required. Ultrasonic debridement after topical local anaesthetic application is a useful non-surgical alternative.

- It is usually necessary to permanently control venous hypertension and congestion by endovenous intervention or surgery once the ulcer has been stabilized by conservative measures.
- Surgery for ulcer excision or skin grafting is only occasionally required. If oedema is not controlled, then the ulcer will not heal but then neither will the surgical wound heal nor the skin graft take. If there is no oedema, then the ulcer should be healing otherwise it is not a venous ulcer.

Failure to heal

- An alternative diagnosis to venous ulceration may be suspected at the outset, but it is usually difficult to distinguish between different causes at first presentation. Associated arterial disease can be assessed from the history of pain and claudication, examination for pulses and investigation by ankle–brachial pressure studies or duplex ultrasound.
- If an ulcer has not demonstrated significant healing within an arbitrary four weeks after implementation of adequate conservative treatment, then it is as well to commence investigation as to possible alternative causes such as peripheral arterial disease, vasculitis or even squamous cell carcinoma. The most definitive procedure is to obtain a generous excisional biopsy from the edge of the ulcer, obtained using a local anaesthetic. Put the specimen into sterile saline rather than formalin and request microbiology in addition to histology.

History

- Bandaged lower limbs are seen in drawings of warriors in caves in the Sahara dating back to before 2500 BC.
- The Edwin Smith Papyrus which dates to about 1600 BC is the oldest known manual of military surgery and describes mechanical compression treatment for legs.
- It is possible that the Old Testament was referring to contemporary management of venous ulceration with the reprimand 'From the sole of your foot to the top of your head there is no

soundness – only wounds and welts and open sores, not cleansed or bandaged or soothed with olive oil'. Isaiah I 6.

- Hippocrates (450–350 BC) treated leg ulcers with tight bandages, described in his *Corpus Hippocraticum*.
- Galen (130–200) used wool and linen compression bandages to prevent blood from pooling in the legs.
- The French physician Guy de Chauliac (1300–1368) treating the Popes in Avignon wrote a treatise on surgery titled *Chirurgia Magna* in which he advocated treatment for venous disease by bandaging.
- William Harvey's discovery of the link between venous stasis and the external pressure resulted in clinical development of laced stockings, elastic bands and tight bandages impregnated with resin.

References

1. Swanson T, Angel D, Sussman G, Cooper R, Haesler E, Ousey K, Carville K et al. International Wound Infection Institute. Wound infection in clinical practice. International consensus update. 2016. https://www.bbraun.com/content/dam/b-braun/global/website/products-and-therapies/wound-management/Docs/askina-calgitrol-ag-scientific-evidence/IWII%20Consensus_Final%20web.pdf.bb-.03454072/IWII%20Consensus_Final%20web.pdf

2. Wittens C, Davies AH, Bækgaard N, Broholm R, Cavezzi A, Chastanet S, de Wolf M, et al. Management of chronic venous disease. clinical practice guidelines of the European Society for vascular surgery. *Eur J Vasc Endovasc Surg* 2015;49:678–37. https://www.researchgate.net/publication/280483468_Editor's_Choice_-_Management_of_Chronic_Venous_Disease_Clinical_Practice_Guidelines_of_the_European_Society_for_Vascular_Surgery_ESVS

3. Mosti G, De Maeseneer M, Cavezzi A, Parsi K, Morrison N, Nelzen O, Rabe E et al. Society for Vascular Surgery and American Venous Forum guidelines on the management of venous leg ulcers: The point of view of the International Union of Phlebology. *Int Angiol.* 2015;34:202–18. https://www.researchgate.

4. NICE guidelines. *Varicose Veins: Diagnosis and Management.* 2013; CG168. https://www.nice.org.uk/guidance/cg168

5. Marsden G, Perry M, Kelley K, Davies AH. Diagnosis and management of varicose veins in the legs: Summary of NICE guidance. *BMJ* 2013;347:f4279–f4279. http://www.bmj.com/content/347/bmj.f4279

6. Gloviczki P, Comerota AJ, Dalsing MC, Eklof BG, Gillespie DL, Gloviczki ML, Lohr JM et al. The care of patients with varicose veins and associated chronic venous diseases: Clinical practice guidelines of the Society for Vascular Surgery and the American Venous Forum. *J Vasc Surg* 2011;53:2S–48S. https://www.ncbi.nlm.nih.gov/pubmed/21536172

7. Australian and New Zealand Clinical Practice Guideline for Prevention and Management of Venous Leg Ulcers 2011. http://www.awma.com.au/publications/2011_awma_vlug.pdf

8. Neumann HA, Partsch H, Mosti G, Flour M. Classification of compression stockings: Report of the meeting of the International Compression Club, Copenhagen. *Int Angiol* 2016;35:122–8. https://www.ncbi.nlm.nih.gov/pubmed/?term=neumann+int+angil+2016

9. Partsch H. Compression for the management of venous leg ulcers: Which material do we have? *Phlebology.* 2014;19;29(1 suppl):140–45. http://www.ncbi.nlm.nih.gov/pubmed/24843100

10. Mosti G, Picerni P, Partsch H. Compression stockings with moderate pressure are able to reduce chronic leg oedema. *Phlebology.* 2012;27:289–96. http://www.ncbi.nlm.nih.gov/pubmed/22090466

11. Mosti G, Partsch H. Improvement of venous pumping function by double progressive compression stockings: Higher pressure over the calf is more important than a graduated pressure profile. *Eur J Vasc Endovasc Surg.* 2014;47:545–9. http://www.ejves.com/article/S1078-5884(14)00008-2/abstract

12. Partsch H. Physics of compression. http://www.conferencematters.co.nz/pdf/PartschPhysics%20of%20Compression.pdf

13. Webster J, Scuffham P, Stankiewicz M, Chaboyer WP. Negative pressure wound therapy for skin grafts and surgical wounds healing by primary intention. *Cochrane Database System Rev* 2014;10: Art. No.: CD009261. http://www.cochrane.org/CD009261/WOUNDS_negative-pressure-wound-therapy-for-acute-surgical-wounds

net/publication/309670926_Evidence-based_S3_guidelines_for_diagnostics_and_treatment_of_venous_leg_ulcers

12 | Direct-vision and ultrasound-guided sclerotherapy

> This chapter includes recommendations from the European Society for Vascular Surgery and European Phlebological Societies.[1, 2]

Direct-vision sclerotherapy

- Direct-vision sclerotherapy can be used to treat telangiectases, reticular veins and small varicose veins, usually on the lower limbs but also on the face, hands, breasts or trunk. The actions of polidocanol or sodium tetradecyl sulphate (STS) used as liquid or foam are discussed in Chapter 5.

Techniques

- Many practitioners prefer liquid sclerosant, however foam is favoured by some. When treating telangiectases and reticular varices, use the lowest effective concentration to reduce the risk of side-effects, usually 0.25%–1% polidocanol or 0.1%–0.5% STS solutions, to be injected through 27 or 31 gauge needles.
- Use a commercial headlamp to better view small veins during treatment. This combines magnification and polarized light that enhances blue to purple colours and eliminates competing glare.
- Devices that use trans-illumination or infrared imaging can assist sclerotherapy for reticular veins that are feeding to telangiectases and which are difficult to see.

- Techniques vary (Figure 12.1). Inject feeder veins first if possible in anticipation that sclerosant will fan out into smaller vessels. Slowly inject no more than the required small volume at low pressure at each site. This avoids overfilling the veins which could lead to their rupture with extravasation or backflow through arterio-venous communications in the skin into small arteries. Too rapid injection is thought by some to predispose to subsequent matting, hyperpigmentation and cutaneous necrosis.
- When injecting larger veins, gently aspirate to confirm that injection is intravascular. For telangiectases, correct needle placement is shown by initial disappearance of the vessel followed by a reactive urticarial response. Stop injecting if there is resistance, blanching of the skin or severe pain indicating that the needle tip is probably not inside the vein. Use the 'air-block' technique to reduce risk of extravasation, as air in the syringe is injected before liquid sclerosant.
- Wait for about six weeks between treatment sessions as it takes about four weeks after injection for inflammation to settle and endofibrosis to occur.
- High-frequency ultrasound has shown that resistant telangiectases and telangiectatic matting are frequently associated with deeper reticular veins or non-saphenous tributaries that are not otherwise visible and which require ultrasound-guided sclerotherapy.

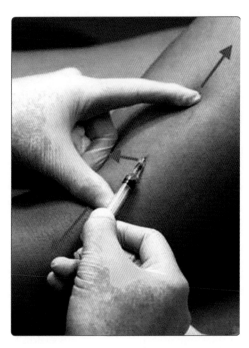

Figure 12.1 A technique for sclerotherapy injections. The left hand is used to give a two- or three-way stretch to the skin to stabilize the target vein for puncture. The left thumb is used as a fulcrum for very precise control of the needle tip. The needle is kept straight and the injecting right hand rests on the patient for stability. The right middle finger, index and thumb hold the syringe while the fourth and fifth fingers control the plunger to aspirate and inject.

Lower limb veins

- For treating telangiectases or reticular veins on the medial thigh or calf, position the patient supine and flat with the limb externally rotated and knee slightly flexed to relax all muscle groups. If small veins are being treated, place the patient semi-reclining. For treating posterior veins, position the patient prone with the foot supported by a pillow to slightly flex the knee.
- Pay attention to small veins running from the lower abdomen to the proximal thigh which need to be sclerosed to achieve best long-term results.

Vulvar veins

- Treatment may be required to relieve symptoms during pregnancy, and is

offered if varices persist after pregnancy.[3] Sclerotherapy with a dilute solution of sclerosant using a fine needle is performed. Compression is achieved by a sanitary pad and bicycle shorts.

Upper limb veins

- Many practitioners prefer to preserve forearm veins for possible later medical use, though there is no reason not to attempt judicious sclerotherapy in selected patients. Some seek treatment for unsightly hand veins; ageing hands show subcutaneous fat loss and skin wrinkles causing veins to become more apparent. Hand rejuvenation can be achieved with a combination of dermal fillers and sclerotherapy.
- Treat prominent hand veins with small volumes (0.5–1 mL) of 0.5%–0.75% polidocanol or 0.2% STS. One to two treatments may be required. Compress after treatment with a bandage for three to four days. Alternatively, inject commercial hyaluronic acid preparations using 0.5–1 mL of filler per hand, depending on the degree of subcutaneous fat loss. Calcium hydroxyapatite and fat are alternatives to fillers. Lasers can be used to resurface skin texture.

Breast veins

- Females may present seeking sclerotherapy for prominent reticular veins or telangiectases on the breasts. Use 0.5%–0.75% polidocanol or 0.2% STS in small volumes. Use a supportive sports undergarment for three to four days after treatment. Alternatively, use a 1064 nm laser system for reticular veins or a 532 nm system for telangiectases.

Superficial laser treatment

- Treatment is usually for Fitzpatrick 1 and 2 skin – white skin, always or usually burns, and never or only occasionally tans. However, Fitzpatrick 3 and above can also be treated with lower fluences. Vascular laser may be appropriate for freckles and lentigines, telangiectases, poor texture, sallow colour, premalignant changes, post acne scarring or fine wrinkling (Figure 12.2). Resurfacing

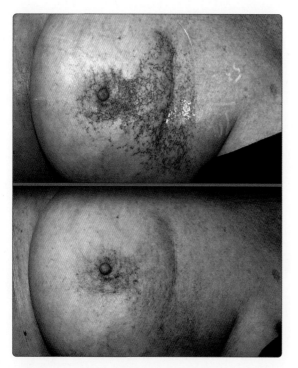

Figure 12.2 Laser treatment for telangiectasia resulting from irradiation for breast cancer, before treatment (above) and one month after treatment (below) Treatment with 532 nm vascular laser (1.2 mm spot size, 10 mj/cm², 15 ms, 5–10 Hz, 10°C contact cooling).

or face-lift is required for medium wrinkling and lax skin common with age.
- Other indications for laser treatment include acne, facial flushing, rosacea, Campbell de Morgan spots, sebaceous hyperplasia, poikiloderma of Civatte, keratosis pilaris rubra and photorejuvenation.
- Patients must avoid the sun for four weeks before and four weeks after treatment for optimal cosmetic outcome.

Ultrasound-guided sclerotherapy

- Ultrasound-guided sclerotherapy (UGS) can be used to treat primary or recurrent saphenous veins, perforators or tributaries as well as some malformations. Histology after foam applied to isolated saphenous vein segments during surgery demonstrates intimal destruction within two minutes and intimal

separation by 15–30 minutes.[4] Fibrosis gradually develops over the next few weeks.
- Advantages for UGS compared to other endovenous procedures or surgery include less discomfort and disturbance of activities and lower initial costs. However, late success rates are lower requiring more frequent repeat treatment at further cost.
- There are disadvantages.
  - Sclerosant and foam bubbles can travel to cause a systemic rather than a local targeted effect.
  - There is a limit as to the dose of sclerosant that can be safely given at any treatment session so that multiple sessions may be required, and each leg frequently needs to be treated separately.
  - Injected veins may remain inflamed for several weeks, and patience is required to allow this to settle.

Ultrasound guidance

- Some practitioners prefer to handle the ultrasound probe in one hand while performing the procedure with the other to allow best coordination. Others prefer to use both hands for the intervention to allow greater dexterity with a sonographer responsible for ultrasound guidance, but this requires good rapport.
- A high-frequency linear array transducer is used, and there is a place for very high-frequency transducers for treating very superficial veins. Hold the transducer to show the vein in either transverse or longitudinal. Some favour the transverse probe approach because it is technically easier to inject smaller veins and because relevant adjacent arteries and nerves can be seen. Others prefer the longitudinal probe approach since it allows flow of sclerosant to be observed along the vein.
- Hold the transducer vertical in the same line of sight. Image the needle and vein simultaneously to ensure the needle is being introduced in the correct plane. The needle appears as a reflective straight line angling towards the vein. Use fine movements to adjust the position of the needle and probe to maintain alignment.

Technique

- Most practitioners now use foam as the sclerosant prepared by the Tessari technique or variations.[5] An alternative is to use liquid sclerosant preceded by a saline flush.[6] Use a long 25 g needle as this is the smallest diameter needle that is readily visualized by B-mode ultrasound. Draw up sclerosant into a 2–5 mL Luer-lock syringe. The ratio of sclerosant to air may vary from 1:3 (wetter foam) which tends to have a longer duration to 1:6 (drier foam) which better displaces blood. Use the foam promptly after preparation to prevent it from degrading.

- Inject at strategic intervals along the veins with the intention to fill the total segment of treated vein with sclerosant foam seen with B-mode ultrasound (Figure 12.3). Some serially inject from above down and some from below upwards, but there is no evidence to favour either. Inject smaller volumes at multiple sites rather than larger volumes at one site to reduce dilution in superficial veins and reduce overflow into deep veins. A European consensus on foam sclerotherapy set an upper limit of 10 mL of foam per treatment session,[2] and the Australasian College of Phlebology recommends a maximum of 20 mL. Larger volumes using CO_2 or O_2/CO_2 mixes may be safer than air.

- As the needle tip contacts the vein, note an indentation on the wall then apply a little extra pressure to pierce the wall. Then aspirate a little blood to ensure correct intravenous needle position before completing foam injection under continuous ultrasound imaging. Alternatively, inject a little foam and use the B-mode image to determine whether injection is intra-luminal, into the wall or peri-venous. Avoid movement and excessive compression to allow the foam to work properly and avoid foam migration into deep veins. Some advocate active ankle flexion movements to expel foam if it is seen to pass into deep veins but this may aspirate more foam. Limit injections adjacent to perforators to reduce risk of spillage into deep veins.

- An innovation has been to supplement venospasm induced by sclerosant with peri-venous compression by normal saline or tumescent anaesthetic fluid, similar to the technique used for endothermal ablation (see Chapter 13).

- Measures described to attempt to prevent foam from escaping into the general circulation include holding the limb elevated, applying compression at the saphenous junction, restricting ambulation for a short time and avoiding the Valsalva manoeuvre by assisting the patient off the table and putting their socks and shoes on for them. However, no regime

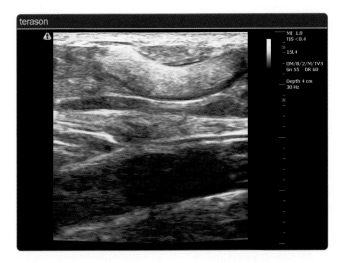

Figure 12.3 Foam in superficial vein after injection for ultrasound-guided sclerotherapy.

has been shown to be effective.[7,8] Release of saphenous junction compression has been associated with two reported foam-related episodes of transient ischaemic attacks.

- An operation report that can be used is shown in the Appendix.

Catheter-directed sclerotherapy

Open cannula technique

- This was introduced to minimize the risk of inadvertent intra-arterial injection. Correct placement of a cannula can be confirmed by aspiration of non-pulsatile venous blood, ultrasound visualization of the cannula tip and injection of normal saline into the vein prior to sclerosant injection.
- A current modified version is to insert multiple cannulas or 23 g butterfly needles while the patient lies supine, then elevate the limb by about 30° to empty the veins prior to injection at each site.

Extended long line echosclerotherapy (ELLE)

- This technique was developed both to reduce the risk of intra-arterial injection and to better treat larger diameter saphenous veins by prolonging exposure of sclerosant to the venous endothelium.[9]
- Make a percutaneous entry for cannulation under local anaesthesia with ultrasound guidance at the most distal accessible level. Insert a short 16–18 g cannula using a tourniquet if necessary. Note spontaneous venous return then flush the cannula with normal saline which is also visualized with ultrasound. Thread a commercial catheter of appropriate length up the vein over a guidewire to 5 cm distal to the saphenous junction. Elevate the limb to about 30° to empty the vein, compress the junction with the probe and inject small increments of foamed sclerosant as the catheter is gradually withdrawn. Inject extra amounts as the catheter passes perforators.

- The technique is further improved by combining catheter foam sclerotherapy with peri-venous tumescence to collapse the vein prior to foam delivery.[10] This reduces the vein calibre and limits blood inflow from tributaries and deep veins so as to allow best effect from sclerosant in a saline environment. A balloon catheter inflated at the upper end can keep sclerosant in the lumen for longer to enhance its action, but can also force it through perforators into deep veins and favour foam bolus migration after releasing the balloon.

General complications

- A multicentre prospective study of over 1000 patients with saphenous reflux treated by foam UGS showed a low rate of mostly mild adverse reactions.[11] Systemic complications are less likely using O_2/CO_2 gas rather than air to make foam.[12]

> ### 12.1 Systemic complications of chemical ablation
> - Allergic or anaphylactic reaction.
> - Neurological disturbances.
> - Visual disturbances.
> - Respiratory symptoms.

Allergic or anaphylactic reaction

- An allergic reaction can range from mild urticaria to anaphylactic shock. Anaphylaxis is an IgE-mediated mast cell activated reaction that occurs within minutes of exposure to the antigen. Anaphylactoid reaction is non-immunoglobulin-mediated mast cell degranulation and does not require previous exposure to an antigen. They have similar clinical manifestations and treatment. Patients should be observed for 20–30 minutes after treatment prior to discharge to detect possible allergic reactions. Wall charts for cardio-pulmonary resuscitation and treatment of anaphylactic shock should be on site in every treatment room.[13,14]

12.2 Acute management of anaphylaxis

- Call for assistance immediately and arrange for an ambulance[12]
- For an older child or adult >50 kg weight, give an intramuscular injection into the mid-lateral thigh of 0.5 mL adrenaline 1:1000.
- If there is an inadequate response in 3–5 minutes or deterioration, administer a second dose or start an intravenous adrenaline infusion as follows:
  - Mix 1 mL of 1:1000 adrenaline in 1000 mL of normal saline.
  - Start infusion at 5 mL/kg/hour (0.1 microgram/kg/minute) or let the drip run freely though a 16–20 G cannula titrating the rate according to the pulse and blood pressure response, turning it down if tachycardia or chest pain develops.
  - Monitor continuously.
  - An intravenous bolus of adrenaline is not recommended due to the risk of cardiac arrhythmia – intramuscular absorption is excellent in minutes.
- If adrenaline infusion is ineffective or unavailable, consider:

- For upper airway obstruction:
  - nebulized adrenaline continuously until responds
  - intubation if skills and equipment are available.
- For persistent hypotension or shock:
  - give 1–2 litres normal saline
  - in an adult patient with cardiogenic shock, especially if taking beta blockers, consider an intravenous glucagon bolus of 1–2 mg.
- For persistent wheeze:
  - bronchodilators: Salbutamol 8–12 puffs of 100 ug using a spacer or 5 mg salbutamol by nebuliser
  - oral prednisolone 1 mg/kg (maximum 50 mg) or intravenous hydrocortisone 5 mg/kg (maximum 200 mg) are frequently given but take hours to act, though they may protect against later rebound attacks
  - H_1 and H_2 blockers may have a role in persistent itching, but care must be taken with sedating antihistamines such as promethazine.

Neurological disturbances

- Neurologic complications including transient ischemic attacks and stroke are rare. Parsi described 13 reported cases of stroke after chemical ablation, four after liquid and nine after foam. There was immediate onset in seven, of which two were liquid and five were foam, while the mean volume was 2.1 mL of liquid and 12 mL of foam.[15]
- Stroke due to paradoxical gas embolism after UGS has an early onset, whereas stroke due to paradoxical thrombus embolism has a delayed onset. Rare instances of stroke after direct-vision sclerotherapy are unlikely to result from paradoxical embolism, and the mechanism is not clear.
- After foam injection, echogenic bubbles invariably appear in the right ventricle. These are probably gas bubbles with no active sclerosant content, but endothelial particles may be released as well. A patent foramen ovale (PFO) is present in 30% of the general population. Transcranial Doppler showed microbubbles passing through the middle cerebral artery after foam UGS in some 14%–42% of patients in one study,[16] and some 60% of patients with great saphenous reflux at rest or after a Valsalva manoeuvre in another,[17] indicating an even higher incidence of PFO in patients with great saphenous reflux.
- Valsalva manoeuvres enhance the likelihood of bubble passage through a PFO. The effect of these as a potential cause of diffuse cortical ischemia leading to impaired cognitive function has not been investigated. Pre-treatment screening for a PFO is justified only for known high risk such as past cryptogenic stroke, severe migraine with aura, sleep apnoea or chronic obstructive pulmonary disease and pulmonary hypertension.

- Right heart signals appear independent of the foam volume, leg elevation, saphenous junction compression or use of CO_2/O_2 rather than air.[8]

Visual disturbances

- Blurred vision or scotomata can develop within a few minutes after treatment but usually resolve within 30 minutes, although they are very likely to recur with subsequent treatment sessions. The incidence is no more than 2%, and all reported events have been transient.[18] They are more frequent with foam than liquid but there is a lower incidence with CO_2 foam.
- These usually affect patients with a previous history of migraine, and may simply be a prodromal phase. Visual disturbances are postulated to result from release of endothelin from the damaged intima,[19] and have been related to the presence of a PFO but not to transient cerebrovascular ischaemia. They can be associated with migrainous paraesthesiae and dysphasia, depending on the extension of cortical spreading depression. Patients may wish to take their usual migraine treatment an hour prior to treatment in the hope of preventing symptoms.

Respiratory symptoms

- The lungs function as a natural filter for foam. Chest pressure, painful chest tightness or coughing lasting for about five minutes occur in about 1%. It is more frequent if large volumes of foam are injected, while frequency is reduced by substituting CO_2 for air. Isotope studies show no evidence of sclerosant deposition in the lungs.

Local complications

- Severe complications are rare. A review of multiple studies reported matting, skin staining or pigmentation in <20% and thrombophlebitis in <5%.[20] Side-effects include bruising, blistering and urticaria. Trapped blood in the treated vein is common and persists for the first few weeks. It is slowly absorbed by the body, and it liquefies by about two weeks so that the vein can be punctured or aspirated using local anaesthetic if required.

> ### 12.3 Local complications of direct vision sclerotherapy
>
> - Venous thrombo-embolism.
> - Intra-arterial injection.
> - Injection ulcer.
> - Nerve injury.
> - Infection.
> - Hyperpigmentation.
> - Matting.
> - Hypertrichosis.
> - Eye splash injury.

Venous thrombo-embolism

- Deep vein thrombosis after direct vision sclerotherapy is probably under-reported, but is not a sufficient threat to warrant routine post-treatment surveillance, unless there is known predisposition such as thrombophilia. Several instances of pulmonary embolism have been reported after direct-vision sclerotherapy.
- Venous thrombo-embolism after UGS is uncommon. Ultrasound review soon after UGS detects deep venous occlusion (either thrombosis or simple sclerosis) in less than 2% of procedures although the risk increases three-fold for veins ≥5 mm diameter and for foam volume ≥10 mL.[21] The patient may then require treatment with anticoagulation until further scans show that any clot is resolving.

Intra-arterial injection

- Intra-arterial injection can occur with any major artery adjacent to a treated vein, and aberrant veins are at high risk. Intra-arterial sclerosant is not in contact with the major artery endothelium for enough time to cause major damage or induce marked vasospasm, and distal occlusion is due to embolism of thrombotic sludge into the microcirculation. Accordingly, treatment is directed to removing thrombus and suppressing the resultant inflammatory reaction.

- Stop injection immediately if there is complaint of pain distal to the treatment site. Treatment can be with a combination of oral steroids – prednisolone 0.5–1 mg/kg slowly reduced for up to several months, systemic anticoagulation – enoxaparin 1.5 mg/kg daily by subcutaneous injection, and consideration of hyperbaric oxygen therapy.[22]
- Demarcation of infarcted tissue initially appears as a purpuric area which may or may not progress to skin breakdown (Figure 12.4), and second intention healing can take several months. Surgical debridement and attempted repair is usually necessary. Amputation may be required.

Injection ulcer

- An injection ulcer (embolia cutis medicamentosa) is thought to result from reflux into arterioles through arterio-venous communications. An ascending arteriole supplies an area of skin, often hexagonal in shape, termed an angiosome which is infarcted if the arteriole is occluded (see Figure 6.16). Subcutaneous perivenous injection of liquid or foamed sclerosant is not considered to be responsible. It appears as a lesion, often about 4 mm diameter with a reticulate edge surrounding a central purpuric region. An ulcer may be avoided by aggressive

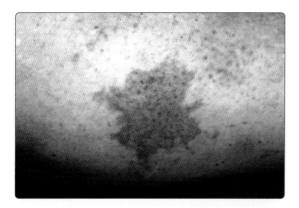

Figure 12.4 Purpuric ischaemic pre-ulcer resulting from local ischaemia after sclerotherapy, which may resolve or may cause skin breakdown.

treatment at the purpuric stage with high-dose oral steroids tapering off over several weeks, a hydrocolloid dressing and compression stocking and anticoagulation with low-molecular weight heparins. An ulcer takes about two to three months to heal and may leave a hyper- or hypo-pigmented scar. Excision of the ulcer leaves a significantly worse cosmetic result and should be avoided.

Nerve injury

- Neuropraxias from needle trauma or bruising are not uncommon, causing some tingling or numbness for up to several months. Sensory nerve injury can involve the saphenous or sural nerves and is debilitating if persistent. Motor nerve damage affecting the posterior tibial or common peroneal nerves is fortunately rare but devastating. Injury should be recognized immediately by severe pain in the distribution of the nerve.

Infection

- Infection is rare as detergent sclerosants are antiseptic, so that routine sterilizing of the skin with an antiseptic is not necessary. Inflammation is almost invariably due to superficial vein thrombosis.

Hyperpigmentation

- Hyperpigmentation with brown staining results from haemosiderin deposition from extravasated red blood cells during the post-treatment inflammatory stage (Figure 12.5). Secondary melanin deposition is also involved. Hyperpigmentation is more likely in patients with a dark complexion and those with higher total body iron stores. It gradually fades so that treatment to bleach the colour with laser should be delayed for at least 12 months, as premature treatment can lead to hypopigmentation or worsening of hyperpigmentation. Minocycline can lead to blue–grey pigmentation after sclerotherapy, and histology shows haemosiderin deposition in the dermis and pigmented macrophages within the sub-endothelial layer of the vein wall.[23]

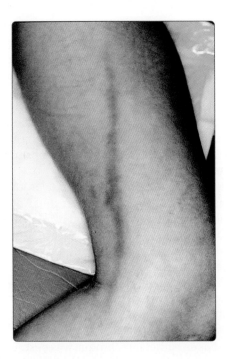

Figure 12.5 Pigmentation along a treated vein after ultrasound-guided sclerotherapy.

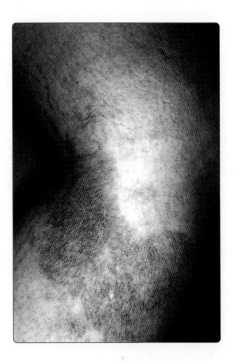

Figure 12.6 Matting after sclerotherapy.

Matting

- Matting refers to the appearance of clusters of fine vessels within superficial layers in the dermis (Figure 12.6). It occurs in about 15% of patients typically appearing about four to six weeks after sclerotherapy, and it can spontaneously resolve. The reason for telangiectatic matting is uncertain, but it may result from inadequate treatment of underlying reflux, hypoxic neovascularization, endothelial injury releasing growth factors, increased flow through dilated arterio-venous shunts or excessive repeated sclerotherapy before inflammation from the first session has settled. It may also be associated with poor technique, and is more likely in obese patients, particularly if taking oestrogens. It is not seen on the hands, face or chest, and rarely occurs in males. It frequently indicates the presence of reflux in a larger proximal underlying vein such that if injection occludes a distal reticular vein but not the proximal segment then blood can reflux to the point of closure and then disperse into the skin to produce the matting. Matting is usually treated with repeat sclerotherapy of the fine vessels and underlying vein, but can also be treated by superficial laser.

Eye splash injury

- Drugs can escape and splash into the eyes if the needle disconnects if improperly fixed to a Luer-lock syringe. Severity of chemical injury is determined by the pH of the solution, contact duration and amount of solution. Sclerosants are mildly alkaline as STS is buffered to pH7.6 and polidocanol to pH6.5–9. However, they are unlikely to penetrate the cornea, as do stronger alkali.
- Eye splash with sclerosants require immediate eye wash, and continuing redness and irritation should lead to slit lamp examination. Severe contamination may warrant irrigation with normal saline until the pH returns to neutral, as monitored with litmus paper. Topical steroids and antibiotics may be needed.

- It is recommended to wear protective eye shields during chemical treatment of veins at all times and to use Luer-lock syringes.

Results

Direct vision sclerotherapy

- One clinical trial found that foam sclerotherapy provided considerably better control of these small veins than using liquid sclerosant,[24] but another showed no difference in side-effects or complications for liquid compared to foam or for polidocanol compared to sodium tetradecyl suphate.[25] There is a need for further studies to compare sclerosants and different concentrations for treating small veins.

Ultrasound-guided sclerotherapy

- Foam had an advantage over liquid for UGS in three randomized trials. There was complete occlusion in 94% with foam compared to 53% with liquid at 90 days in one,[24] elimination of reflux in 69% and 27%, respectively, at three months in another[25] and occlusion in 53% and 12%, respectively, at two years in the third.[26]
- A study comparing conventional surgery and foam UGS for great saphenous reflux showed occlusion rates at two years to be 79% and 65%, respectively.[28]
- Studies comparing EVLA and foam UGS for great saphenous reflux have shown occlusion rates at one year to be 93% and 74%, respectively,[29] and 97% and 51%, respectively.[30]
- Occlusion rates are maintained long-term in some 75% of tributaries, 50% of treated great saphenous veins and 30% of treated small saphenous veins.[31] Accordingly, patients should be warned that repeat treatment may be required for the presenting venous disease, much less new disease. There is a lower cost for initial treatment for UGS when compared to endovenous thermal ablation, but this advantage is lost over the long term due to the more frequent need for repeat treatment.[32, 33]

History

- The introduction of sclerotherapy has been attributed to Zollikofer in Switzerland in 1682, Debout and Chassaignac in 1853 and Desgranges in 1854, but it would seem that the first systematic use of the technique was by Joseph Pierre Pétrequin (1809–76) working as surgeon-in-chief at the Hôtel Dieu in Lyon.
- Modern sclerotherapy was developed by Karl Sigg, Raimon Tournay, George Fegan and John Hobbs, stressing the need for the empty vein technique and prolonged compression after treatment.
- The current technique for foam sclerotherapy was promoted by brothers Juan and Antonio Cabrera in the mid-1990s and by Alain Monfreux in 1997. Lorenzo Tessari, Attilio Cavezzi and Alessandro Frullini reported a technique in 2001 for a simple method to make foam using two disposable syringes and a three-way tap.[5]
- Ultrasound-guided sclerotherapy was first described by Michel Schadeck in 1986.[34] The first open catheter technique was described by Louis Grondin in 1992.[35] The ELLE technique was described by Kurosh Parsi in 1997.[9]

References

1. Wittens C, Davies AH, Bækgaard N, Broholm R, Cavezzi A, Chastanet S, de Wolf M et al., Management of chronic venous disease. Clinical practice guidelines of the European Society for Vascular Surgery. *Eur J Vasc Endovasc Surg* 2015;49:678–737. https://www.researchgate.net/publication/280483468_Editor's_Choice_-_Management_of_Chronic_Venous_Disease_Clinical_Practice_Guidelines_of_the_European_Society_for_Vascular_Surgery_ESVS

2. Rabe E, Breu FX, Cavezzi A, Coleridge Smith P, Frullini A, Gillet JL, Guex JJ et al.; Guideline Group. European guidelines for sclerotherapy in chronic venous disorders. *Phlebology* 2014;29:338–54. http://journals.sagepub.com/doi/abs/10.1177/0268355513483280

3. Van Cleef J-F. Treatment of vulvar and perineal varicose veins. *Phlebolymphology* 2011;18:38–43. http://www.phlebolymphology.org/treatment-of-vulvar-and-perineal-varicose-veins/

4. Orsini C, Brotto M. Immediate pathologic effects on the vein wall of foam sclerotherapy. *Dermatol Surg* 2007;33:1250–4. http://www.ncbi.nlm.nih.gov/pubmed/?term=Orsini+C%2C+Brotto+M.+Immediate

5. Tessari L, Cavezzi A, Frullini A. Preliminary experience with a new sclerosing foam in the treatment of varicose veins. *Dermatol Surg* 2001;27:58–60. http://www.ncbi.nlm.nih.gov/pubmed/11231246

6. Myers KA, Clough AM. Ultrasound-guided sclerotherapy using liquid sclerosant after preliminary saline flush. *Veins Lymphatics* 2014;3:1–4. http://www.pagepressjournals. org/index.php/vl/article/view/vl.2014.1933/2723

7. Parsi K. Paradoxical embolism, stroke and sclerotherapy. *Phlebology* 2012;27:147–67. http://www.ncbi.nlm.nih. gov/pubmed/21890881

8. Hill D, Hamilton R, Fung T. Assessment of techniques to reduce sclerosant foam migration during ultrasound-guided sclerotherapy of the great saphenous vein. *J Vasc Surg* 2008;48:934–9. http://www.ncbi.nlm.nih. gov/pubmed/?term=Hill+D%2C+Hamilton+R%2C+Fung+T

9. Parsi K. Catheter-directed sclerotherapy. *Phlebology* 2009;24:98–107. http://www.ncbi.nlm.nih.gov/ pubmed/19470860

10. Cavezzi A, Mosti G, Di Paolo S, Tessari L, Campana F, Urso SU. Ultrasound-guided peri-saphenous tumescence infiltration improves the outcomes of long catheter foam sclerotherapy combined with phlebectomy of the varicose tributaries. *Veins Lymphatics* 2015;4:1. http://www.pagepressjournals.org/index.php/vl/ article/view/vl.2015.4676/5613

11. Gillet JL, Guedes JM, Guex JJ, Hamel-Desnos C, Schadeck M, Lauseker M, Allaert FA. Side-effects and complications of foam sclerotherapy of the great and small saphenous veins: A controlled multicentre prospective study including 1025 patients. *Phlebology* 2009;24:86. http:// www.varicoseveins.ie/wp-content/uploads/2011/11/ complications-of-foam-sclerotherapy.pdf

12. Morrison N, Neuhardt DL, Rogers CR, McEown J, Morrison T, Johnson E, Salles-Cunha SX. Incidence of side-effects using carbon dioxide-oxygen foam for chemical ablation of superficial veins of the lower extremity. *Eur J Vasc Endovasc Surg* 2010;40:407–13. http://www.ncbi.nlm.nih.gov/pubmed/20547080

13. Anaphylaxis: Emergency management for health professionals. *Australian Prescriber* 2011;34:124. https:// www.nps.org.au/australian-prescriber/articles/ anaphylaxis-wallchart

14. ANZCOR Guideline 8 – Cardiopulmonary Resuscitation (CPR). http://www.hpw.qld.gov.au/SiteCollection Documents/AnzcorGuideline8CPRJan16.pdf

15. Parsi K. Venous gas embolism during foam sclerotherapy of saphenous veins despite recommended treatment modifications. *Phlebology* 2011;26:140–7. https://www. ncbi.nlm.nih.gov/pubmed/21087951

16. Morrison N, Neuhardt DL. Foam sclerotherapy: Cardiac and cerebral monitoring. *Phlebology* 2009;24:252–9. http://www.ncbi.nlm.nih.gov/pubmed/19952381

17. Wright DD, Gibson KD, Barclay J, Razumovsky A, Rush J, McCollum CN. High prevalence of right-to-left shunt in patients with symptomatic great saphenous incompetence and varicose veins. *J Vasc Surg* 2010;51:104–7. http://www.sciencedirect.com/ science/article/pii/S0741521409016218

18. Willenberg T, Smith PC, Shepherd A, Davies AH. Visual disturbance following sclerotherapy for varicose veins, reticular veins and telangiectasias: A systematic literature review. *Phlebology* 2013;28:123–31. https:// www.ncbi.nlm.nih.gov/pubmed/23761921

19. Gillet JL, Donnet A, Lausecker M, Guedes JM, Guex JJ, Lehmann P. Pathophysiology of visual disturbances occurring after foam sclerotherapy. *Phlebology* 2010;25:261–6. http://www.ncbi.nlm.nih. gov/pubmed/20870875

20. Jia X, Mowatt G, Burr JM, Cassar K, Cook J, Fraser C. Systematic review of foam sclerotherapy for varicose veins. *Br J Surg* 2007;94:925–36. http://www.ncbi.nlm. nih.gov/pubmed/?term=Jia+X%2C+Mowatt+G%2C +Burr+JM%2C+Cassar+K%2C+Cook+J%2C+Fraser+ C.+Systematic

21. Myers KA, Jolley D. Factors affecting the risk of deep venous occlusion after ultrasound-guided sclerotherapy for varicose veins. *Eur J Vasc Endovasc Surg* 2008;36:602–5. http://www.ncbi.nlm.nih.gov/pub med/?term=Myers+KA%2C+Jolley+D.+Factors+affe cting

22. Parsi K, Hannaford P. Intra-arterial injection of sclerosants: Report of three cases treated with systemic steroids. *Phlebology*. 2016;31:241–50. http://www.ncbi.nlm.nih. gov/pubmed/25837790

23. Star P, Choy C, Parsi K. Black veins: A case of minocycline-induced pigmentation post-sclerotherapy and a review of literature. *J Cutaneous Pathol* 2017;44:83–92. http://onlinelibrary.wiley.com/doi/10.1111/cup.12824/ abstract

24. Alòs J, Carreño P, López JA, Estadella B, Serra-Prat M, Marinel-Lo J. Efficacy and safety of sclerotherapy using polidocanol foam: A controlled clinical trial. *Eur J Vasc Endovasc Surg* 2006;31:101–7. http://www.ncbi. nlm.nih.gov/pubmed/?term=Al%C3%B2s+J%2C+Ca rre%C3%B1o+P%2C+L%C3%B3pez+JA%2C+Estadell a+B%2C+Serra-Prat+M%2C+Marinel-Lo+J.+Efficacy

25. Rao J, Wildemore JK, Goldman MP. Double-blind pros pective comparative trial between foamed and liquid polidocanol and sodium tetradecyl sulfate in the treatment of varicose and telangiectatic leg veins. *Dermatol Surg* 2005;31:631–5. http://www.ncbi.nlm.nih. gov/pubmed/?term=Rao+J%2C+Wildemore+JK%2C +Goldman+MP.+Double-blind

26. Rabe E, Otto J, Schliephake D, Pannier F. Efficacy and safety of great saphenous vein sclerotherapy using standardised polidocanol foam (ESAF): A randomised controlled multicentre clinical trial. *Eur J Vasc Endovasc Surg* 2008;35:238–45. http://www.ncbi.nlm.nih.gov/ pubmed/17988905

27. Ouvry P, Allaert FA, Desnos P, Hamel-Desnos C. Efficacy of polidocanol foam versus liquid in sclerotherapy of the great saphenous vein: A multicentre randomised controlled trial with a 2-year follow-up. *Eur J Vasc Endovasc Surg* 2008;36:366–70. http://www.ncbi.nlm.nih.gov/pubmed/18524643

28. Shadid N, Ceulen R, Nelemans P, Dirksen C, Vcraart J, Schurink GW, van Neer P, vd Kley J, de Haan E, Sommer A. Randomized clinical trial of ultrasound-guided foam sclerotherapy versus surgery for the incompetent great saphenous vein. *Br J Surg* 2012;99:1062–70. http://www.ncbi.nlm.nih.gov/pubmed/?term=Shadid+N%2C+Ceulen+R%2C+Nelemans+P

29. Gonzalez-Zeh R, Armisen R, Barahona S. Endo-venous laser and echo-guided foam ablation in great saphenous vein reflux: One-year follow-up results. *J Vasc Surg* 2008;48:940–6. http://www.ncbi.nlm.nih.gov/pubmed/?term=Gonzalez-Zeh+R%2C+Armisen+R%2C+Barahona+S

30. Venermo M, Saarinen J, Eskelinen E, Vähäaho S, Saarinen E, Railo M, Uurto I, Salenius J, Albäck A; Finnish Venous Study Collaborators. Randomized clinical trial comparing surgery, EVLA and ultrasound-guided foam sclerotherapy for the treatment of great saphenous varicose veins. *Br J Surg* 2016;26:1438–1444. http://www.ncbi.nlm.nih.gov/pubmed/27561823

31. Myers KA, Jolley D, Clough A, Kirwan J. Outcome of ultrasound-guided sclerotherapy for varicose veins: Medium-term results assessed by ultrasound surveillance. *Eur J Vasc Endovasc Surg* 2007;33:116–21. http://www.ncbi.nlm.nih.gov/pubmed/?term=Myers+KA%2C+Jolley+D%2C+Clough+A%2C+Kirwan

32. Brittenden J, Cotton SC, Elders A, Tassie E, Scotland G, Ramsay CR, Norrie J et al. Clinical effectiveness and cost-effectiveness of foam sclerotherapy, EVLA and surgery for varicose veins: Results from the Comparison of LAser, Surgery and foam Sclerotherapy (CLASS) randomised controlled trial. *Health Technol Assess* 2015;19:27. http://www.ncbi.nlm.nih.gov/pubmed/25858333

33. Marsden G, Perry M, Bradbury A, Hickey N, Kelley K, Trender H, Wonderling D, Davies AH. A cost-effectiveness analysis of surgery, endothermal ablation, ultrasound-guided foam sclerotherapy and compression stockings for symptomatic varicose veins. *Eur J Vasc Endovasc Surg* 2015;50:794–801. http://www.ncbi.nlm.nih.gov/pubmed/26433594

34. Schadeck M. Doppler et echotomographie dans la sclerose des veines saphenes. *Phlebologie* 1986;39:697–716. http://www.ncbi.nlm.nih.gov/pubmed/3538068

35. Grondin L, Soriano J. Duplex-echosclerotherapy, in the quest for the safe technique. In *Phlebologie 92*. Raymond-Martimbeau P, Prescott R, Zummo M, Eds. 1992; 828–33. Paris: John Libbey Eurotext.

APPENDIX 12.A

A worksheet used for ultrasound-guided sclerotherapy.

Patient: Date:

Referring doctor: UR number:

Treating doctor: Sonographer:

Right leg.
Sclerosant -
Concentration   %
Volume   ml
Diameter vein   mm
Length vein   cm

Left leg.
Sclerosant -
Concentration   %
Volume   ml
Diameter vein   mm
Length vein   cm

Right   Left

Veins treated.

Procedure:

Post-operative instructions:

13 Endovenous ablation and cyanoacrylate closure

This chapter incorporates recommendations from the European Society for Vascular Surgery, Society for Vascular Surgery, and American Venous Forum.[1,2]

Preparation

- Endovascular procedures can be performed in a hospital operating suite but are conveniently performed as an out-patient.
- For endovenous thermal ablation (ETA), initially prepare the patient away from the procedure room. Use ultrasound to mark the full length of the veins to be treated with a cross-mark at the saphenous junction and distal end with the limb in the same position as used for subsequent treatment. Marker pens are sterile.
- Prior to ETA, many practitioners then apply 10% topical lignocaine gel along the length to reduce discomfort from later injections of tumescent anaesthetic. In addition, many apply a vasodilator gel at the distal end for all procedures requiring needle access to increase the vein diameter and to reduce the risk of vasospasm. Cover the site with an adhesive wrap and leave it for 30 minutes. The amount of local anaesthetic applied is not sufficient to contribute to lignocaine toxicity.
- The patient is transferred to the procedure room and placed on an adjustable tilt-table. Position the limb for best access for the great saphenous vein with the patient rolled 45° to the side of the vein supported by a pillow under the buttock, and for the small saphenous vein with the patient prone. Tilt the table 20°–30° feet downwards to fill the veins for a difficult vein puncture.

Needle vein access

- Prepare the limb with antiseptic and isolate the operation field with sterile drapes. Choose the insertion site for a point where the vein is relatively close to the skin. Inject a bleb of 1% lignocaine, make a very small stab if necessary with an 11 blade and puncture the vein under ultrasound guidance with an angiogram needle attached to a 3 mL syringe, confirmed by drawback of blood. Newer systems allow direct puncture without a skin incision. Make multiple serial entry punctures if necessary if there is vein tortuosity. Venous spasm may thwart attempts at puncture. Secure access by inserting a 5F sheath (F = French, 1F = 1/3 mm or diameter = F/3 mm – e.g. a 9F sheath is 3 mm diameter).
- If required, feed an 0.035inch safety-J guidewire up the vein with ultrasound guidance, and while the sonographer shows the saphenous junction, pass the wire up to the junction but not through into the deep vein. Then flatten the table or tilt into reverse Trendelenburg.
- Inject tumescence fluid if this technique is chosen, perform the intervention, and at

completion apply pressure to the puncture site until bleeding stops. When all veins have been treated, clean the limbs, apply stockings and mobilize the patient.

Tumescent anaesthesia

- ETA can be performed under general anaesthesia, spinal anaesthesia or femoral nerve block, but tumescent anaesthesia is the preferred technique as it allows early ambulation. Sedation before or during treatment is optional.
- Tumescent anaesthesia involves injecting dilute anaesthetic solution around the length of the treated vein. The result is to prevent pain, provide a heat sink to protect surrounding tissue, separate adjacent nerves and arteries, and compress the vein to improve contact between vein wall and probe, thus allowing treatment of large diameter veins.
- Make up a fresh solution shortly before use.
  - Normal saline – 1000 mL of 0.9% NaCl solution.
  - Lignocaine – 500 mg (50 mL of 1% lignocaine solution).
  - Adrenaline – 1 mg (1 mL of 1:1,000 solution of adrenaline).
  - Sodium bicarbonate – 12.5 mEq (12.5 mL of an 8.4% NaH_2CO_3 solution.
- The manufacturer's maximum recommended dose of 7 mg/kg of lignocaine with adrenaline is contained in 700 mL of this solution. Store in a refrigerator at 4°C to reduce pain during infusion. The anaesthetic effects last for up to 18 hours.
- Adrenaline-induced vasoconstriction reduces the rate of systemic absorption of lignocaine, and peak plasma levels do not occur until 12–14 hours following injection so that signs of toxicity may not appear until well into the post-operative period. Fortunately, absorption is usually slower than the rate of metabolism and excretion.

Technique

- Infuse with ultrasound guidance into the saphenous space through a long 25-gauge needle and consider using a mechanical pump.

Use the laser fibre or radiofrequency probe or leave the guidewire in place to provide a target on ultrasound to gauge the depth of injection. If a tributary is being treated by EVLA, then infuse into the perivenous tissue with a volume sufficient to separate the vein from the skin by about 1 cm on ultrasound; usually sufficient that the guide-wire is no longer palpable through the skin.

- Inject approximately 15 mL of anaesthetic fluid into the saphenous compartment at each interval along the saphenous vein depending on how far the previous injection has tracked up the vein. Take care at the saphenous junction to ensure that there is complete closure of the vein.
- During infusion, identify the saphenous nerve during treatment of the great saphenous vein and sural nerve during treatment of the small saphenous vein, particularly for distal puncture. This ensures that the nerve is separated from the vein by anaesthetic fluid thus minimizing the likelihood of nerve damage during activation of the thermal probe.
- While infusing tumescent anaesthetic, hold the probe in transverse to show the full width of the saphenous compartment during injection (Figure 13.1), or in longitudinal to show the anaesthetic fluid tracking up along the saphenous sheath (Figure 13.2).

Endovenous laser ablation

- The technique is used to treat saphenous veins, incompetent perforators and relatively straight major tributaries. The saphenous veins treated are the great, small, anterior accessory and posterior accessory saphenous veins.
- EVLA is used to destroy a vein by passing an optical fibre up the vein so that laser energy generates heat within the lumen. The aim is to cause maximum damage to the inner layers attempting not to perforate the vein or damage surrounding tissues.
- Commercial systems are available in a range of frequencies. Optimal laser settings allow laser energy to be directed precisely to the target chromophore, thereby avoiding damage to healthy tissue. The predominant chromophore is haemoglobin for the lower

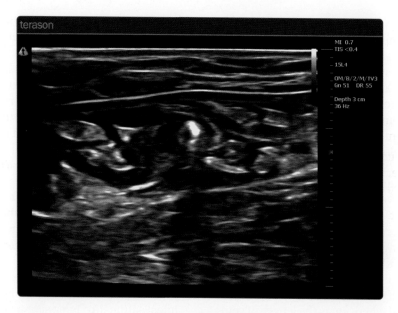

Figure 13.1 Ultrasound image in transverse of tumescent anaesthetic being injected into the saphenous compartment.

wavelengths (810, 940, 980 nm) and water for the higher wavelengths (1320, 1470, 1500 nm). This is considered to result in different modes of action and different side-effects, with less pain using the higher wavelengths, as the primary chromophore is water in the vein wall requiring less energy to achieve vein closure and with fewer vein perforations.[3]

- Thrombotic occlusion results from temperatures of up to 1200–1400°C at the laser probe tip. However, the temperature at the outer vein wall is in the order of 35–50°C

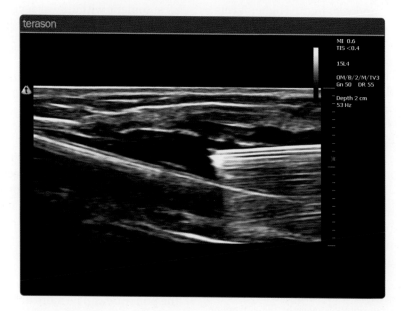

Figure 13.2 Ultrasound image in longitudinal of tumescent anaesthetic being injected into the saphenous compartment.

depending on the power setting, and heat dissipates rapidly away from the vein resulting in only a small risk of perivenous thermal damage. The vein wall is injured directly by thermal damage from absorbed photon energy, and to a much lesser degree indirectly by steam generated by heating the small amount of blood within the vein and by the heated blood itself.

- The original laser fibres were bare-tipped but radial fibres are now preferred to promote uniform delivery of laser energy and reduce the incidence of vein wall perforations.
- Each commercial laser system has variable control of power and a recommended rate of probe withdrawal. Energy is measured in Joules (J). The linear endovenous energy density (LEED – J/cm) and fluence (J/cm^2) can be calculated where cm is the length of vein treated.
- LEED > 80 J/cm and <95 J/cm appear to provide optimal efficacy for successful ablation with the lowest rates of complications and side-effects using lasers of shorter wavelengths. LEED < 50 J/cm is associated with lower closure rates, although longer wavelength lasers appear to give as good efficacy whilst minimizing side-effects with LEED>50 J/cm and <80 J/cm.[4] Higher levels are required for larger diameter veins and lower levels with radial and hooded fibre tips.[1]
- There is need for randomized trials to evaluate the variables that can be controlled by the operator, including the amount of laser energy, rate of energy (power setting), wavelength and fibre design.

Technique for saphenous veins[*]

- Pass a 45 cm or 60 cm sheath with dilator up the vein over a guidewire, if used, to the saphenous junction. Confirm the position by straightening the J of the wire by the dilator; the dilator protrudes 2 cm beyond

the sheath so that leaving it in this position ensures that the sheath is 2 cm below the junction. Alternatively, use a short sheath, advance the fibre alone up the vein and straighten the leg or apply external compression if the catheter or fibre will not pass to help it to advance. Ultrasound helps identify if the guidewire or laser fibre is jamming against a valve, kink or tributary allowing external manipulation to straighten the vein.

- Exchange the guide wire for the laser fibre, connect the fibre to the laser machine, set the power level to the manufacturers recommendations and measure the length of vein to be treated.
- Adjust the tip of the fibre by ultrasound to be 2 cm below the junction (Figure 13.3), inject saline through a side-arm to show flow on ultrasound to further confirm the correct position, and look for light illumination through the skin below the junction. Activation of the laser produces bubbles at the tip that can help to confirm its position (Figure 13.4).
- After tumescent anaesthesia, activate the laser and withdraw at the manufacturer recommended rate. This can be performed using an automatic withdrawal device.

13.1 Precautions

- Check the position of the tip to ensure that it is below the saphenous junction by:
  - direct ultrasound imaging
  - light from the tip beam visible through the skin
  - marking at the puncture site is the same as the measurement before insertion.
- On withdrawal of the laser, confirm it is fully intact and that no laser fibre remains in the patient.

Technique for tributaries

- The puncture can be more difficult due to the short distance below the skin with a tendency to insert the needle to one side of the vein.

---

[*] Approved training for all of the techniques described is mandatory. No responsibility is taken by the authors or publishers for use of these summaries as a basis to perform the procedures.

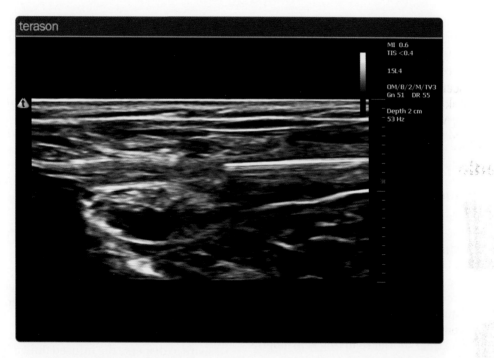

Figure 13.3 Ultrasound image of a laser fibre positioned just below the sapheno-femoral junction.

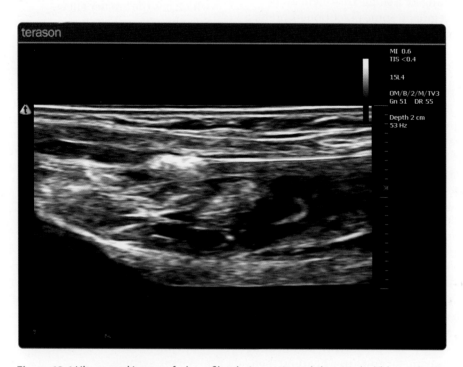

Figure 13.4 Ultrasound image of a laser fibre being activated showing bubbles at the tip.

- It is possible to negotiate curves and angles up to 90°, sometimes assisted by a catheter with a curved tip.
- Take care to separate the vein and skin with tumescent anaesthetic fluid to eliminate any risk of skin burns. There should be sufficient fluid between vein and skin surface so that the guidewire is not palpable.

Radiofrequency ablation

Technique

- Advance a 7F catheter up the vein to 2 cm from the saphenous junction to where treatment will begin using ultrasound guidance.[5] Deliver perivenous anaesthesia as previously described.
- The procedure uses a segmental ablation technique that heats a full 7 cm vein length at 20-second intervals. Alternatively, there is the option to treat shorter refluxing vein lengths with a 3 cm catheter.
- Two treatment cycles are delivered to the first segment. Then for each subsequent segment, markings on the catheter shaft allow precise repositioning for a single treatment cycle to the next segment. Some practitioners prefer a double pass.

Steam ablation

- The technique has the potential to treat both saphenous veins and tributaries.[6] After needle puncture of the vein under ultrasound guidance and placement of a sheath, a 5F catheter is used that can be threaded up even tortuous saphenous veins usually without the need for a guidewire, and the tip is positioned 3 cm distal to the saphenous junction. For tributaries, an 18 g catheter is used for larger veins and 20 g for smaller veins. Tumescent anaesthetic is injected as for the other endo-thermal techniques. Steam which is super-heated to 120°C under pressure is produced by a generator and administered in pulses through side holes as it is slowly withdrawn to directly heat the vein wall. A recommended regime is to give five pulses (two non-heating to clear the catheter and three heating) then as the catheter is withdrawn in 1 cm intervals, two pulses/cm for veins up to 7 mm, three pulses/cm for larger veins and four or more pulses at focal dilatations. Heat accumulates so that it is advised to pause for 5–10 seconds every ten pulses. Heating is stopped as the catheter and sheath are removed 2 cm before the distal end of the treated vein, with a 5-second cooling time to prevent a skin burn. Post-operative management indicated is as for the other endothermal techniques.

Mechanical Occlusion Chemically Assisted (MOCA)

Principles

- MOCA is designed to introduce a sclerosant solution into a target vein for infusion through a catheter, with sclerosant action on the intima enhanced by a rapidly-rotating wire to disperse the infused fluid and to damage the vessel wall. Animal studies show that the combination of mechanical and sclerosant injury causes greater damage to the vein than either alone, but it is not clear which has the greater effect.[7]
- Specific advantages are that there is no chance of injury to adjacent nerves, there is no need for tumescent anaesthesia, there is minimal discomfort during the operation unless it snags on the vein wall, and less post-procedure discomfort compared to ETA.
- However, the rotating tip can catch the vein at an entering tributary or even on a valve cusp causing severe pain, and this may require injection of local anaesthetic at the site to allow it to be tugged free.

Operating system

- The components are:
  - A cartridge unit incorporating a 45 cm or 60 cm working length catheter in which is an 0.035-inch diameter wire with an angled dispersion tip that can be extruded from or withdrawn back into the catheter.
  - A handle unit containing a 9V DC battery-operated motor drive that rotates the wire.
  - A 5 mL syringe.

- The units are locked together to allow simultaneous infusion of liquid sclerosant from the syringe while the motor drive unit rotates the wire and dispersion tip at 3500 r/min.
- Wire rotation is activated by a trigger while at the same time the syringe is simultaneously depressed using a single-handed technique.
- Either STS or polidocanol is used, usually diluted to 1.5%–2% to provide 8–10 mL volume of sclerosant delivered in two lots of 4–5 mL. Some practitioners are prepared to use greater volumes.

Technique

- Prepare the limb, puncture the vein with an angiogram needle and pass a guidewire to allow insertion of a short 4–5F sheath or 16 g catheter.
- Pass the catheter and wire to the saphenous junction, assemble the system, withdraw the catheter to 2 cm distal to the saphenous junction then retract the catheter to expose a 3 cm length of the angled dispersion tip.
- Activate the trigger to commence wire rotation for approximately five seconds to induce proximal venous spasm. Injection during this stage will eject saline used to prime the catheter rather than sclerosant.
- Activate the trigger and slowly withdraw the catheter and wire at 1–2 mm/s while the sclerosant is injected at a rate to empty the 5 mL syringe by the time that one-half of the length of vein is traversed. Attach a fresh syringe and recommence the procedure to treat the remaining vein.
- On approaching the puncture site in the vein, cease wire rotation and withdraw the dispersion tip back into the catheter, cease infusion, disassemble the unit and remove the catheter system and sheath together.
- Do not compress the vein while the wire is rotating as this may cause the wire to snag on a side branch, valve or vein wall. If this occurs, cease rotation, tug the dispersion tip back into the catheter to free it from the vein before recommencing the procedure.

Cyanoacrylate closure (CAC)

Principles

- Early results indicate that the venous CE system is effective. It avoids the use of thermal energy so there is virtually no risk of nerve injury. It does not require tumescent local anaesthesia avoiding the immediate discomfort of multiple injections and potential reaction to anaesthetic agents. Some patients have reservations about a risk of embolisation of material and concerns as to long-term stability of the glue. In addition, CE is proving to cause an appreciable incidence of inflammation along the treated vein.
- Rapid closure may avoid the need for subsequent compression or travel restrictions, and allows early return to normal activities.

Technique

- Use 5% dextrose instead of saline on the preparation tray to avoid inadvertent polymerization.
- Prepare the patient position as previously described. Access the target vein and pass a 180 cm 0.035-inch safety-J guidewire up the vein to the saphenous junction. Advance a 5F sheath and dilator over the guidewire to the junction, remove the guidewire and dilator and flush the system. Position the introducer tip 5 cm caudal to the saphenous junction. Attach the dispenser needle to a syringe, extract adhesive from its vial into the syringe and purge air from the syringe.
- Calculate the total amount of adhesive to be delivered as a function of the vein treatment length. This varies according to the system used. If the vein diameter is greater than 6 mm, sufficient amounts of CA are needed to ensure adequate vein occlusion. One manufacturer cites a maximum of 8.7 mL per patient while another states that there is no upper limit.
- Remove the dispenser tip and connect the system to the catheter. Lock the syringe into place within the dispenser gun taking care not to kink the catheter. Prime the catheter

by pulling the trigger on the dispenser gun to advance the adhesive to within 3 cm of the distal catheter tip but not beyond.

- Remove the flushing syringe from the introducer, insert the primed catheter into the introducer and advance to the mark on the catheter. Pull the introducer back caudal by another 5 cm, advance the catheter cephalad and lock the introducer to the catheter to expose the catheter tip at 5 cm caudal to the saphenous junction. With the ultrasound probe in transverse just cephalad to the catheter tip, apply adequate pressure to compress the saphenous junction.
- One technique injects 0.1 mL aliquots of adhesive into the vein by pulling the trigger of the dispenser gun once and holding and counting to 3 seconds after the trigger pull to completely inject the 0.1 mL of adhesive. Immediately pull back 1 cm and deliver another 0.1 mL of adhesive to the vein with an additional trigger pull again holding the dispenser counting for three seconds after the trigger pull. Following this second injection, within three seconds pull back the connected introducer catheter by 3 cm and maintain transverse compression with the ultrasound probe for a minimum of three minutes. In addition, apply light pressure caudal to the transducer. Holding the ultrasound probe in transverse, compress the vein caudal to the previous injection and cephalad to the catheter tip and deliver 0.1 mL of adhesive into the vein by pulling the trigger of the dispenser gun once and holding for 3 seconds. Following this injection, again immediately pull back the connected introducer catheter by 3 cm and maintain transverse compression of the ultrasound probe for a minimum of 30 seconds. Again, apply light pressure caudal to the transducer. Repeat these steps down the entire length of the target vein to 5 cm cephalad to the access site. Ultrasound clearly identifies the intravenous cyanoacrylate (Figure 13.5).
- Another technique uses continuous infusion with a slow steady rate of catheter withdrawal in the anticipation that a continuous column of glue is less likely to recanalize. This is made possible by the cyanoacrylate for this procedure has far lower viscosity, but it is

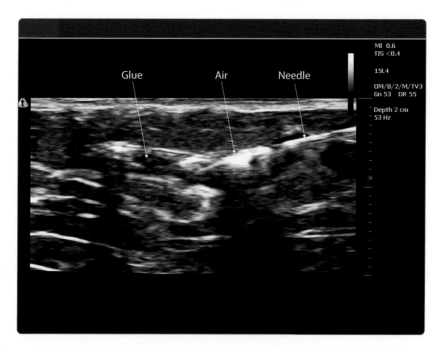

Figure 13.5 Ultrasound image of cyanoacrylate glue being injected into a saphenous vein.

not known whether this increases the risk of embolization.

- Remove the introducer catheter and apply pressure for as long as necessary to achieve haemostasis. Confirm vein closure along the treated segment with ultrasound.

Treatment of tributaries

- Tributaries can be treated by direct-vision sclerotherapy, by UGS or by phlebectomy under local anaesthesia. The saphenous vein distal to the puncture site is also treated by ultrasound-guided sclerotherapy.
- This can be concurrent with any of these techniques to avoid multiple treatment sessions, or performed subsequently at any interval from one to several weeks later. The National Institute for Health and Clinical Excellence (NICE) has provided a guideline for interventional treatment:[8] 'If incompetent varicose tributaries are to be treated, consider treating them at the same time'. However, others are of an opinion that waiting for two weeks or more can allow some veins to disappear allowing more limited treatment, and other veins that persist to decrease in size making their subsequent management by UGS more effective and associated with less post-treatment inflammation.

Management after treatment

- Walk for 15 minutes immediately after treatment and at least 15 minutes per day for the next few days. Maintain normal daytime activities and avoid standing still for long periods. Resume normal exercise activities within 24–36 hours.

Ultrasound surveillance

- A check ultrasound scan may be arranged within a week after treatment to ensure that the treated vein is occluded, determine whether any further veins require treatment and exclude small risk of deep vein occlusion.
- Early post-operative scans look for deep vein thrombosis or sclerosis, but routine scanning

for this reason alone is not cost-effective. Thrombosis is shown by venodilation and initial hypo-echogenic occlusion, while sclerosis results in venoconstriction and hyper-echogenic filling. In addition, the upper end for occlusion of a saphenous vein treated by endovenous techniques can be assessed, and whether secondary thrombosis extends into adjacent deep veins.

- Each post-treatment ultrasound scan notes whether the vein is occluded, absent or patent, and whether there is reflux in any patent segments. If tributaries are treated subsequently by foam sclerotherapy, then it is not uncommon for ultrasound to demonstrate foam within the occluded saphenous vein, but the significance of this is not known.

Complications

- Local side-effects are more often a result of concomitant or subsequent UGS or phlebectomy for tributaries.
- Phlebitis is common following ETA, but this does not represent infection and does not require treatment with antibiotics. Treated veins become clinically inflamed in up to 15% of patients after CE, and this then takes about two weeks to settle. Inflammation can be managed with compression and a non-steroidal anti-inflammatory drug, which may be given before treatment. More serious local complications include skin burns or nerve injury, and arterio-venous fistula has been reported after EVLA. There has been at least one recorded case of stroke after EVLA.
- Thrombus extension beyond the saphenous junction into the adjacent deep vein is referred to as Endovenous Heat-Induced Thrombus (EHIT).[9] It does not have the same risk of pulmonary embolism as spontaneous saphenous vein thrombosis, clinical sequelae are rare and the thrombus usually retreats with serial ultrasound examinations. EHIT is classified as EHIT-1 if at the saphenous junction, EHIT-2 if occluding <50% of the deep vein, EHIT-3 if 50%–99% deep vein occlusion and EHIT-4 if complete deep vein occlusion. Most practitioners start anticoagulation

for EHIT-3 or EHIT-4 until thrombus is seen to retract, although it is not known if this is effective for preventing pulmonary embolism.

- Damage to the saphenous or sural nerves can occur after ETA, and this usually returns to normal within weeks to months although persisting numbness is an occasional late complication. Damage can rarely occur to nerves behind the knee causing motor damage after ETA.
- Infection is rare after ETA due to the sterilizing effect of heat from the probe, and inflammation is almost invariably due to superficial vein thrombosis, but there is a track of thrombus for a nidus for bacteria, allowing possible suppuration along a considerable length of vein. Systemic features of infection warrant aggressive treatment with antibiotics and possible drainage.
- There have been reports of lost guidewires ending in the right ventricle, broken laser fibres in the vein left after EVLA and wires caught and requiring surgical removal after MOCA.
- Retinal damage to the patient or staff from laser injury if the fibre breaks or if the laser is activated when the laser is outside of the body is a serious but very rare complication.

Results

Endovenous thermal ablation

- The literature has consistently shown no more than about 10% recurrence rate at one year or more after EVLA.[10] A multicentre study showed better than 90% closure at three years for RF.[5] The clinical CEAP class and vein diameter have been the strongest predictors of outcome.[3]
- A randomized trial of EVLA compared to surgery for great saphenous reflux showed identical initial technical success rates but with quicker return to work and normal activity for endothermal treatment (about four days versus 14 days).[11,12]
- A randomized trial of EVLA compared to surgery for small saphenous reflux showed better technical success (96% versus 72%)

again with quicker return to work and normal activity.[13]

- Trials comparing EVLA and RF showed identical early occlusion rates but with less bruising and post-operative pain for the RF procedure.[14,15]
- A randomized clinical trial for great saphenous vein EVLA showed that there was less pain and better quality of life using a longer wave length (1470 nm) laser system than a shorter wave length (910 nm), although treatment success and adverse event rates were similar.[16]
- The most frequent sites for recurrence after ETA of the great saphenous vein are recanalization (30%) and development of anterior thigh vein reflux (20%).[17]
- A study has shown no difference in post-procedural pain, quality of life or bruising scores, with occlusion in all patients at one year for compression against no compression after ETA.[18]
- A randomized trial comparing steam and laser ablation for great saphenous reflux showed similar one-year occlusion rates (92% and 96%, respectively), less post-procedure pain and earlier return to normal activities.[19]

MOCA

- Early technical success rates are good[20,21] but longer follow-up studies are required.

Cyanoacrylate closure

- The initial study by Almeida and colleagues reported 38 patients with great saphenous reflux treated by CAC followed for up to 24 months.[22] Neither perivenous tumescent anaesthesia nor graduated compression stockings were used. It was concluded that the procedure was feasible, safe and effective.
- A multicentre American study of 222 patients with great saphenous reflux randomized to cyanoacrylate closure or RF showed that the CAC technique was non-inferior to RF at three months and that both showed good safety profiles.[23]

- A multicentre European trial reported results for CAC of 70 great saphenous veins. Neither tumescent anaesthesia nor post-interventional compression stockings were used and varicose tributaries remained untreated for at least three months. Cumulative 12-month survival free from recanalization was 92.9%. A phlebitic reaction occurred in 11.4%, with a median duration of 6.5 days, but no serious adverse event occurred.[24]
- A Turkish trial studied 310 patients with great saphenous reflux treated with CAC or EVLA. The one-year closure rate for CAC was 95.8%. Operative time was shorter (15 ± 2.5 vs. 33.2 ± 5.7, respectively) and periprocedural pain was less (3.1 ± 1.6 vs 6.5 ± 2.3, respectively) for CAC.[25]
- An American study reported early outcome for 70 veins treated including great, small, and anterior accessory saphenous veins up to 20 mm diameter.[26] Compression stockings were not used and side-branches were not treated. All veins were occluded at one month, and the mean time to return to work and normal activities was less than three days. Phlebitis in the treatment area or side-branches occurred in 20%, but completely resolved in all but one patient by one month.
- A single-centre study of 57 legs treated for great saphenous reflux in Hong Kong showed a 78.5% closure rate at one year.[27] Mean vein diameter ≥ 8 mm was a significant predictor for recanalization.
- A study from The Netherlands shows that it is feasible to use CAC to treat incompetent perforators.[28]
- Unlike the follow-up for ETA which invariably shows that occluded treated veins disappear within 12 months, veins do not disappear after CAC and remain much the same size as immediately after treatment.

Templates

- Sample operation report forms are shown in the Appendix (Chapter 12).

References

1. Wittens C, Davies AH, Bækgaard N, Broholm R, Cavezzi A, Chastanet S, de Wolf M. et al. Management of chronic venous disease. Clinical practice guidelines of the European Society for vascular surgery. *Eur J Vasc Endovasc Surg* 2015;49:678–737. https://www.researchgate.net/publication/280483468_Editor's_Choice_-_Management_of_Chronic_Venous_Disease_Clinical_Practice_Guidelines_of_the_European_Society_for_Vascular_Surgery_ESVS

2. Gloviczki P, Comerota AJ, Dalsing MC, Eklof BG, Gillespie DL, Gloviczki ML, Lohr JM et al. The care of patients with varicose veins and associated chronic venous diseases: Clinical practice guidelines of the Society for Vascular Surgery and the American Venous Forum. *J Vasc Surg* 2011;53:2S–48S. https://www.ncbi.nlm.nih.gov/pubmed/21536172

3. Van der Velden SK, Lawaetz M, De Maeseneer MG, Hollestein L, Nijsten T, van den Bos RR. Predictors of recanalization of the great saphenous vein in randomized controlled trials 1 year after endovenous thermal ablation. *Eur J Vasc Endovasc Surg.* 2016;16:234–41. http://www.ncbi.nlm.nih.gov/pubmed/?term=Van+der+Velden+SK%2C+Lawaetz+M%2C+De+Maeseneer+MG%2C+Hollestein+L%2C+Nijsten+T%2C+van+den+Bos+RR.+Predictors+of+Recanalization+of+the+Great+Saphenousmal

4. Cowpland CA, Cleese AL, Whiteley MS. Factors affecting optimal linear endovenous energy density for endovenous laser ablation in incompetent lower limb truncal veins: A review of the clinical evidence. *Phlebology* 2017;32:299-306. http://www.ncbi.nlm.nih.gov/pubmed/?term=Cowpland+CA%2C+Cleese+AL%2C+Whiteley+MS.+Factors+affecting+optimal+linear+endovenous+energy+density+for+endovenous+laser+ablation+in+incompetent+lower+limb+truncal+veins+-+A+review+of+the+clinical+evidence.+Phlebology.+2016

5. Proebstle TM1, Alm J, Göckeritz O, Wenzel C, Noppeney T, Lebard C, Pichot O, Sessa C, Creton D; European Closure Fast Clinical Study Group. Three-year European follow-up of endovenous radiofrequency-powered segmental thermal ablation of the great saphenous vein with or without treatment of calf varicosities. *J Vasc Surg* 2011;54:146–52. http://www.ncbi.nlm.nih.gov/pubmed/21439757

6. Milleret R. Obliteration of Varicose Veins with Super heated Steam. *Phlebolymphology* 2011;18:174–81. http://www.phlebolymphology.org/obliteration-of-varicose-veins-with-superheated-steam/

7. Boersma D, van Haelst ST, van Eekeren RR, Vink A, Reijnen MM, de Vries JP, de Borst GJ. Macroscopic

and histologic analysis of vessel wall reaction after mechanochemical endovenous ablation using the ClariVein OC device in an animal. *Eur J Vasc Endovasc Surg* 2017;53:290–8. https://model.www.ncbi.nlm.nih.gov/pubmed/28025005

8. NICE quidelines. Varicose veins: Diagnosis and management. [CG168] July 2013. https://www.nice.org.uk/guidance/cg168

9. Harlander-Locke M, Jimenez JC, Lawrence PF, Derubertis BG, Rigberg DA, Gelabert HA, Farley SM. Management of endovenous heat-induced thrombus using a classification system and treatment algorithm following segmental thermal ablation of the small saphenous vein. *J Vasc Surg* 2013;58:427–32. http://www.jvascsurg.org/article/S0741-5214(13)00188-2/fulltext

10. Myers KA, Jolley D. Outcome of endovenous laser therapy for saphenous reflux and varicose veins: Medium-term results assessed by ultrasound surveillance. *Eur J Vasc Endovasc Surg* 2009;37:239–45. https://www.ncbi.nlm.nih.gov/pubmed/18993093

11. Carradice D, Mekako A, Mazari FA, Samuel N, Hatfield J, Chetter IC. Clinical and technical outcomes from a randomized clinical trial of endovenous laser ablation compared with conventional surgery for great saphenous varicose veins. *Br J Surg* 2011;98:1117–23. http://www.ncbi.nlm.nih.gov/pubmed/21638277

12. Carradice D, Mekako AI, Mazari FA, Samuel N, Hatfield J, Chetter IC. Randomized clinical trial of endovenous laser ablation compared with conventional surgery for great saphenous varicose veins. *Br J Surg* 2011;98:501–10. http://www.ncbi.nlm.nih.gov/pubmed/21283981

13. Samuel N, Carradice D, Wallace T, Mekako A, Hatfield J, Chetter I. Randomized clinical trial of endovenous laser ablation versus conventional surgery for small saphenous varicose veins. *Ann Surg* 2013;257:419–26. http://www.ncbi.nlm.nih.gov/pubmed/23160149

14. Nordon IM, Hinchliffe RJ, Brar R, Moxey P, Black SA, Thompson MM, Loftus IM. A prospective double-blind randomized controlled trial of radiofrequency versus laser treatment of the great saphenous vein in patients with varicose veins. *Ann Surg* 2011;254:876–81. http://www.ncbi.nlm.nih.gov/pubmed/21934487

15. Rasmussen LH, Lawaetz M, Bjoern L, Vennits B, Blemings A and Eklof B. Randomized clinical trial comparing endovenous laser ablation, radiofrequency ablation, foam sclerotherapy and surgical stripping for great saphenous varicose veins. *Br J Surg* 2011;98:1079–87. http://www.ncbi.nlm.nih.gov/pubmed/21725957

16. Malskat WS, Giang J, De Maeseneer MG, Nijsten TE, van den Bos RR. Randomized clinical trial of 940- versus 1470-nm endovenous laser ablation for great saphenous vein incompetence. *Br J Surg* 2016;103:192–8. http://www.ncbi.nlm.nih.gov/pubmed/2666152

17. O'Donnell TF, Balk EM, Dermody M, Tangney E, Iafrati MD. Recurrence of varicose veins after endovenous ablation of the great saphenous vein in randomized trials. *J Vasc Surg Venous Lymphat Disord.* 2016;4(1):97–105. http://www.ncbi.nlm.nih.gov/pubmed/26946904

18. Ayo D, Blumberg SN, Rockman CR, Sadek M, Cayne N, Adelman M, Kabnick L, Maldonado T, Berland T. Compression vs no compression after endovenous ablation of the great saphenous vein: A randomized controlled trial. *Ann Vasc Surg* 2017;38:72–77. http://www.ncbi.nlm.nih.gov/pubmed/27554689

19. Van den Bos RR, Malskat WS, De Maeseneer MG, de Roos KP, Groeneweg DA, Kockaert MA, Neumann HA, Nijsten T. Randomized clinical trial of endovenous laser ablation versus steam ablation (LAST trial) for great saphenous varicose veins. *Br J Surg.* 2014; 101:1077–83. https://www.ncbi.nlm.nih.gov/pubmed/24981585

20. Boersma D, van Eekeren RRJP, Werson DAB, van der Waal RIF, Reijnen MMJP, de Vries JPPM. Mechanochemical endovenous ablation of small saphenous vein insufficiency using the ClariVein device: One-year results of a prospective series. *Eur J Vasc Endovasc Surg* 2013;45:299–303. http://clarivein.com/clarivein/wp-content/uploads/2016/04/2.-Boersma-et-al-2013-Eur-J-Vasc-Endovasc.pdf

21. Tang TY, Kam JW, Gaunt ME. ClariVein® - Early results from a large single-centre series of mechano-chemical endovenous ablation for varicose veins. *Phlebology.* 2017;32:6–12. http://www.ncbi.nlm.nih.gov/pubmed/?term=Tang+TY%2C+Kam+JW%2C+Gaunt+ME

22. Almeida JI, Javier JJ, Mackay EG, Bautista C, Cher DJ, Proebstle TM. Two-year follow-up of first human use of cyanoacrylate adhesive for treatment of saphenous vein incompetence. *Phlebology.* 2015;30:397–404. http://www.ncbi.nlm.nih.gov/pubmed/24789750

23. Morrison N, Gibson K, McEnroe S, Goldman M, King T, Weiss R, Cher D, Jones A. Randomized trial comparing cyanoacrylate embolization and radiofrequency ablation for incompetent great saphenous veins (VeClose). *J Vasc Surg.* 2015;61:985–94. http://www.ncbi.nlm.nih.gov/pubmed/?term=Morrison+N%2C+Gibson+K%2C+McEnroe+S%2C+Goldman+M%2C+King+T%2C+Weiss+R%2C+Cher+D%2C+Jones+A.+Randomized+trial+comparing+cyanoacrylate+embolization+and+radiofrequency+ablation+for+incompetent+great+saphenous+veins

24. Proebstle TM, Alm J, Dimitri S, Rasmussen L, Whiteley M, Lawson J, Cher D, Davies A. The European multicenter cohort study on cyanoacrylate embolization of refluxing great saphenous veins. *J Vasc Surg Venous Lymphat Disord.*

2015;3:2–7. http://www.ncbi.nlm.nih.gov/pubmed/26993674

25. Bozkurt AK, Yılmaz MF. A prospective comparison of a new cyanoacrylate glue and laser ablation for the treatment of venous insufficiency. *Phlebology.* 2016;31(Suppl):106–13. https://www.ncbi.nlm.nih.gov/pubmed/26916777

26. Gibson K, Ferris B. Cyanoacrylate closure of incompetent great, small and accessory saphenous veins without the use of post-procedure compression: Initial outcomes of a post-market evaluation of the VenaSeal System (the WAVES Study). *Vascular* 2017;25:149–156. https://www.ncbi.nlm.nih.gov/pubmed/27206470

27. Chan YC, Law Y, Cheung GC, Ting AC, Cheng SW. Cyanoacrylate glue used to treat great saphenous reflux: Measures of outcome. *Phlebology.* 2017;32:99–106. http://www.ncbi.nlm.nih.gov/pubmed/?term=Chan+YC%2C+Law+Y%2C+Cheung+GC%2C+Ting+AC%2C+Cheng+SW.+Cyanoacrylate+glue+used+to+treat+great+saphenous+reflux%3A+Measures+of+outcome.+Phlebology.

28. Toonder IM, Lam YL, Lawson J, Wittens CH. Cyanoacrylate adhesive perforator embolization (CAPE) of incompetent perforating veins of the leg, a feasibility study. *Phlebology.* 2014:19;29(1 suppl):49–54. http://www.ncbi.nlm.nih.gov/pubmed/?term=Toonder+IM%2C+Lam+YL%2C+Lawson+J%2C+Wittens+CH.+Cyanoacrylate+adhesive

Appendix 13.A

Endovenous Laser Ablation

Patient: Date:

Referring Doctor: UR Number:

Treating Doctor: Sonographer:

Right leg:

Time for laser	secs
Laser energy	joules
Length of vein	cm
Diameter trunk	mm
Diameter junction	mm
Rate of withdrawal	mm/sec

Left leg:

Time for laser	secs
Laser energy	joules
Length of vein	cm
Diameter trunk	mm
Diameter junction	mm
Rate of withdrawal	mm/sec

Right   Left

Volume of lignocaine 0.1 ml

Veins treated:

Procedure:

Post-operative instructions:

Radiofrequency Ablation

Patient: Date:

Referring Doctor: UR Number:

Treating Doctor: Sonographer:

Right leg:
Diameter junction   mm
Diameter of vein   mm
Length of vein   cm
Number of passes:

Left leg:
Diameter junction   mm
Diameter of vein   mm
Length of vein   cm
Number of passes:

Volume of lignocaine 1 ml

Veins treated:

Procedure:

Postoperative instructions:

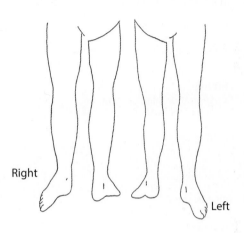

Right

Left

MOCA

Patient: Date:

Referring Doctor: UR Number: 26258

Treating Doctor: Sonographer:

Right leg:
Concentration of sclerosant %
Volume of sclerosant   ml
Diameter of vein   mm
Length of vein   cm
Procedure duration   mins

Left leg:
Concentration of sclerosant %
Volume of sclerosant   ml
Diameter of vein   mm
Length of vein   mins

Right   Left

Veins treated:

Procedure:

Postoperative instructions:

Cyanoacrylate Embolisation

Patient: Date:

Referring Doctor: UR Number:

Treating Doctor: Sonographer:

Right leg:
Diameter junction   mm
Diameter of vein   mm
Length of vein   cm

Volume of chemical   ml

Left leg:
Diameter junction   mm
Diameter of vein   mm
Length of vein   cm

Volume of chemical   ml

Procedure duration: minutes

Veins treated:

Procedure:

Post-operative instructions:

Right   Left

14 Surgery for lower limb varicose disease

This chapter discusses options for surgery directed to superficial tributaries, saphenous veins and perforating veins. Deep venous surgery will be discussed in Chapter 15.

Primary great saphenous reflux

- Great saphenous surgery is now performed less frequently than endovenous treatment.
- Surgery involves *high ligation* to divide the proximal great saphenous vein with or without *stripping* to remove the great saphenous vein, either antegrade through its full length from ankle to groin or retrograde from groin to knee.
- Surgery is contraindicated if the great saphenous vein is the major collateral for patients with deep vein occlusion.
- Pre-operative ultrasound scanning to plan the extent of surgery is mandatory.

Choice of technique

- The best technique is that which gives the lowest incidence of recurrence in the treated territory and the least risk of side-effects or complications. True recurrence in the treated territory is most frequently due to reconnections in the groin, either from angiogenesis in response to damaged tissue or foreign material termed neovascularization, or to reconnection of low abdominal and pelvic tributaries to thigh veins from 'frustrated venous drainage'.
- High ligation alone is less invasive, quicker and simpler to perform than ligation and stripping, leading to an easier recovery.

However, high ligation alone is associated with a higher incidence of recurrence through connections from proximal tributaries to the great saphenous vein and thigh tributaries, and has now been largely abandoned. It may have a place if ultrasound has shown anterior or posterior accessory saphenous reflux without great saphenous reflux, particularly if associated with large varices to be managed by phlebectomy. High ligation of the great saphenous vein at the time of endovenous treatment does not improve results.

- A belief that high ligation alone preserves the vein for future use as an arterial bypass graft if occlusive arterial disease develops has been negated by the finding that long-term patency rates for arterial bypass grafting with a diseased vein are poor.[1] Arterial disease co-existing with varicose disease takes priority for current management.
- High ligation and stripping from the ankle to groin was favoured in the past but has now been largely abandoned due to the high incidence of damage to the below-knee saphenous nerve.
- High ligation and stripping from the groin to knee is now the most widely performed procedure. It is important to then control reflux in the below-knee great saphenous vein by other techniques, such as ultrasound-guided sclerotherapy.

High ligation

- Flush ligation at the sapheno-femoral junction together with ligation of the superficial epigastric, circumflex iliac, superficial external pudendal and thigh tributaries that form the *crosse* is the standard technique (Figure 14.1).

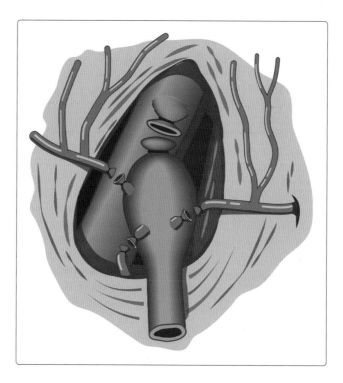

Figure 14.1 Flush high ligation of the great saphenous vein with ligation of all tributaries at the upper end.

Blunt dissection in the groin by retraction rather than dividing tissues is advised to reduce stimulation of angiogenesis and to avoid damage to lymphatics.

Variations of high ligation

- Several variations have been used to attempt to reduce neovascularization or reconnections from proximal veins.[2]

Distal ligation of tributaries

- Some consider that it is important to dissect tributaries to well away from the great saphenous vein to be ligated at their secondary junctions to lengthen the distance for reconnections to develop (Figure 14.2). However, the extra dissection increases local trauma and the likelihood of neovascularization.

Eliminating the saphenous stump

- The ligated stump can be subjected to chemical or thermal trauma to destroy stump

endothelial cells that might stimulate angiogenesis but the benefit has yet to be confirmed. By applying a side-clamp to the common femoral vein, the upper end of the great saphenous vein can be divided flush, then oversewn to avoid a ligated stump being left. Alternatively, the stump can be buried with a running suture.

Barrier techniques

- A prosthetic or anatomical physical barrier can be interposed between the ligated stump and adjacent superficial veins to prevent neovascular veins from developing. A polytetrafluoroethylene (PTFE) patch proved to be an effective barrier at mid-term. Closure of the cribriform fascia and interposition of a silicone patch have also been successful in reducing recurrence rates, although some complications have been reported directly related to the silicone patch.[3] A more complex barrier technique is to use a flap of pectineus fascia.

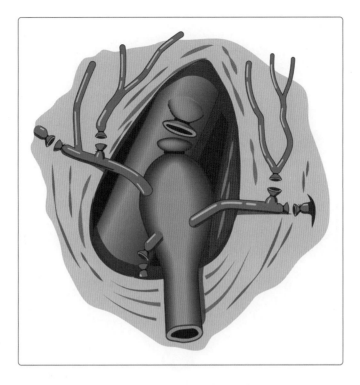

Figure 14.2 Flush high ligation of the great saphenous vein with ligation of all tributaries at their secondary divisions.

Disadvantages are an increased risk of infection and subsequent scarring.

Low ligation of the great saphenous vein

- Although the advantages of high ligation and stripping compared to high ligation alone have been confirmed by many studies, the importance of ligating all tributaries in the groin has always been assumed but never proven.[2] Some feel that it is better to keep these veins in the circulation and ligate the great saphenous vein distal to epigastric and perineal veins to preserve physiologic drainage and to prevent development of connections to thigh tributaries (Figure 14.3).

Stripping

- Several techniques have been used in the past including external stripping, threading an extraluminal ring down over the vein, or cryotherapy to destroy the vein. However, internal stripping is now almost universal. It is usual practice to favour *inversion stripping* also termed *perforation-invagination (PIN) stripping* turning the vein inside out from proximal to distal to reduce bleeding from tributaries and minimize the risk of trauma to the saphenous nerve. It is necessary to avoid missing a duplicated saphenous vein or mistaking an accessory saphenous vein for the great saphenous vein.

- Bleeding along the length of the stripped vein can lead to a column of blood to cause recurrence of reflux due to *strip tract recanalization*.[4] Avulsed tributaries provide a source of endothelial cells to invade the strip tract. Bleeding along the track is reduced by tumescent injection of an anaesthetic solution along the vein, or by an arterial occlusion thigh tourniquet. Results for surgery have been improved by using tumescence to allow ambulatory high ligation and stripping.

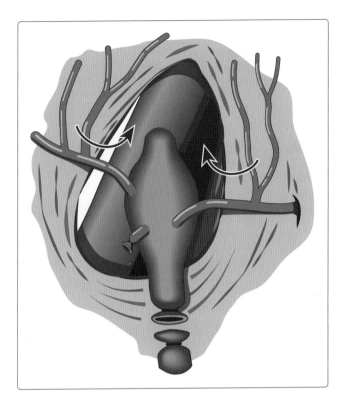

Figure 14.3 Ligation of the great saphenous vein below tributaries draining from the low abdomen and pelvis but above tributaries draining to the thigh.

Results

- High ligation alone is associated with recurrence in the treated territory in about two-thirds of limbs at five years, whereas high ligation and stripping is associated with recurrence in up to 20% at three years.[5]

Complications

- Injury to the saphenous nerve or its branches can result from avulsion while stripping the adjacent vein particularly below knee or to division while avulsing varices. It occurs in up to 10% of stripping operations even if confined to above-knee, but most resolve. Persisting severe anaesthesia or paresthesiae are uncommon, but can lead to litigation.
- Injury to lymphatics can also result from dissection in the groin, particularly from repeat surgery, with dissection through fixed scar tissue, or to avulsion from stripping the adjacent vein. This can result in a lymph collection or lymph fistula in the groin early on, which can be slow to resolve, or to lymph-oedema, which is a rare but devastating complication.
- Inadvertent stripping of the femoral artery instead of the great saphenous vein has been reported.

Primary small saphenous reflux

- Surgery is still favoured by some surgeons to treat small saphenous reflux, but many practitioners now prefer endovenous techniques. Repeat surgery for recurrent small saphenous reflux to remove the saphenous stump or other connections is technically demanding and prone to complications from damage to the popliteal vein or adjacent nerves.
- Pre-operative ultrasound scanning is mandatory to show whether the sapheno-popliteal junction is present, its exact location if so, and

other variations in anatomy, so as to allow the incision to be placed correctly. Intra-operative ultrasound may be the way for the future.

- Surgery is primarily directed toward dividing the sapheno-popliteal junction. A survey of members of the Vascular Surgical Society of Great Britain and Ireland found that most surgeons performed flush ligation, few extensively exposed the popliteal vein unless surgery was for recurrent disease, about one-half avulsed or excised as much vein as possible within the operation field, although approximately one-quarter simply ligated the vein and only 15% routinely stripped the vein.[6] Practice patterns in other countries are probably similar.

The operation

- Surgery is usually performed under general anaesthesia, although spinal anaesthesia or nerve blocks can be used. Most surgeons operate with the patient prone, and this requires intubation for general anaesthesia. A transverse popliteal fossa incision is favoured by most but this incision can be disfiguring particularly for a high ligation producing a scar above the knee crease.
- Each surgeon has a favoured technique.
  - Flush ligation and division requires precise identification of the junction. It is important not to leave a stump particularly if it includes a tributary.
  - Excision of the terminal small saphenous vein within the operation field is preferred by many to eliminate tributaries near the junction that could contribute to recurrence. Care must be taken to identify and ligate gastrocnemius veins if they drain to the SSV, to reduce avenues for revascularization.
  - Retrograde stripping to mid-calf or further can be performed, now favouring invagination stripping. There is no good evidence as to whether stripping reduces recurrence rates or increases risk of sural nerve damage, or whether invagination reduces the incidence of nerve injury.
  - Antegrade stripping from the ankle is no longer considered to be an alternative.

Results

- A small number of prospective studies that used ultrasound for surveillance after small saphenous surgery show disturbingly high recurrence rates, as high as 40%–50%.[5,7]
- Ultrasound studies have shown that recurrence after small saphenous surgery is most often due to persistent connections between the popliteal vein and residual small saphenous vein

Complications

- Nerve injury after venous surgery is the most common reason for medicolegal claims in vascular surgical practice.[8] A survey from the Vascular Surgical Society of Great Britain and Ireland found that nerve injury is perceived to be more likely after small saphenous surgery compared to great saphenous surgery.[6] Damage to the sural nerve during small saphenous surgery probably results from straying away from the vein during dissection.

Phlebectomy

Hook phlebectomy

- This is performed by avulsion through stab incisions teasing out lengths of vein using a variety of commercially available hooks. This may be part of the operation for ligation with or without stripping, but is now also frequently performed to deal with tributaries after endovenous treatment for saphenous reflux, and occasionally as the sole procedure. It is referred to as ambulatory phlebectomy if performed as an outpatient. Distinction is made between *stab phlebectomy* with a scalpel and *microphlebectomy* sometimes even with a 19G needle.
- Careful marking of varices with an indelible ink pen before operation allows precise placement of the small incisions for access to the veins.
- The procedure can be performed using tumescent anaesthesia or multiple injections of local anaesthetic. For best cosmetic results, incisions must be placed in the line of skin

tension which is essentially oblique between the joints and transverse behind the knee. The small stabs are best left open to allow drainage or closed with adhesive tape to aid healing without scarring, and suture closure should be avoided as it increases scarring.

- If extensive phlebectomies are planned in patients under long-term anticoagulation, bridging should be considered to avoid bleeding complications.

Transilluminated powered phlebectomy

- Transilluminated powered phlebectomy is an alternative to hook phlebectomy. An endoscopic transilluminator is inserted under the skin to illuminate vein clusters, and a suction resector device with guarded blades is introduced through the same or another incision. Tumescent anaesthesia (see Chapter 4) is instilled through the illuminated device for hydro-dissection to define the operative plane, and the varices are macerated at an optimum oscillation frequency of 500 r/min and removed by suction. Direct vision reduces the risk of missed veins. Once completed, tumescent anaesthesia is again introduced to minimize bleeding, and the incisions are closed with adhesive tape.
- Studies suggest that this is a quicker procedure than hook phlebectomy with greater cosmetic satisfaction due to fewer incisions and possible reduced pain, but it has a potential for damage to subcutaneous fat, lymphatics and sensory nerves and a higher incidence of haematomas.[9,10]

ASVAL

- Ablation Sélective des Varices sous Anesthésie Locale (ASVAL) or French acronym for tributary varices phlebectomy under local anesthesiae, is a procedure favoured by some to remove varices but preserve the saphenous vein. It is held that disease commences in varices and not in the saphenous veins, the 'ascending theory'. If the saphenous vein has not yet been affected, then it is believed that there is no need to interfere

with it, and if there is secondary involvement then it can recover. Thus, only the 'varicose reservoir' is removed.

- Patients with limited disease progression and mild ultrasound abnormalities are most likely to benefit from this approach. A prospective study with one-year follow-up found that treatment with single phlebectomies of a large tributary was able to abolish great saphenous reflux in 50% of patients and to relieve symptoms in 66% of patients.[11]
- Evidence for long-term outcome is required due to apprehension as to high late recurrence rates.

Perforating veins

- Saphenous surgery will frequently correct perforator reflux by load reduction unless there is coexistent deep venous reflux, so that it is unusual to combine saphenous stripping with perforator ligation at the same operation if there is no deep reflux. Posterior tibial perforators join the posterior arch vein rather than the main trunk of the great saphenous vein, and surgery to remove the great saphenous vein in the calf will not address these perforators. Interrupting perforators has more support if there is associated deep venous reflux.
- Traditional surgical technique to divide incompetent perforators, for example on the medial aspect of the calf, was through a long incision to expose the veins, either superficial to the deep fascia which is the *Cockett operation*[*] or deep to the fascia which is the *Linton operation*[†]. The procedures were associated with a high incidence of wound breakdown and are now considered to be of historical interest.
- These were replaced with sub-fascial endoscopic perforating vein surgery (SEPS) with a small incision just below the knee to allow insertion of an endoscope through which a cutting device could divide the perforators.[12] For many, this has been associated with a high incidence of failure to detect and control perforators.

---

[*] Frank Cockett (1916–2014), was a British surgeon born in Australia.

[†] Robert Linton (1900–1979), was an American surgeon born in Scotland.

- Currently most would treat superficial reflux then allow up to several months before reassessing perforators. However, large perforators especially when associated with skin complications are less likely to regain tone and become competent. If treatment of perforators is required then it is usually performed by endovascular techniques.

Recurrent varicose veins

- Ultrasound scanning usually shows a complex picture that is not suited to simple repeat ligation and stripping. Endovenous techniques, particularly using ultrasound-guided sclerotherapy or endovenous thermal ablation, have replaced open surgery, particularly for recurrence in previously treated segments. The results of repeat surgery are considerably worse than for primary surgery, and the incidence of complications such as wound infection and breakdown, nerve injuries and lymphatic damage are much higher.[13]

Other surgical techniques

External valvuloplasty

- This operation is intended to eliminate reflux at the sapheno-femoral junction and preserve the great saphenous vein. The rationale depends on the descending theory of aetiology. Pre-operative ultrasound identifies suitable patients with sapheno-femoral junction incompetence.
- The sapheno-femoral junction is exposed, all tributaries in the region are ligated and the proximal 5 cm are dissected free. An intraoperative test milking blood distally confirms valvular incompetence. A polyester mesh is wrapped around the vein as a cuff and tightened, then fixed in position with prolene sutures. Successful correction of reflux is confirmed by the milking technique. Results have not been convincing.

CHIVA

- Cure Conservatrice et Hémodynamique de l'Insuffisance Veineuse en Ambulatoire (CHIVA) is an alternative surgical approach that allows the saphenous vein to be preserved. It is based on correcting descending venous reflux. The rationale is to restore flow from the most superficial to deepest venous networks.[14]
- The concept is to divide the lower limb venous system into three compartments based on their relationship to the superficial and deep fascia. Tributaries are designated N3 and lie superficial to the superficial fascia, saphenous veins are N2 and lie deep to the superficial fascia and deep veins are N1 deep to the deep fascia. All are connected by perforating veins providing a hierarchy for normal flow from N3 to N1. Flow is abnormal if there is flow at any level from a deeper to a more superficial compartment through what is referred to as an *escape point*. A connection that allows flow from superficial to deep is a *re-entry point*. The segment in between is a *shunt*. The aim is to excise diseased superficial veins by phlebectomy, to ligate all escape points to favour re-entry points and to preserve the saphenous vein.
- A *closed shunt* has both escape and re-entry points and the surgical treatment is by ligation of tributaries and all escape points, termed a CHIVA 1 operation. The most common example would be high ligation of the great saphenous vein and varices in a patient with sapheno-femoral incompetence and varicose veins, to restore normal drainage through thigh and calf perforators (Figure 14.4).
- An *open shunt* occurs if there is no re-entry point so that a two stage CHIVA 2 operation is required, with preliminary ligation of tributaries then delay while waiting for re-entry perforators to develop, after which the escape points can be ligated. A common example is segmental reflux in the mid great saphenous vein with a competent sapheno-femoral junction draining through mid-thigh perforators (Figure 14.5).
- A *by-passing shunt* directs flow around an obstruction and this should be preserved with no place for surgery. An example is superficial tributaries acting as collaterals around a femoral vein occlusion (Figure 14.6).

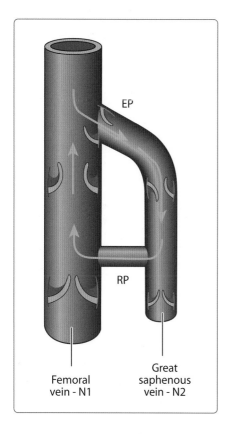

Figure 14.4 CHIVA – closed shunt.

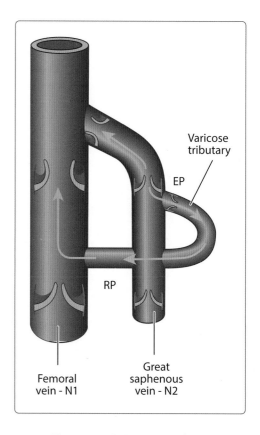

Figure 14.5 CHIVA – open shunt.

- A Cochrane review concluded that 'The CHIVA method reduces recurrence of varicose veins and produces fewer side-effects than vein stripping. However, we based these conclusions on a small number of trials with a high risk of bias as the effects of surgery could not be concealed and the results were imprecise due to low number of events. New RCTs are needed to confirm these results and to compare CHIVA with approaches other than open surgery'.[15]

History

- Hippocrates (460–370 BC) did not recommend excision but rather compression following multiple punctures, and he also believed in cautery.[16] Aulus Cornelius Celsus (25 BC–50 AD) of Rome was probably one of the first to operate on varicose veins, with a detailed description in his book *De Medicina*

although it is not known for certain if he was a doctor. He made multiple incisions four fingerbreadths apart then touched the vein with cautery, grasped it and extracted as much as possible, double clamping and dividing the vein between ligatures. Roman surgeons carried scalpels with blunt handles that could be used for dissecting varicose veins, a procedure that was done without anaesthesia.

- Galen (131–201) described treatment for varicose veins by phlebectomy, making 3–6 incisions with a hook and then bandaging the leg. Oribasius of Pergamum (325–405), a Byzantine physician, described details of surgery for varicose veins of the legs, included shaving and bathing the leg, marking with small incisions and excising the varicose veins with hooks along the leg through small incisions.

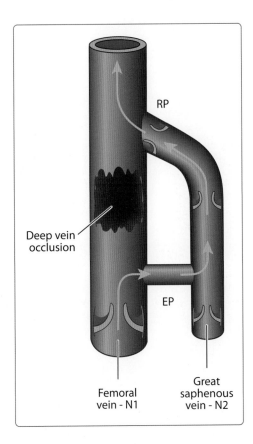

Figure 14.6 CHIVA – by-passing shunt.

- The Byzantine Greek physician Paulus Aegineta (625–690) was perhaps the first to describe ligation of the great saphenous vein in his book *De Re Medica Libri Septem* (*Medical Compendium in Seven Books*). Al-Zahrawi (936–1013) from Córdoba in Spain is believed to have been the first to use the stripping method to treat varicose veins.
- In Germany, Bernhard von Langenbeck described neovascularisation after vein ligation in 1861. Otto Madelung was probably the first to strip the great saphenous vein, reported in 1884, followed by Friedrich Trendelenburg in 1890.
- In America, Charles Mayo and William Babcock promoted saphenous stripping in the early 1900s, Robert Muller developed hook phlebectomy in the 1960s and Andreas Oesch described inversion stripping in the 1990s.

- Claude Franceschi, working in Paris, developed the CHIVA technique in 1988.

References

1. Panetta TF, Marin ML, Veith FJ, Goldsmith J, Gordon RE, Jones AM, Schwartz ML, Gupta SK, Wengerter KR. Unsuspected pre-existing saphenous vein disease: An unrecognized cause of vein bypass failure. *J Vasc Surg.* 1992;15:102–10. https://www.ncbi.nlm.nih.gov/pubmed/1728668

2. De Maeseneer MG. Strategies to minimize the effect of neovascularization at the saphenofemoral junction after great saphenous vein surgery: An overview. *Phlebolymphology* 2006;13:207. http://www.phlebolymphology.org/strategies-to-minimize-the-effect-of-neovascularization-at-the-saphenofemoral-junction-after-great-saphenous-vein-surgery-an-overview/

3. De Maeseneer MG, Philipsen TE, Vandenbroeck CP, Lauwers PR, Hendriks JM, De Hert SG, Van Schil PE. Closure of the cribriform fascia: An efficient anatomical barrier against postoperative neovascularisation at the saphenofemoral junction? A prospective study. *Eur J Vasc Endovasc Surg* 2007;34:361–6. http://www.ncbi.nlm.nih.gov/pubmed/17513142

4. Ostler AE, Holdstock JM, Harrison CC, Price BA, Whiteley MS. Strip-tract revascularization as a source of recurrent venous reflux following high saphenous tie and stripping: Results at 5-8 years after surgery. *Phlebology* 2015;30:569–572. https://www.ncbi.nlm.nih.gov/pubmed/?term=Ostler+AE%2C+Holdstock+JM%2C+Harrison+CC%2C+Price+BA%2C+Whiteley+MS

5. van Rij AM, Jiang P, Solomon C, Christie RA, Hill GB. Recurrence after varicose vein surgery: A prospective long-term clinical study with duplex ultrasound scanning and air plethysmography. *J Vasc Surg.* 2003;38:935–43. http://www.ncbi.nlm.nih.gov/pubmed/14603197

6. Winterborn RJ, Campbell WB, Heather BP, Earnshaw JJ. The management of short saphenous varicose veins: A survey of the members of the vascular surgical society of Great Britain and Ireland. *Eur J Vasc Endovasc Surg.* 2004;28:400–403. https://www.ncbi.nlm.nih.gov/pubmed/15350563

7. Smith JJ, Brown L, Greenhalgh RM, Davies AH. Randomised trial of pre-operative colour duplex marking in primary varicose vein surgery: Outcome is not improved. *Eur J Vasc Endovasc Surg.* 2002;23:336–43. http://www.sciencedirect.com/science/article/pii/S1078588402916072

8. Sam RC, Silverman SH, Bradbury AW. Nerve injuries and varicose vein surgery. *Eur J Vasc Endovasc Surg* 2004;27:113–20. http://www.ejves.com/article/S1078-5884(03)00552-5/abstract

9. National Institute for Health and Care Excellence (NICE). Transilluminated powered phlebectomy for varicose veins. 2004; IPG37. https://www.nice.org.uk/guidance/IPG37/chapter/1-Guidance

10. Franz RW, Hartman JF, Wright ML. Treatment of varicose veins by transilluminated powered phlebectomy surgery: A 9-year experience. *Int J Angiol* 2012;21:201–8. https://www.ncbi.nlm.nih.gov/pmc/articles/PMC3578615/

11. Biemans AA, van den Bos RR, Hollestein LM, Maessen-Visch MB, Vergouwe Y, Neumann HA, de Maeseneer MG, Nijsten T. The effect of single phlebectomies of a large varicose tributary on great saphenous vein reflux. *J Vasc Surg Venous Lymphat Disord*. 2014;2:179–87. https://www.ncbi.nlm.nih.gov/pubmed/26993185

12. Gloviczki P, Bergan JJ, Rhodes JM, Canton LG, Harmsen S, Ilstrup DM. Mid-term results of endoscopic perforator vein interruption for chronic venous insufficiency: Lessons learned from the North American subfascial endoscopic perforator surgery registry. The North American Study Group. *J Vasc Surg*. 1999;29:489–502. http://www.ncbi.nlm.nih.gov/pubmed/10069914

13. De Maeseneer M. Surgery for recurrent varicose veins: Toward a less-invasive approach? *Perspect Vasc Surg Endovasc Ther* 2011;23:244–9. http://www.ncbi.nlm.nih.gov/pubmed/21810818

14. Franceschi C, Cappelli M, Ermini S, Gianesini S, Mendoza F, Passariello F, Zamboni P. CHIVA: Hemodynamic concept, strategy and results. *Int Angiol* 2016;35:8–30. https://www.ncbi.nlm.nih.gov/pubmed/26044838

15. Bellmunt-Montoya S, Escribano J, Dilme J, Martinez-Zapata M. CHIVA method for the treatment of chronic venous insufficiency. *Cochrane Database System Rev* 2015;6: Art. No.: CD009648. DOI: 10.1002/14651858.CD009648.pub3. http://www.cochrane.org/CD009648/PVD_chiva-method-for-the-treatment-of-varicose-veins

16. Perrin M. History of venous surgery. *Phlebolymphology* 2011;18 and 2012;19 http://www.phlebolymphology.org/history-of-venous-surgery-1/; http://www.phlebolymphology.org/history-of-venous-surgery-2/; http://www.phlebolymphology.org/history-of-venous-surgery-3/

15 Chronic deep venous disease

Chronic deep venous disease can be due to venous obstruction, reflux or both. Clinical features consequent on past deep vein thrombosis constitute the post-thrombotic syndrome.

Pathogenesis

- Deep venous obstruction usually results from past thrombosis with or without extrinsic compression, and recanalization after deep vein thrombosis causes secondary deep venous reflux. Primary deep venous reflux is due to non-functional 'floppy' valves or congenital absence of valves.

Post-thrombotic syndrome

- The post-thrombotic syndrome can occur as a long-term complication of deep vein thrombosis due to persisting obstruction or to loss of valve function from damage after recanalization. Venous hypertension and congestion cause bursting pain in the calf or thigh during exercise relieved by leg elevation referred to as *venous claudication*. The limb then develops oedema, venous eczema, lipo-dermatosclerosis and potential ulceration. Clinical examination may reveal suprapubic collateral varices. Investigation is required to show the site and extent of disease in the femoro-popliteal, ilio-femoral or ilio-caval segments.
- Secondary inflammation from residual post-thrombotic changes may also be involved, with increased levels of inflammatory cytokines or adhesion molecules such as interleukin-6 and intercellular adhesion molecule-1 (ICAM-1) which may further damage venous valves.

- The condition is more likely to develop in older or obese patients, those with a more proximal first deep vein thrombosis, after a second or multiple deep vein thromboses in the same leg, and if anticoagulation for the initial deep vein thrombosis has been inadequate.
- Following deep vein thrombosis, reflux associated with recanalization is demonstrated in some 20% of patients by one week and approximately two-thirds by one year. About one-half of these have residual partial or complete obstruction. The natural history of deep vein thrombosis is further discussed in Chapter 22.
- Typically, the more proximal and extensive the deep vein thrombosis, the more severe are the symptoms of the post-thrombotic syndrome, but the outcome is unpredictable. Approximately 60% of patients recover from deep vein thrombosis without residual symptoms, 40% have some degree of the post-thrombotic syndrome and 5% have severe symptoms. Symptoms usually occur within the first six months but can develop up to two years after the acute event. Absence of symptoms by then makes it highly unlikely that a patient will develop the post-thrombotic syndrome.
- Deep venous reflux may involve the full length of the limb or one or more venous segments. The degree to which flow is restricted by obstruction depends on the number, location, and extent of diseased segments. Flow is maintained through collateral veins, but even extensive collateral development fails to compensate for severe stenosis or obstruction. The collateral circulation across an occluded femoral vein is through the rich

deep femoral vein circulation, and this is much greater than collaterals bypassing an occluded iliac vein.

Investigations

- Conservative treatment is not influenced by the location and extent of underlying disease but only by clinical severity, and investigation beyond routine ultrasound examination is required only if intervention is being considered.[1]

Ultrasound

- Ultrasound is required to show the sites and extent of disease, while valve morphology and function can be assessed by B-mode imaging and B-flow studies.
- Deep venous reflux is defined as reversed flow for more than one second after distal augmentation. A short segment of reflux in the common femoral or popliteal veins opposite the corresponding saphenous junctions is not pathological deep reflux but simply blood passing to the superficial veins.
- It was hoped that the amplitude and duration of deep reflux demonstrated by spectral analysis from duplex ultrasound might relate to the severity of venous disease and risk of complications, but this proved not to be the case. Presumably, these are just a function of the venous volume held in varices.
- Intravascular ultrasound (IVUS) with access from the common femoral vein has been found to be invaluable in some specialist centres for assessment of ilio-caval stenosis.

CT venography

- CT venography shows thrombus that is often eccentric, partly adherent to the vein wall, and partly recanalized, with a heterogeneous lumen and intraluminal strands. The vein may be thick-walled, small and retracted and finally replaced by a fibrous cord. Multiple collateral veins are commonly seen.[2]

Venography

- Ascending venography identifies post-thrombotic changes in deep veins and collateral patterns. Descending venography determines whether there is axial reflux when considering deep venous reconstruction and the most suitable site for an operation.

Laboratory investigations

- Specialist units routinely measure physiological variables by air plethysmography, ambulatory venous pressures, arm/foot venous pressure differential and femoral vein pressure (see Chapter 10). However, there is poor correlation between clinical outcome and pre-operative haemodynamic assessment, so that selection of suitable patients should be largely on clinical grounds. Obstruction and reflux are frequently associated, and there is no investigation that clearly identifies which is more important. Air plethysmography before and after surgery allows quantitative measurement of early and late success, and serial pressure measurements can be used for the same purpose.

Surgery for deep venous reflux

- Most patients are managed by conservative measures.[3,4] Treatment for reflux in superficial veins is frequently sufficient to relieve deep venous load. Deep vein valve surgery is reserved for patients with severe complications in whom compression treatment and superficial vein ablation, where feasible, has failed to resolve the problem. Surgery to restore deep vein valve function is restricted to a few specialist centres since the indications are few, the techniques are demanding and the results are uncertain.
- The aim is to place a functioning valve in the femoral or popliteal vein. Relative contraindications include inactivity, a stiff ankle or severe thrombophilia. Success at operation is confirmed by a simple *strip test* showing that milking cannot allow blood to pass distally across the reconstructed valve.

Intra- and post-operative risk of thrombosis is controlled by prolonged anticoagulation.

Valve interposition

- A new valve introduced from elsewhere can be used if the native valve has been damaged or destroyed due to the post-thrombotic syndrome, or if valves are absent due to the rare congenital state of valve agenesis.

Vein valve transplantation

- A patient with femoro-popliteal reflux can be treated with a short segment of axillary vein containing a valve, placed as an interposition graft in the proximal femoral vein or popliteal vein (Figure 15.1).

Venous transposition

- An incompetent deep venous tract can be divided then anastomosed to another vein that has a competent proximal valve. For example, a refluxing femoro-popliteal vein could be divided at its proximal end and anastomosed to the great saphenous or deep femoral vein (Figure 15.2). However, ultrasound shows favourable anatomy in no more than about 20% of candidates.

Construction of a new valve

- Techniques have been devised to create a valve-like structure from adjacent veins. Synthetic grafts, homografts and cryopreserved allografts and a bioprosthetic valve made from small intestinal submucosa have been used.

Valve repair

- Valve repair can be considered in patients with redundant valves that prolapse but are not damaged. This is usually associated with venous dilation. It is sufficient to repair just one valve in a diseased segment of the deep venous system for a successful outcome.

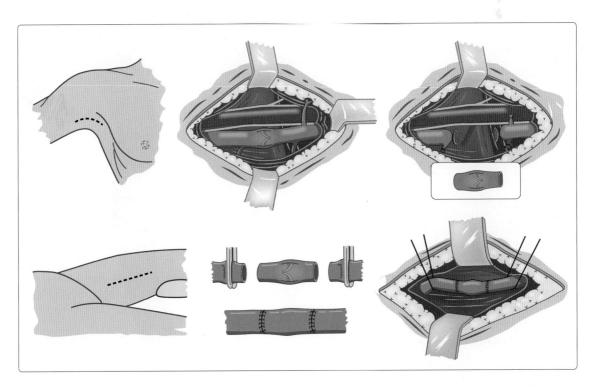

Figure 15.1 Technique for transplantation of a working valve from a segment of axillary vein into a lower limb deep vein. The donor site for the axillary vein segment is shown on the upper row. The recipient site for transplantation into the femoral vein is shown on the lower row, where the anastomosis is depicted in the centre.

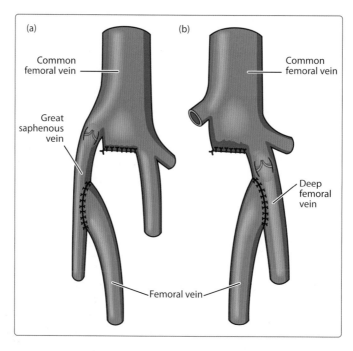

Figure 15.2 Techniques for vein transposition below a functioning valve in (a) the great saphenous vein or (b) the deep femoral vein.

Internal valve repair

- This was the first technique used in 1968. One or more valves can be directly repaired under vision through open venotomy (Figure 15.3). The valve is exposed through a longitudinal, transverse, T-shaped or trap-door incision. About 20% of redundant valve cusp length is sutured to the vein wall with fine polypropylene sutures to plicate the valve and restore cusp apposition. It is best performed on the valve in the femoral vein just below the deep femoral junction. The advantages of internal valvuloplasty are that it offers an anatomically precise repair since it is carried out under direct vision so that results are more lasting. The disadvantages are that it is time-consuming, is not feasible for multiple site repairs and needs postoperative anticoagulation.

External valve repair

- The aim is to reduce vein dissection and the risk of venous dilatation which can complicate open repair. Various techniques can be

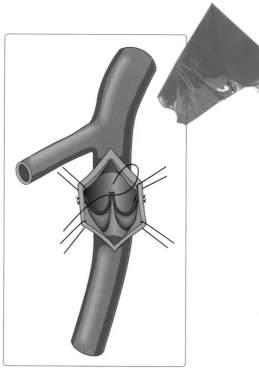

Figure 15.3 Technique for internal valvuloplasty using very fine sutures to plicate the base of the valve to tighten valve closure.

used to place rows of sutures along the valve cusp insertion lines to narrow the angle between valve attachments so as to tighten valve cusps and to restore good apposition (Figure 15.4). Advantages are that it avoids venotomy with no need for postoperative anticoagulation, the technique needs less time and multiple site repairs can be undertaken, such as the femoral and deep femoral veins at the groin and the popliteal and posterior tibial veins at the knee.

New valve formation

- Techniques have been devised to create a new monocuspid or bicuspid valve by dissection to raise a flap of intima and fashion it to the shape of a valve.

Valve restoration

- Valve function can be restored by bringing the cusps into apposition by external cuffing, banding or wrapping (Figure 15.5). The

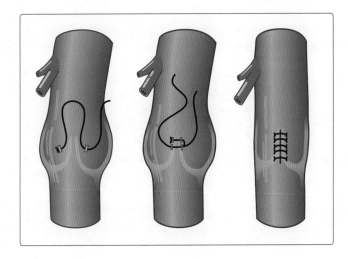

Figure 15.4 Technique for external valvuloplasty using very fine sutures to plicate the base of the valve from the outside to tighten valve closure.

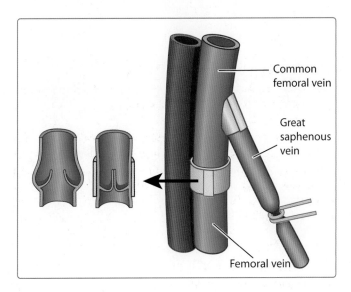

Common femoral vein

Great saphenous vein

Femoral vein

Figure 15.5 Placement of an external cuff to narrow a vein to restore valve apposition.

promise held for treatments involving circumferential reduction of vein diameter has not materialized in clinical practice.

Results

- Evidence from observational studies strongly supports these procedures. However, a Cochrane review concluded that 'no evidence was found for benefit or harm of valvuloplasty in the treatment of patients with deep venous insufficiency secondary to primary valvular incompetence. ... Trials investigating the effects of other surgical procedures on deep veins are needed. Until the findings of such trials become available, the benefit of valvuloplasty remains uncertain'.[5]

Intervention for chronic deep venous obstruction

Endovenous stenting

- Balloon dilatation and stenting are now the favoured technique for treating intractable complications from severe stenosis or occlusion of the inferior vena cava, the iliac veins, and the common femoral vein where conservative management has failed.[3] Selection of suitable patients is determined by the degree of impairment, initially assessed by clinical features and haemodynamic studies followed by good imaging with venography, CTV, MRV and intravenous ultrasound, if available. Ascending venography is required to determine the best patent distal vein to be the site for access.
- Stenoses are dilated by a 15–16 mm balloon, always followed by placement of one or more self-expanding stents (Figure 15.6). Gianturco Z stents have been favoured for large diameter veins such as the inferior vena cava, Wallstents have been used for inferior vena cava, pelvic veins and larger thigh veins and various self-expanding stents are used for medium-sized veins.
- Access is by percutaneous puncture or open exposure of the vein. The patient may require subsequent treatment to correct deep venous reflux or superficial venous disease. Long-term anticoagulation is required to reduce the risk of thrombosis.

Surgical bypass

- This is now only considered if endovascular treatment has failed. Unilateral iliac

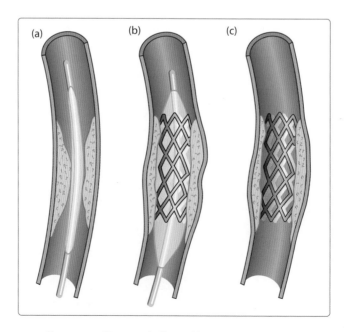

(a)   (b)   (c)

Figure 15.6 Iliac vein balloon dilatation and stenting.

vein occlusion can be treated by passing the contralateral great saphenous vein through a suprapubic tunnel to anastomose end-to-end or end-to-side to the common femoral vein of the occluded side (see Palma operation – Figure 15.7). It is necessary to have a patent contralateral ilio-femoral venous segment and a patent caval run-off, an adequate ipsilateral venous system with a patent deep femoral vein, preferably with an open or partially recanalized femoral vein, a patent and competent great saphenous vein on the recipient side with a minimal diameter of 4–5 mm and no varicosities.

- A femoral vein occlusion can be treated by implanting the ipsilateral great saphenous vein end-to-side into the popliteal vein (the May–Husni procedure – Figure 15.8).
- Synthetic material such as polytetrafluoroethylene can be used to bypass iliac or inferior vena caval occlusions. It may be necessary to excise redundant flaps and fibrous strictures.

- All operations require a temporary arteriovenous fistula to increase flow to attempt to prevent thrombosis. This can be made between the posterior tibial artery and vein. The fistula is usually closed by eight weeks after the bypass surgery.

Results

- The risk of early post-stent thrombosis is less than 5%. Late cumulative patency rates for stenting are in the order of 60%–80%, with best results for non-thrombotic stenosis or obstruction such as the May–Thurner syndrome and worst for the post-thrombotic syndrome.[5,6] Venous clinical severity scores and quality of life measurements are improved after stenting in more than 70% of patients, with rates for ulcer healing of more than 50%.[7]
- The long-term results of venous bypass grafts are less favourable, with late degeneration a problem with autologous vein grafts and obstruction likely with either vein or synthetic grafts.

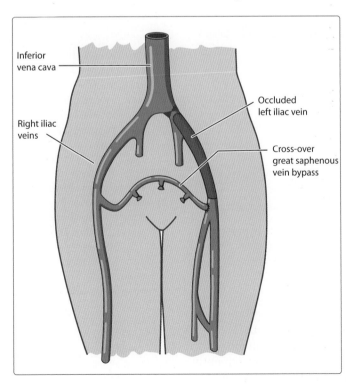

Figure 15.7 A femoro-femoral cross-over vein bypass graft (Palma operation).

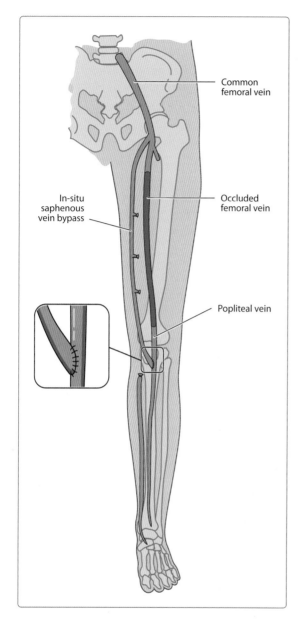

Common
femoral vein

In-situ
saphenous
vein bypass

Occluded
femoral vein

Popliteal vein

Figure 15.8 A femoro-popliteal vein bypass graft
(May–Husni operation).

History

- Palma and Esperon described the femoro-femoral cross-over bypass in 1958.[8]
- Warren and Thayer described sapheno-popliteal bypass in 1954. It was subsequently developed by Frileux et al. in France, Husni in the USA and May in Austria.[9–12]

- Internal and external valve repair surgery were both introduced by Robert Kistner.[13]
- Venous valve transfer was developed by Syde Taheri.[14]

References

1. Perrin M. Investigations in post-thrombotic syndrome according to clinical status. *Phlebolymphology* 2009;16:277–82. http://www.phlebolymphology. org/investigations-in-postthrombotic-syndrome-according-to-clinical-status/

2. Ghaye B, Szapiro D, Willems V, Dondelinger RF. Pitfalls in CT venography of lower limbs and abdominal veins. *Am J Roentgenol* 2002;178:1465–71. http://www.ajronline.org/doi/full/10.2214/ajr.178.6.1781465

3. Eklof BG, Kistner RL, Masuda EM. Venous bypass and valve reconstruction: Long-term efficacy. *Vasc Med* 1998;3:157–64. http://vmj.sagepub.com/content/3/2/157.full.pdf

4. Perrin M. History of venous surgery (3). *Phlebolymphology* 2012;19:59–67. http://www.phlebolymphology.org/history-of-venous-surgery-3/

5. Goel R, Abidia A, Hardy SC. Surgery for deep venous incompetence. *Cochrane Database System Rev* 2015; 2. Art. No.:CD001097. DOI:http://www.cochrane.org/CD001097/PVD_surgery-for-deep-venous-incompetence

6. Raju S, Neglen P. High prevalence of non-thrombotic iliac vein lesions in chronic venous disease: A permissive role in pathogenicity. *J Vasc Surg* 2006;44:136–43. https://www.ncbi.nlm.nih.gov/pubmed/16828437

7. Raju S, Neglén P. Percutaneous recanalization of total occlusions of the iliac vein. *J Vasc Surg* 2009;50:360–8. http://www.jvascsurg.org/article/S0741-5214(09)00197-9/fulltext?mobileUi=0

8. Palma EC, Esperon R. Vein transplants and grafts in surgical treatment of the postphlebitic syndrome. *J Cardiovasc Surg* 1960;1:94–107.

9. Warren R, Thayer TR. Transplantation of the saphenous vein for postphlebitic stasis. *Surgery* 1954;35:867–76.

10. Frileux C, Pillot-Bienayme P, Gillot C. Bypass of segmental obliterations of ilio-femoral venous axis by transposition of saphenous vein. *J Cardiovasc Surg* 1972;13:409–14.

11. Husni EA. Clinical experience with femoropopliteal venous reconstruction. In *Venous Problems*. Bergan JJ, Yao JST, Eds. 1978; 485–91. Chicago: Yearbook Medical Publishers, Inc.

12. May R. The femoral bypass. *Int Angiol* 1985;4:435–40.

13. Kistner RL. Surgical repair of a venous valve. *Straub Clin Proc* 1968;34:41–3.

14. Taheri SA, Lazar L, Elias S, Marchand P, Heffner R. Surgical treatment of postphlebitic syndrome with vein valve transplant. *Am J Surg* 1982;144:221–24.

16 Venous compression syndromes

These syndromes are infrequent but usually affect otherwise healthy young individuals. Venous obstruction leads to features of venous congestion with collateral formation. Repetitive damage to a vein predisposes to thrombosis.[1] Clinical diagnosis is confirmed by imaging with ultrasound, CT or MR venography, and occasionally by conventional venography (see Chapter 10). Management involves conservative, endovascular or open surgical options.

Thoracic outlet syndrome (TOS)

The anatomy of the thoracic outlet has been described in Chapter 2.[1]

Pathology

- Magnetic resonance imaging shows that compression affects nerves in 70%, veins in 65% and arteries in 40%, with frequent combinations of two or all three. Various bony or muscular abnormalities can cause TOS, and compression usually occurs in the costoclavicular space.
  - A cervical rib or its fibrous extension arises from C7 and passes to the first rib. It runs along the anterior border of the scalenus medius muscle immediately under the artery. It is present in less than 1% of individuals, 50% are bilateral and fewer than 10% cause symptoms.
  - Congenital abnormalities of the first rib are less common. The most frequent is first rib atresia leaving an exostosis on the second rib at the scalenus anterior insertion.

- A past fractured clavicle or first rib.
- Fibrosis of the scalenus anterior and medius muscles can cause compression where the neurovascular bundle passes through the interscalene triangle, as can the costoclavicular ligament or fibromuscular bands.
- Repetitive trauma leads to progressive fibrous stenosis in the vein wall and surrounding tissues. Arterial compression can cause turbulent flow, post-stenotic dilatation, intimal disruption, aneurysm formation, thrombosis or embolism. Nerve compression usually affects the lower brachial plexus roots causing medial arm symptoms.

Subclavian vein thrombosis

- Subclavian vein compression can lead to acute thrombosis known as the *Paget–Schroetter syndrome*[*] or *effort thrombosis*. Thrombus can propagate into the axillary or more proximal veins, and can lead to pulmonary embolism. Unlike lower limb deep vein thrombosis, it is not a result of influences such as underlying coagulation disorders, surgery or direct trauma. It is usually precipitated by physical activities with overuse of the dominant arm provoked by overhead activities associated with work or sports activities such as swimming or throwing. It particularly affects healthy young people with long necks and droopy shoulders.

---

* Sir James Paget (1814–1899), English surgeon and pathologist, described the condition in 1875. Leopold von Schroetter (1837–1908), Austrian physician, independently described the condition in 1884.

Clinical features

Venous compression

- Venous compression may remain asymptomatic due to a collateral circulation or cause congestion with arm pain and swelling, hand cyanosis and enlarged shoulder and chest wall collaterals.
- Subclavian vein thrombosis can occur with or without prior symptoms causing marked oedema with heaviness and prominent surface veins in the arm and hand made worse by strenuous physical activity using the arm.

Nerve and arterial compression

- Neurological features include pain around the shoulder and neck, and referred pain, sensory disturbance or weakness down the medial upper extremity.
- Arterial stenosis, occlusion or embolism can cause coldness or vasospasm in the hand or severe distal ischaemia. An arterial aneurysm presents with a tender pulsatile mass in the neck.
- The *military brace* manoeuvre with the arms elevated and shoulders forced back then opening and closing the hands 20 times (Figure 16.1) is used to induce arterial compression. It causes pallor of the hand, loss

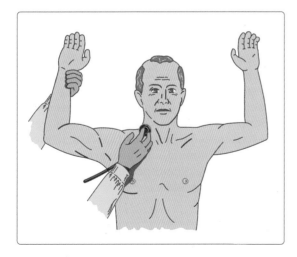

Figure 16.1 The military brace manoeuvre to demonstrate the thoracic outlet syndrome.

of the radial pulse and sometimes a bruit at the base of the neck. Although it has a high incidence of false-positive results in normal subjects, a negative test virtually excludes vascular involvement.

Investigation

- The most useful investigation is vascular ultrasound, examining both arteries and veins and always scanning both upper limbs. However, ultrasound examination of the thoracic outlet is technically demanding, while contrast-enhanced CT or MR angiography are accurate and diagnostic. A plain chest X-ray is the best way to demonstrate a cervical rib.

Ultrasound examination

Protocols for scanning

- Examine the patient seated or standing so that the shoulder girdle is relaxed and falls under gravity to improve access. Examine the subclavian and axillary artery and vein through anterior suprasternal, supraclavicular and infraclavicular windows to show extrinsic compression on B-mode and increased Doppler velocities. The vessels are easier to see with the arm abducted and scanned from an axillary approach, but can be scanned through an anterior window.
- Provocative positions for examination for the thoracic outlet syndrome are non-specific but include:
  - *Military brace* position (see above)
  - *Adson's manoeuvre* with the arms dependent, neck extended and head turned to the ipsilateral side, and the patient asked to hold a deep breath
  - abduction to 90° or 180°
  - any position that brings on symptoms

Upper limb venous thrombosis – direct evidence

- Inability to compress a vein diagnoses distal thrombosis, but the subclavian and more proximal veins cannot be compressed by the probe due to obstruction by ribs and the clavicle. There is no flow with occlusive thrombosis and only peripheral flow around a central non-occlusive thrombus.

- Fresh intraluminal clot is echolucent while old thrombus is increasingly echogenic, although this feature is highly dependent on image quality and instrument settings.
- The vein diameter increases from the bulk of thrombus in the acute phase then gradually shrinks to become smaller than normal in the chronic phase.
- The wall thickness gradually increases with time.

Upper limb venous thrombosis – indirect evidence

- Diminished or loss of phasic flow with respiration or little or no response to the Valsalva manoeuvre suggests obstruction proximal to the examination site. However, a normal spectral Doppler signal cannot exclude thrombosis since there may be only partial thrombosis in more proximal veins or extensive collaterals. Loss of change of diameter with a sniff test suggests thrombosis.
- Superficial chest wall veins enlarge if they are acting as collaterals, and large deep veins acting as collaterals may be seen adjacent to the thrombosed vein.

CT and MR imaging

- These studies are highly accurate for detecting axillary–subclavian vein occlusion or focal stenosis. They can be performed at rest and with the arm elevated into provocative positions. They provide good information as to the presence and size of collateral veins and chronicity of thrombus.

Treatment

Subclavian vein stenosis

- Conservative treatment is directed towards improving posture and strengthening supportive muscles. Vascular compression frequently requires surgical thoracic outlet decompression by removing the first rib and cervical rib, or dividing the scalenus anterior muscle and fibromuscular bands. Cervical

sympathectomy can also be performed to relieve secondary vasospasm.

Subclavian vein thrombosis

- The aims are to prevent extension of thrombosis and risk of embolism and to attempt to minimize long-term sequelae. Initial treatment is by prompt anticoagulation as for lower limb deep vein thrombosis. Thrombosis detected early can be managed by thrombolysis under venographic control followed by vein balloon dilatation and stenting (see Chapter 15).
- Subsequent treatment is then usually by surgical decompression of the thoracic outlet (see above) to maintain drainage if the vein has been re-opened or to facilitate a collateral circulation if the main vein remains occluded. This is usually performed within three months of the onset and is of less value for long-standing occlusions.

Arterial or brachial plexus compression

- Arterial injury usually requires surgical repair with a bypass graft although early presentation can be treated by an endoluminal stent-graft. Nerve root compression is likely to be managed by non-surgical means.

Nutcracker syndrome

Pathogenesis

- The typical nutcracker syndrome (renal vein entrapment syndrome) results from compression of the left renal vein between the aorta and superior mesenteric artery, sometimes referred to as the *anterior nutcracker* (Figure 16.2).[2] Less frequently, the left renal vein is compressed by the third part of the duodenum. A retro-aortic or circum-aortic renal vein can be compressed between the aorta and vertebral body, referred to as the *posterior nutcracker*. The left renal vein can be compressed by a pancreatic tumour, retroperitoneal tumour or fibrosis, or para-aortic lymphadenopathy. Predisposing factors may be renal ptosis, abnormal high course of the left renal vein or abnormal origin of the

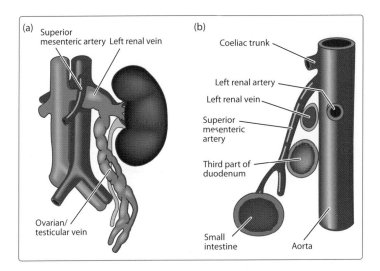

Figure 16.2 Anatomy of the nutcracker syndrome. (a) Anterior view. (b) Lateral view.

superior mesenteric artery. This causes collateral pathways to open to drain the left kidney with partially obstructed or reversed flow in the left renal vein.

- Variations of normal anatomy should be considered. The aortic to superior mesenteric artery angle is variable but is smaller in patients with this syndrome. The left renal vein is 6–10 cm long and its average normal diameter is 4–5 mm. Unlike the right renal vein, it receives the left adrenal, left gonadal, ureteric and lumbar veins. These tributaries normally have valves preventing reflux, and if they are functioning, then they allow renal congestion to develop, whereas if they are absent or lose their function then they act as collaterals to decompress the left kidney.

Clinical features

- The nutcracker syndrome has a wide spectrum of clinical presentations and is frequently not recognized until late. The severity varies from asymptomatic haematuria to severe pelvic congestion. It can occur at any age, although most frequently in the 15–30 age group, it is slightly more common in women and may first become apparent during pregnancy. It is more common in lean subjects or after weight loss, since a fat pad

normally supports the aorto-mesenteric angle. Progressive development of collaterals can result in gradual spontaneous improvement, particularly in children as they grow older.

- Haematuria is the most common symptom, occasionally with resultant anaemia, and may only be evident after exertion in athletes. This varies from microhaematuria and proteinuria to macrohaematuria. Cystoscopy may show bleeding from the left ureter.

- Left renal vein congestion can cause left flank or lower quadrant pain occasionally radiating to the outer thigh and buttock, exacerbated by standing or walking. Ovarian vein congestion can cause pelvic congestion syndrome.

- Reflux in the left testicular vein can cause left-sided varicocoele or left testicular pain. Connection through pelvic veins may be associated with varicosities in the perineum and lower limbs.

Investigation

- Urinalysis and urine cytology and culture are required. Abdominal ultrasound is usually the first investigation, and ratios have been defined for renal vein diameters and flow

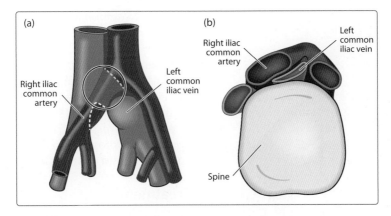

Figure 16.3 The pathologic anatomy of iliac vein compression for the classic left-sided May–Thurner syndrome due to localized compression of the proximal left common iliac vein by the right common iliac artery. (a) Anterior view. (b) Transverse section.

velocities, but findings are not definitive. Imaging techniques include CT, MR or digital subtraction angiography, and trans-catheter venography allows pressure gradient measurements although these can be misleading. Cystoscopy and retrograde pyelography are of value.

- Imaging shows that the hilar portion of the left renal vein and left gonadal vein are distended. Dilated collaterals may be seen including varicosities around the renal pelvis, upper ureter and calyx. There may be a delayed nephrogram. Changing positions can make the appearances more obvious.
- Imaging shows other causes of haematuria such as renal tumours or arteriovenous malformations.

Treatment

- Conservative treatment is recommended for mild haematuria, particularly in young patients. If intervention is warranted, then the objective is to reduce outflow obstruction. Stenting of the renal vein should be considered first. Reported complications of stenting include stent migration, thrombosis and late stent stenosis. Anticoagulation is recommended. This may be followed by embolization of the left gonadal vein, provided it can be shown that it is not an outflow conduit.

- Other procedures that have been described include nephropexy, with excision of renal varicosities, left renal vein bypass or transposition around the aorta, left gonadal vein to IVC anastomosis, renal auto-transplantation or even nephrectomy.

Iliac vein compression – May–Thurner syndrome

Pathogenesis

- The May–Thurner syndrome* (iliac vein compression syndrome) usually results from compression of the left common iliac vein between the right common iliac artery and the sacral promontory or fifth lumbar vertebra just before the ilio-caval junction (Figure 16.3).[3,4] Less common variants include compression of the right common iliac vein by the right common iliac artery or compression of the left iliac vein by the left internal iliac artery (Figure 16.4). Repetitive trauma from arterial pulsations leads to intraluminal webs, channels and spurs, which predispose to iliac vein thrombosis.

---

* Rudolf Virchow reported the condition in 1851, but the definitive description was by R May and J Thurner in 1957.[5]

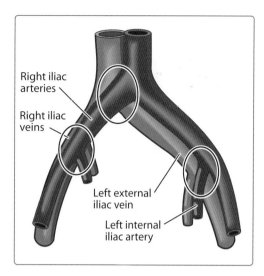

Figure 16.4 Less common variants of elongated compression of the right common iliac vein by the right common iliac artery, or compression of the more distal left iliac vein by the left internal iliac artery.

Clinical features

- Luminal compression by more than 50% can be demonstrated in some 20% of asymptomatic healthy individuals, and the degree of compression can vary through the day. Clinical manifestations are far less frequent and occur more often in women than men as the artery becomes more tortuous. Presentation may be chronic with features of varicose disease, or acute with ilio-femoral venous thrombosis. Examination may reveal suprapubic collaterals.

Investigations

- The diagnosis can be made by trans-abdominal ultrasound but this is technically challenging and a negative study does not exclude the condition. The patient should be fasting but may need intravenous fluids to fill the veins, and imaging during a Valsalva manoeuvre can improve the appearance.
- CT and MR venography both have high sensitivity and specificity to identify venous compression and pelvic venous collaterals and for ilio-femoral thrombosis. The most common venous collateral pathways are ascending lumbar, pre-sacral, trans-pelvic and abdominal wall veins. MR venography

can also demonstrate intra-luminal pathology and flow direction in iliac and collateral veins.
- Ascending venography by femoral vein puncture is accurate for detecting stenosis and measuring its severity, but it is invasive and only required if intervention is contemplated. A pressure gradient >2 mm Hg is held to be diagnostic. Intravascular ultrasound shows changes in the vein wall.

Treatment

- Conservative treatment with compression stockings is usually sufficient for pain and swelling in the absence of venous thrombosis. Initial treatment for deep vein thrombosis is with anticoagulation and compression stockings. Endovascular stenting or rarely open surgical treatment may be required, as described in Chapter 15.

Popliteal vein compression

- Popliteal vein compression is seen in approximately 25% of healthy individuals.[6] Clinical popliteal vein entrapment may be isolated or combined with popliteal arterial entrapment. There is no apparent anatomical abnormality in many patients, and compression has been related to muscular calves or obesity without demonstrable pathology other than from the popliteal fat pad. There can be anatomical displacement by the medial head of the gastrocnemius muscle due to anomalous insertion to the medial femoral condyle, and rarely from the popliteus muscle or lateral head of gastrocnemius. There is frequent secondary saccular dilatation above and below the obstructing site.
- The condition can lead to calf pain and oedema, is occasionally a cause of venous stasis skin complications and predisposes to deep vein thrombosis, particularly during and after surgery due to prolonged hyperextension of the knee. Compression is position-dependent and usually occurs with active plantar-flexion with a fully extended knee.
- Clinical suspicion can be confirmed by ultrasound, CT or venography, with

provocative manoeuvres such as extending the knee, passive ankle dorsiflexion or standing on tip-toes, although these changes are frequently seen in subjects without symptoms. Popliteal vein pressure measurements can be useful to select patients likely to benefit from treatment.

- CT or MR venography provide additional information as to anatomical abnormalities such as abnormal muscle insertions and fibrous bands. Contrast MR allows for extended scanning time to provide images performed with stress manoeuvres such as plantar flexion.

- Positional ascending venography remains the definitive diagnostic test. Pressure measurements can also be obtained to detect venous hypertension and to show pressure variations in response to positional changes.

- Patients can be managed with compression stockings. Anticoagulation is required for acute DVT. Treatment for severe symptomatic compression is by surgical decompression through a posterior approach to the popliteal vein, with or without partial division of muscle bands.

References

1. Butros SR, Liu R, Oliveira GR, Ganguli S, Kalva S. Venous compression syndromes: Clinical features, imaging findings and management. *Br J Radiol* 2013;86: Epub. https://www.ncbi.nlm.nih.gov/pmc/articles/PMC3798333/

2. Kurklinsky AK, Rooke TW. Nutcracker phenomenon and nutcracker syndrome. *Mayo Clin Proc* 2010;85:552–9. http://www.mayoclinicproceedings.org/article/S0025-6196(11)60346-7/abstract

3. Brinegar KN, Sheth RA, Khademhosseini A, Bautista J, Oklu R. Iliac vein compression syndrome: Clinical, imaging and pathologic findings. *World J Radiol* 2015;7:375–81. https://www.ncbi.nlm.nih.gov/pmc/articles/PMC4663376/

4. Raju S. Iliac vein outflow obstruction in 'primary' chronic venous disease. *Phlebolymphology* 2008;15:12–6. http://www.phlebolymphology.org/iliac-vein-outflow-obstruction-in-primary-chronic-venous-disease/

5. May R, Thurner J. The cause of the predominantly sinistral occurrence of thrombosis of the pelvic veins. *Angiology* 1957;8:419–27. https://www.ncbi.nlm.nih.gov/pubmed/13478912

6. Raju S, Neglen P. Popliteal vein entrapment: A benign venographic feature or a pathologic entity? *J Vasc Surg* 2000;31:631–41. http://www.sciencedirect.com/science/article/pii/S0741521400678254

17 Other venous disorders

Chronic pelvic venous disorder

- This condition is also referred to as pelvic venous congestion syndrome, and can cause chronic debilitating pelvic pain in women. It results from dilation of ovarian or pelvic veins causing venous reflux and congestion. Ovarian vein reflux is held by some to increase the likelihood of lower limb varicose veins by connections across the groin.[1,2]

Pathogenesis

- Ovarian vein dilation can be detected in up to 10% of asymptomatic women. Pathological reflux most often affects the left ovarian vein but can also be present in the right ovarian vein. Reflux can occur in internal iliac venous tributaries, but only about 10% of these have venous valves, so that there is reflux in the veins even in healthy subjects, and the clinical relevance of pelvic vein reflux is frequently uncertain.
- There is a probable hormonal basis as it is more prevalent in younger multiparous women, is rarely diagnosed in nulliparous and almost never in post-menopausal women. The vascular capacity of ovarian veins increases during pregnancy by some 60 times which persists for months after delivery.
- Ovarian vein entrapment has also been attributed to retroperitoneal fibrosis or major vein stenosis, and pelvic congestion can result from the nutcracker syndrome (see Chapter 16). Testicular vein reflux in the male can be associated with a varicocoele.

Clinical features

- Presentation is so varied that the underlying cause is frequently not immediately appreciated. A dull aching deep pelvic pain is usually worse at the end of the day, after exercise, with prolonged standing or after heavy lifting, and is usually improved by lying down. Pain is often worst during menstruation and during intercourse. There may be bladder irritation or stress incontinence.
- Patients may have atypical varicose veins in the vulva, buttocks or upper medial thigh. Many patients are diagnosed after finding ovarian vein reflux during ultrasound examination for lower limb varicose veins.

Investigation – ultrasound

- Trans-abdominal ultrasound is used to establish the diagnosis, and trans-vaginal ultrasound is sometimes indicated. Reflux shown by ultrasound may affect more than one pelvic venous system so that it is necessary to examine both ovarian veins and the internal iliac venous system. Pelvic varices appear as tortuous, dilated veins in the uterine adnexae or besides the ureter. Ultrasound may also show refluxing veins passing across the inguinal region to lower limb varices, although this does not mean that they are the cause of lower limb varicose disease.
- Absence of pelvic varices during supine ultrasound or during laparoscopy when the veins are compressed under peritoneal insufflation does not exclude pelvic varices.

Technique

- This is not part of a routine examination for lower limb venous disease and if requested requires the patient to be fasted and examined either standing or in reverse Trendelenburg.
- For the left side find the left renal vein as it crosses the aorta and trace it out to where it is joined by the left ovarian vein passing vertically upwards. For the right side find the inferior vena cava and trace it down to where the right ovarian vein joins at an angle.
- Test for reflux either spontaneous or induced by epigastric compression. If spontaneous, this may be arrested by iliac fossa compression. If ovarian vein reflux is demonstrated, measure diameters in the proximal and distal segments – the vein is probably abnormal if >6 mm diameter. Use colour Doppler to scan the pelvic floor looking for varicosities. Test the iliac veins for reflux.

Investigation – venography

- CT or MR venography can differentiate primary pelvic venous congestion from other causes of pelvic pain and help plan for treatment. Catheter-directed venography is usually reserved for the time of endovascular treatment. Diagnostic criteria are ovarian vein dilatation, uterine venous enlargement, congestion of the ovarian plexus, retrograde filling of the main internal iliac vein and at least one gluteal, ischiatic or obturator tributary, and contrast filling of pelvic veins across the midline and of vulvo-vaginal and thigh varicosities.

Treatment

- Past treatment by open or laparoscopic ovarian vein ligation has been superseded by endovascular treatment with trans-catheter embolization and sclerotherapy of the refluxing veins.
- Treatment is appropriate for most patients diagnosed with this syndrome. However, it is debatable whether it is warranted for patients with lower limb varicose veins shown to be associated with connections from pelvis veins without pelvic symptoms. Vulval veins are considered to be best treated by sclerotherapy and lower limb veins by conventional methods.
- Internal iliac, internal pudendal, obturator and ischial vein tributaries may also need to be treated and this may require separate sessions. Access for percutaneous catheterization is either from the left common femoral or right internal jugular vein for most veins. Angled catheters such as the Cobra catheter are useful to traverse the left renal vein to access the left ovarian vein. Target veins are occluded with 4–6 coils after which a sclerosant such as 3% STS mixed with contrast is injected to thrombose the vein.
- Complications of coil embolization are few but include migration of coils into the renal vein or pulmonary circulation, and local thrombophlebitis causing acute pain and possible subsequent perivenous fibrosis causing chronic pain. There are no adverse effects on subsequent pregnancy, although recurrent ovarian vein reflux is likely.
- Technical results are good, although careful interrogation of all potentially affected veins as well as the left ovarian vein, and of anatomical variants such as duplicated ovarian veins, is necessary. However, 10%–20% of patients remain symptomatic after treatment, and good results require careful exclusion of other causes for symptoms before intervention.[2]

Hepato-portal venous diseases

Pathogenesis

- Disease can affect the hepatic arterial and portal venous circulation passing to the liver, the intrahepatic circulation or the hepatic venous circulation leaving the liver.

Portal vein thrombosis

- Portal or splenic vein thrombosis is due to coagulation disorders, malignancy or intra-abdominal sepsis. An infected umbilical vein catheter is a cause in infants. The portal vein can be obstructed by pancreatic disease or hepatocellular carcinoma. It can be absent due to developmental anomalies.

Cirrhosis

- Alcoholic liver disease can lead to cirrhosis and superimposed hepatocellular carcinoma. Alcohol damages hepatocytes by its metabolic products stimulating an inflammatory response through cytokines, tissue factors and immune mechanisms.[3,4]
- Cirrhosis can be a late sequel of infection with hepatitis B or C. Both chronic hepatitis B and C progress to cirrhosis in about 2% per annum, and patients with the acute disease may not be diagnosed.
- Other causes of cirrhosis include fatty liver, autoimmune hepatitis, primary biliary cirrhosis and haemochromatosis.
- Tissue fibrosis and vaso-active substances increase resistance in the sinusoids and terminal portal venules to cause portal hypertension. Blood is shunted away from the liver to diminish hepatic reserve. Toxic substances from the intestine pass directly to the systemic circulation through porto-systemic venous collaterals. Visceral venous congestion causes ascites and splenomegaly.

Non-cirrhotic portal fibrosis

- Non-cirrhotic portal fibrosis (idiopathic portal hypertension) is characterized by portal hypertension and splenomegaly, but with preserved liver function and patent hepatic and portal veins.[5] The condition probably results from a genetically-based auto-immune injury.

Budd–Chiari syndrome

- The Budd–Chiari syndrome* results from total or partial occlusion of two or more major hepatic veins and/or the intra-hepatic or supra-hepatic inferior vena cava.[6] Budd–Chiari is classified as primary when the obstruction is due to primary venous thrombosis, stenosis or webs, and secondary if due to extrinsic compression. Common causes include myeloproliferative disease and inherited or acquired hypercoagulable states (see Chapter 20), but the cause may not be apparent.

---

* George Budd (1808–1882), an English physician. Hans Chiari (1851–1916), an Austrian pathologist.

- The condition is very uncommon. In the West, Budd–Chiari is more frequent in young women and is most often due to pure hepatic vein occlusion. In contrast, in Asia it is more predominant in middle-aged men, and pure inferior vena cava or combined inferior vena cava and hepatic vein occlusion predominate.
- Once liver venous outflow is compromised, sinusoidal and portal pressures increase and portal venous flow decreases, and some 15% of patients develop portal vein thrombosis. Presentation can be acute or chronic, with painful hepatomegaly, ascites, hepato-renal failure, coagulopathy and portal hypertension.

Mesenteric inflammatory veno-occlusive disease

- This is a condition of unknown aetiology where inflammatory changes in veins of the bowel and mesentery result in bowel ischaemia in the absence of any arteritis. It usually requires surgical resection and has a high mortality.

Paroxysmal nocturnal haemoglobinuria

- This rare acquired defect in the erythrocyte membrane is associated with intra-abdominal venous and cerebral venous thrombosis. It leads to haemolytic anaemia, haemoglobinuria, abdominal pain and venous thrombo-embolism. Treatment is bone marrow transplant or a complement inhibitor.

Portal hypertension

- Portal hypertension may be:[5]
  - prehepatic – portal vein thrombosis, occlusion or absence
  - intrahepatic – cirrhosis or idiopathic non-cirrhotic portal fibrosis
  - post-hepatic – the Budd–Chiari syndrome
- Portal hypertension is defined by a pressure gradient between the portal vein and inferior vena cava >5 mm Hg. It is initially associated with well-preserved liver function compared to the Budd–Chiari syndrome.

Porto-systemic collaterals

- These are potential sites for anastomosis between portal and systemic venous tributaries. They can lead to varices which may rupture causing bleeding, particularly oesophageal varices. There are four main groups (Figure 17.1).

Gastro-oesophageal

- Oesophageal – in the wall of the oesophagus.
- Para-oesophageal – located outside the oesophagus.
- Coronary – in the lesser omentum.
- Gastric – at the postero-superior aspect of the fundus.

Para-umbilical

- These can arise from the left portal vein and drain through the epigastric veins into the external iliac veins.

- They can also connect with subcutaneous vessels on the anterior abdominal wall around the umbilicus creating the *caput medusae.*

Spleno-renal

- These pass from the splenic hilum to left renal vein.

Inferior mesenteric

- Inferior mesenteric – veins of the haemorrhoidal plexus connect superior haemorrhoidal veins in the portal venous system with middle and inferior haemorrhoidal veins which drain into the internal iliac vein.
- Meso-caval – between the inferior mesenteric vein and inferior vena cava through lumbar and retroperitoneal veins.
- Mesenterico-renal – between the superior mesenteric vein and right and left renal veins.

Clinical presentations

Gastrointestinal haemorrhage

- Bleeding can result from rupture of submucosal porto-systemic varices in the lower oesophagus, or cardia and fundus of the stomach. This occurs in some 50% of patients with cirrhosis and has an immediate mortality rate of >10%. There is an approximate 50% risk of re-bleeding and 50% mortality within 1–2 years without treatment.

Ascites

- Ascites often occurs secondary to cirrhosis. It is usually a relatively early presentation and may be precipitated by fluid retention, heart failure or intraperitoneal malignancy.

Hepatic encephalopathy

- The liver normally detoxifies products from the digestive tract. Shunting blood flow from the portal to systemic circulation, either through collaterals or a surgical connection, can cause a toxic neurological deficit from ammonia and other breakdown products of protein metabolism. Spontaneous development has an insidious onset with intellectual deterioration, while advanced stages can lead to coma.

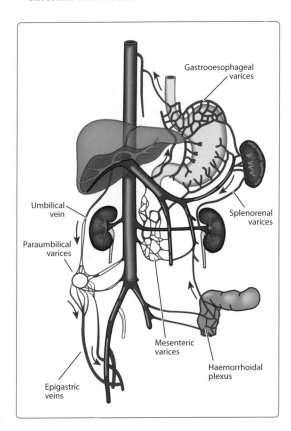

Figure 17.1 Potential sites for anastomosis between intra-abdominal portal and systemic venous tributaries.

Hepato-renal syndrome

- This severe complication of advanced liver disease can be precipitated by shock, infection, surgery, large volume paracentesis or nephrotoxic drugs. It results from intense splanchnic vasodilatation causing reduced effective blood volume leading to renal vasoconstriction. The process is reversible with treatment.

Splenomegaly and hypersplenism

- This is common and can lead to thrombocytopenia, leukopenia and even haemolytic anaemia.

Endocrine dysfunction

- Hypothyroidism, and feminization and hypogonadism in males are features of liver disease due to failure to metabolize pituitary hormones.

Coagulation disorders

- Increased risk of bleeding in liver disease results from failure to synthesize coagulation factors. Despite prolonged coagulation times, patients have at least the same clotting potential as normal subjects and should be anticoagulated as appropriate.

Investigation

Ultrasound

- Ultrasound is used to assess vascular changes, plan for interventional treatment and perform surveillance after intervention. It should be possible to identify all hepato-portal veins and hepatic arteries. Normal portal venous flow is towards the liver (hepatopetal). Flow in the hepatic artery and branches is in the same direction and it can be difficult to distinguish between them with colour Doppler. Portal venous flow is continuous, with respiratory phasicity, while hepatic veins also show superimposed triphasic flow due to right heart systole.
- Portal venous flow becomes biphasic with moderate liver disease and eventually is directed away from the liver (hepatofugal).

Portal hypertension will cause dilation of the portal vein and tributaries with development of collaterals, while portal vein thrombosis may show as a filling defect. Many collateral veins can be seen on ultrasound. The Budd–Chiari syndrome results in abnormal or absent flow in the hepatic veins with intra-hepatic collaterals.

- B-mode can be used to distinguish the type of liver disease with moderate accuracy.
  - Diffuse liver disease due to cirrhosis – nodular liver surface and texture.
  - Non-cirrhotic portal fibrosis – diffuse texture.
  - Fatty infiltration – increased parenchymal echogenicity.
  - Liver tumours – B-mode to detect a tumour and colour Doppler to assess its vascularity.
- Ultrasound is used to measure spleen size and demonstrate ascites.

Endoscopic ultrasound

- This allows very close imaging of the portal vein as well as biliary tree and pancreas. It may be combined with endoscopic pancreatic cannulation and sphincterotomy or pancreatic biopsy.

Venography

- CT and MR findings in the Budd–Chiari syndrome include changes in liver morphology with patchy enhancement related to stasis in the sinusoids and portal vein, an enlarged caudate lobe, compressed inferior vena cava, absent hepatic veins and ascites. The acute syndrome may show acute thrombosis of the inferior vena cava and portal vein. MR angiography is useful to show the vascular changes. Either can demonstrate collaterals.
- Catheter venography is required prior to endovascular interventions. It precisely defines anatomy, provides haemodynamic information through pressure measurements and allows histologic studies from transcatheter liver biopsy. Access to the hepatic veins is through an internal jugular or common femoral vein approach.

Treatment

- Medical measures are the first line of treatment. Interventions that may be required are bleeding control, surgical or transhepatic porto-systemic shunting or liver transplantation.

Porto-systemic shunting

- This has been the traditional technique to decompress the portal venous circulation and prevent recurrence of haemorrhage from varices. However, it is a major operation, with appreciable mortality, it can cause encephalopathy and it interferes with the ability to use vessels to anastomose for liver transplantation.
- Various techniques are available. The portal vein, superior mesenteric vein or splenic vein is anastomosed to the inferior vena cava or a major tributary such as the left renal vein.

Percutaneous transjugular intrahepatic porto-systemic shunting (TIPS)

- TIPS has largely replaced surgical shunting, with percutaneous insertion of a stent between a large branch of the hepatic and portal venous systems.
- TIPS is equivalent to side-to-side portocaval shunting. It does not interfere with subsequent ability to perform liver transplantation. It can be complicated by hepatic encephalopathy.
- TIPS may be definitive treatment for portal hypertension but it has a high restenosis rate, and is now mostly used as a temporary measure while waiting for transplantation.
- Liver function may improve and hepatic haemodynamics may return towards normal after TIPS due to hypertrophy of remaining non-cirrhotic liver tissue.

Liver transplantation

- Transplantation has become widely accepted as the definitive treatment for advanced liver disease as immunosuppression techniques have become more effective.

Selection of treatment

- Primary bleeding is not usually an indication for prophylaxis by operative intervention. Active bleeding requires volume resuscitation, correction of coagulopathy, antibiotics for concurrent primary bacterial peritonitis, vasoconstrictors such as vasopressin and balloon tamponade with a Sengstaken–Blakemore tube. Endoscopic techniques are then used to sclerose or ligate varices.
- Indications for shunting or TIPS include intractable variceal haemorrhage, recurrent variceal bleeding after failure of endoscopic treatment, refractory ascites or the Budd–Chiari syndrome. Contraindications to shunting or TIPS include progressive liver failure, coagulopathy, pulmonary hypertension or severe hepatic encephalopathy.

Chronic cerebrospinal venous insufficiency (CCSVI)

- Zamboni and colleagues postulated that multiple sclerosis is caused by impaired cerebral venous drainage due to narrowing or occlusion of the azygos and internal jugular veins.[7] This proposal has been refuted by others.[8] Opponents claim that the incidence of these anomalies is small and no different to that in the normal population, and that treatment proposed is ineffective and potentially dangerous.
- Multiple sclerosis is an inflammatory disease of unknown cause where activated immune cells invade the central nervous system to cause inflammation and disseminated nervous tissue sclerosis. The current belief is that it is probably an auto-immune disease. The proposed basis for CCSVI as a causative factor is that restricted outflow leads to breakdown of the brain/blood barrier, extravascular iron deposition and development of local inflammation and fibrosis analogous to lower limb skin changes due to chronic venous hypertension.
- Normal physiology is that the internal jugular vein (IJV) is the predominant pathway for unidirectional outflow when a subject is

supine, whereas flow is redirected to the vertebral veins (VVs) in the upright position.

- Impaired outflow is held to be due to:
  - stenosis, collapse or twisting of the vein
  - an abnormal valve, septum, flap or membrane
  - atresia, hypoplasia or agenesis
- It has been considered that these represent developmental truncular malformations (see Chapter 1). However, this has been disputed by Thibault, who has proposed an alternative theory that the abnormal obstructive venous lesions are caused by an acquired inflammatory/thrombotic process that may have an infective aetiology.[9]
- Morphology of the neurological disorder is demonstrated by MR imaging, and the venous abnormalities are shown by ultrasound or MR venography confirmed by direct invasive venography if treatment is contemplated. Zamboni's studies used duplex ultrasound for extracranial IJVs and VVs with the subject supine and sitting and transcranial Doppler ultrasound.
- Diagnosis was made by ultrasound findings of reflux or absence of flow in any of the jugular, vertebral or deep cerebral veins, IJV stenosis, loss of the normal cerebral drainage and change of flow from the IJV to vertebral vein on assuming the upright position.
- Treatment when feasible consists of balloon dilatation with or without stenting of IJVs in the neck. However, multiple studies have failed to find an association between cerebral venous pathology and multiple sclerosis, and trials of treatment have failed to show benefit.

Superior vena cava syndrome

- Obstruction of flow through the superior vena cava (SVC) can result from lung cancer, mediastinal lymphomas and other tumours, thrombosis complicating a central vein catheter or other devices or vascular diseases such as aortic arch aneurysm or mediastinal fibrosis. Collateral venous return is through the azygos, internal mammary and long thoracic veins.

- Symptoms include dyspnoea, dysphagia, cough and naso-pharyngeal obstruction. Examination shows distended neck and chest wall veins, arm and face swelling and cyanosis. A chest X-ray may show a mediastinal mass, but contrast CT or MR provide the diagnosis.
- Treatment is with endovascular angioplasty, stenting or thrombolysis.

Popliteal vein aneurysms

- Venous aneurysms are rare and most affect popliteal veins. The jugular or saphenous veins can become aneurysmal, with the rarest being those involving the femoral, caval, forearm or portal veins.[10]

Pathology

- A vein is usually defined as aneurysmal if it is at least twice the diameter of the normal vein, as opposed to ectasias which have diameters more than 50% greater than normal size. Approximately 75% are saccular and 25% are fusiform. The wall shows loss of elastic fibres and smooth muscle cells in the media, with proliferation of elastic, muscle and connective tissue in the intima. They are usually lined by thrombus which can be a source for pulmonary embolism.
- Their cause is uncertain, but they do not appear to be a manifestation of varicose disease. They may be late congenital malformations.

Clinical features

- The sex incidence is equal and most often affect patients aged 50–60 years. Most are asymptomatic and detected on routine investigation for varicose veins, but they may present with pulmonary or paradoxical embolism, which has been reported in 70%–80% of patients if left untreated. Other presentations can be with pain and a mass in the popliteal fossa, pain secondary to tibial nerve compression or superficial vein thrombosis. Physical examination can appear to be normal unless the aneurysm is large.
- Ultrasound detects an aneurysm and shows its diameter and extent, shape and presence and amount of mural thrombus. Colour

Doppler ultrasound may show swirling with augmentation, and spectral Doppler may then even show aliasing. CT and MR imaging may be used, and conventional venography has its advocates.

Treatment

- Asymptomatic aneurysms greater than 2 cm in diameter and all symptomatic aneurysms should be treated by operation, as thrombus in larger aneurysms can detach to cause pulmonary embolism, particularly for saccular aneurysms. Smaller asymptomatic aneurysms can be managed expectantly with a low risk of embolism, although anticoagulation alone is ineffective.
- A prophylactic temporary inferior vena cava filter should be considered prior to surgery, particularly if ultrasound shows free-floating thrombus. Catheter-directed thrombolysis before open surgical repair can also be considered to reduce risk of intra-operative embolism.
- Surgical repair can be performed through a posterior popliteal approach, although exposure must allow preliminary proximal control. Saccular aneurysms can be repaired by partial excision and removal of thrombus, then lateral venorrhaphy. Fusiform aneurysms may require a vein patch or vein bypass. Post-surgical anticoagulation is required for several months.

Venous trauma

Mechanisms

- Venous trauma most often occurs in the extremities, but may involve major veins in the thorax or abdomen. Venous injuries can be iatrogenic, blunt trauma in accidents or from gun and knife injuries.
- A fractured long bone can injure an adjacent vein, as can posterior dislocation of the knee, and popliteal vessel injury occasionally complicates knee surgery.
- Complete transection can allow vessel spasm to arrest bleeding, whereas partial damage may prevent venous spasm to allow persistent haemorrhage.

- Most venous injuries are discovered during surgical exploration for an arterial injury; isolated venous injuries are usually only detected if there is active bleeding, and many other venous injuries are not detected at the time, although they may present later with a post-thrombotic syndrome.

Treatment

- Bleeding and soft tissue trauma can make it difficult to identify injured arteries and veins prior to their treatment, and this may necessitate extending the wound or making an incision away from the injury to gain control. A tourniquet may have been required but should be removed as soon as possible.
- Venous injuries found during exploration for associated arterial injury should be repaired if the patient is haemodynamically stable and the repair itself will not significantly delay treatment of associated injuries or destabilize the patient's condition.
- Lateral venorrhaphy that does not significantly narrow the lumen or panelled grafts appear to be the best options for repair. Interposition vein grafts consistently have poor results, and synthetic grafts are the least desirable option. Fasciotomy to prevent compartment syndrome should be considered, particularly when there is a combined arterial and venous injury. The need for anticoagulation to reduce the risk of subsequent thrombosis is balanced against the risk of bleeding in a trauma patient.
- Definitive repair should not be attempted in unstable patients. Venous ligation in conjunction with leg elevation, compression stockings and liberal use of fasciotomies offer similar results to repair.
- The prognosis is largely determined by concurrent nerve and arterial injuries, but there are late sequelae of pain and swelling due to impaired venous outflow, even after technically successful venous repair.

Arteriovenous fistulae

- An arteriovenous fistula (AVF) is an abnormal connection between an artery and a vein and can occur at any site in the body. Congenital AVFs from arterio-venous malformations are described in Chapter 26. AVFs result from trauma or disease, or may be surgically created for haemodialysis.

Aetiology

- A traumatic AVF can be accidental from blunt or penetrating trauma, or iatrogenic from needle biopsy, arterial puncture or intravenous catheter insertion. Cases have been reported following endovenous laser ablation.
- AVF due to disease can result from a neoplasm such as renal carcinoma, or aneurysms such as rupture of an abdominal aortic aneurysm into the inferior vena cava.
- A haemodialysis fistula is formed either by direct anastomosis between artery and vein in an extremity, termed a native arteriovenous fistula, or by a synthetic or vein graft between the two, termed a prosthetic haemodialysis access arteriovenous graft. Adjacent vessels used are the radial artery and cephalic vein at the wrist (Brescia–Cimino fistula) or brachial artery and cephalic or basilic vein at the cubital fossa.

Clinical manifestations

- Clinical features are a pulsatile swelling if close to the surface, machinery murmur with auscultation and reduced pulse rate with digital occlusion of the AVF (Branham's sign).
- Complications include high-pressure arterial flow entering veins through an AVF in the limbs leading to thin-walled varicosities, bleeding such as with haematuria from a renal AVF, reduced distal perfusion causing ischaemia and high-output heart failure from a large AVF.

Investigation

- Some are inaccessible to ultrasound examination, such as cerebral, spinal cord, pulmonary or coronary AVFs. However, AVFs affecting the extremities or viscera are well-suited to detection and assessment by ultrasound.
- Ultrasound shows:
  - low-resistance flow in the supplying artery
  - high-velocity arterialized waveform in the draining vein
  - turbulent high-velocity flow signal in the AVF
- Angiography is usually required prior to treatment.

Treatment

- Surgical separation and repair of the vessels.
- Endovascular cover by an intra-arterial stent-graft.
- Endovascular coil embolization.

History

- Galen of Pergamon (129–c.200/216) considered that the liver rather than the heart was the most important organ, stating that 'the liver is the source of the veins and the principal instrument of sanguification'. He argued that the heart was of secondary importance since it was not the site of production of the humours. He also considered that 'the spleen serves to purify the liver'. This opposed the teachings of Aristotle (384–322 BC) who had considered that the heart was more important, and also that that 'the heart is the origin of the nerves'.
- The Persian physician Avicenna (980–1037) attempted to reconcile these views in his book *The Canon of Medicine*. He observed that 'physicians regard the liver as the seat of manufacture of the dense part of the humours', but that 'all agree that the brain and the liver each receive their power of life, natural heat and breath from the heart'.
- William Harvey (1578–1657) was more fulsome in his opinion that 'the spleen causes one to laugh', although he referred to the liver as 'noble' and the spleen 'ignoble'.
- Canadian physician Sir William Osler (1849–1919) first described an axillary vein aneurysm in 1915.
- William Hunter first described the superior vena cava syndrome in a patient with a syphilitic aortic aneurysm in 1757.
- Georg Eduard von Rindfleisch (1836–1908), German pathologist, had associated venous pathology with multiple sclerosis in 1863.

References

1. Asciutto G. Pelvic vein incompetence: A review of diagnosis and treatment. *Phlebolymphology* 2012;19:84–90. http://www.phlebolymphology.org/pelvic-vein-incompetence-a-review-of-diagnosis-and-treatment/

2. Meissner MH, Gibson K. Clinical outcome after treatment of pelvic congestion syndrome: Sense and nonsense. *Phlebology* 2015;30:73–80. https://www.ncbi.nlm.nih.gov/pubmed/25729071

3. Huang Y, Yang SS, Kao JH. Pathogenesis and management of alcoholic liver cirrhosis: A review. *Hepat Med* 2011;3:1–11. https://www.ncbi.nlm.nih.gov/pmc/articles/PMC3846480/

4. Gao B, Bataller R. Alcoholic liver disease: Pathogenesis and new therapeutic targets. *Gastroenterology* 2011;141:1572–1585. https://www.ncbi.nlm.nih.gov/pmc/articles/PMC3214974/

5. Khanna R, Sarin SK. Non-cirrhotic portal hypertension – Diagnosis and management. *J Hepatology* 2014;60:421–41. http://www.sciencedirect.com/science/article/pii/S0168827813006077

6. Ferral H, Behrens G, Lopera J. Budd-Chiari syndrome. *Am J Roentgen* 2012;199:737–745. http://www.ajronline.org/doi/full/10.2214/AJR.12.9098

7. Zamboni P, Galeotti R, Menegatti E, Malagoni AM, Tacconi G, Dall'Ara S, Bartolomei I, Salvi F. Chronic cerebrospinal venous insufficiency in patients with multiple sclerosis. *J Neurol, Neurosurg Psychiatry* 2009;80:392–9. http://jnnp.bmj.com/content/80/4/392.full

8. Valdueza JM, Doepp F, Schreiber SJ, van Oosten BW, Schmierer K, Paul F, Wattjes MP. What went wrong? The flawed concept of cerebrospinal venous insufficiency. *J Cereb Blood Flow Metab* 2013;33:657–68. https://www.ncbi.nlm.nih.gov/pmc/articles/PMC3652697/

9. Thibault PK. Multiple sclerosis: A chronic infective cerebrospinal venulitis? *Phlebology* 2012;27:207–18. http://hiihoo.mbnet.fi/ccsvi/thibault%20tutkimus.pdf

10. Flekser RL, Mohabbat W. Popliteal vein aneurysms: The diagnostic and surgical dilemma. *Vasc Dis Mgmt* 2015;12:E26–32. http://www.vasculardiseasemanagement.com/content/popliteal-vein-aneurysms-diagnostic-and-surgical-dilemma

18 Lymphoedema – pathology and clinical features

Written with Neil Piller

This chapter includes recommendations from the International Society of Lymphology, National Lymphoedema Network and Union Internationale de Phlebologie.[1–3]

Pathogenesis and classification

- Lymphoedema is chronic progressive swelling in a region due to excessive build-up of protein-rich interstitial fluid. It develops when the lymphatic load is consistently greater than the lymphatic transport capacity in a specific lymphatic territory.
- *Low-output lymphoedema* occurs when the lymphatic system's ability to transport is reduced. This may be primary due to congenital lymphatic dysplasia or secondary due to lymphatic damage or obliteration through surgery, irradiation or chronic inflammation.
- *High-output lymphoedema* can develop when there is an increased load on an otherwise normal system. This may be caused by lower limb varicose disease with peripheral oedema or phlebo-lymphoedema, or general medical conditions such as hepatic cirrhosis causing ascites or nephrotic syndrome causing anasarca. Transport capacity through intact lymphatics is overwhelmed by an excessive burden of capillary filtrate. Lymphatic transport is normal in the early stages but long-standing high-output lymphatic failure causes gradual secondary functional deterioration of draining lymphatics. This reduces their transport capacity even if the underlying disease is corrected, and the lymphatic system eventually fails.

Primary lymphoedema

- Primary lymphoedema has various manifestations. It is a truncular lymphatic malformation due to a developmental abnormality causing hypoplasia or aplasia of lymphatic vessels, lymphatic valvular incompetence or functional defects (see Chapters 1 and 26). It affects females more often than males and the estimated prevalence is 1 in 6000 individuals. It usually affects lower limbs, but can involve the upper limbs, genitalia, trunk or face.
- It is usually an autosomal-dominant genetic condition inherited from either parent or resulting from spontaneous mutation.[4] Most appear sporadically, but variable penetrance means that familial cases can be missed. Traditionally, it has been classified by age of onset into three types.

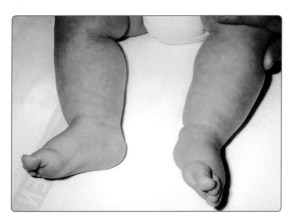

Figure 18.1 Primary lymphoedema in an infant – Milroy's disease.

Type 1 – Lymphoedema congenita – Milroy's disease*

- This is responsible for about 3% of primary lymphoedemas. It is present from birth or apparent by one year of age, generally presents first with foot oedema, usually affects females and progresses from being unilateral to bilateral (Figure 18.1). The genitals may be involved and there can be upslanting toenails, papillomatosis, prominent leg veins, urethral abnormalities and hydrocoele in males, intestinal lymphangiectasias, cholestasis, lymphopenia and impaired cell-mediated immunity due to reduced lymphocyte transport. Lymphatics may be hypoplastic but generally show functional impairment of absorption at the level of the initial lymphatics.
- This is a familial autosomal-dominant disorder with poor penetrance due to mutation in the FLT4 gene located on chromosome 5 which codes for the vascular endothelial growth factor receptor 3 (VEGFR-3), a tyrosine kinase receptor specific for lymphatic vessel function.

Type II – Lymphoedema praecox – Meige disease[†]

- This accounts for 80% of primary lymphoedemas. It becomes clinically evident in females during puberty, often after trauma or infection or with body mass change, and before about the age of 35 years, suggesting that oestrogen plays a role in its pathogenesis. Lymphatics are hypoplastic and reduced in number. It usually presents in one lower limb but becomes bilateral in 50%, and the arms and face can be affected. It may be associated with the yellow-nail syndrome.
- It is autosomal dominant and can be due to mutation of the FOXC2 gene of the forkhead family located on chromosome 16. The same gene mutation is involved in the yellow-nail, distichiasis lymphoedema and lymphoedema-ptosis syndromes (see below).

Type III – Lymphoedema tarda

- This appears after about 35 years of age and is uncommon. The legs are most often affected but the arms and other areas may also be involved. It is thought to be most often caused by impaired valve function with increased numbers of dilated tortuous lymphatics which can be similar to those seen in lipoedema.

Associated conditions

- *Yellow-nail syndrome* is a rare genetic disorder that develops around puberty characterized by yellow thickened curved nails and arrested nail growth. Lymphoedema of the arms and legs is associated with bronchiectasis and pleural effusion. It is associated with FOXC2 gene mutation.
- *Distichiasis lymphoedema syndrome* is hereditary lymphoedema present at birth due to avalvulia and lymph reflux. Patients have double eyelashes (distichiasis) which can range from a few extra lashes to a full double row that arise from the Meibomian glands on the posterior lamella of the tarsal

---

* William Milroy (1855–1942), professor of Medicine and Hygiene at Omaha Medical College in Nebraska, reported the occurrence of congenital hereditary lymphedema in six generations of an afflicted family in 1892.

† Described by H. Meige in 1898.

plate. Oedema most often affects the legs, and associated anomalies include short stature, webbed neck, vertebral abnormalities, spinal arachnoid cysts, cleft palate, ptosis, haemangiomas, thoracic duct abnormalities and cardiac defects. It is an autosomal dominant genetic disorder associated with FOXC2 mutation.

- *Lymphoedema-ptosis syndrome* is an extremely rare genetic disorder that usually occurs around puberty and is characterized by lymphoedema of the lower limbs and ptosis.
- *Hypotrichosis lymphoedema telangiectasia syndrome* is characterized by hair loss during infancy, lymphoedema in the lower limbs developing in puberty and telangiectasia particularly on the palms and soles. It is associated with a mutation of the transcription factor gene SOX18.
- *Hennekam syndrome* is a rare congenital syndrome of intestinal and other lymphangiectases, facial anomalies and intellectual disability.
- *Emberger syndrome* is childhood-onset lymphoedema. It is associated with congenital deafness, neck webbing and generalized warts, and it usually precedes acute myeloid leukemia. Children with lower limb and genital lymphoedema should be screened for haematological abnormalities.
- *Dahlberg Borer Newcomer syndrome* is a rare autosomal X-linked recessive genetic condition characterized by lymphoedema, hypoparathyroidism, cardiac valve prolapse, progressive kidney failure and very short distal phalanges of the fingers.
- *Intestinal lymphangiectasia* is due to oedematous thickening of the small intestinal wall associated with protein-losing enteropathy, ascites, pleural effusion, peripheral oedema, diarrhea and immunodeficiency. This can lead to generalized oedema from hypoalbuminemia due to increased pressure and loss of water-soluble proteins throughout the gastrointestinal lymphatic system, with malabsorption of dietary long-chain fatty acids. It can be primary (Waldham's disease) or secondary due to chronic inflammation in the intestinal wall and subsequent involvement of the lymphatic system.
- Primary lymphoedema may be associated with several genetic multisystem disorders including *Noonan syndrome, Turner syndrome* and *Klippel–Trénaunay syndrome*.

Clinical differentiation of primary lymphoedemas

- Current opinion suggests that there is a greater range of presentations of primary lymphoedema than presented above, leading to an even more complex pathway for classification.[5]
  - The initial presentation should establish whether the patient has a known syndrome such as the Noonan or Turner syndromes.
  - If not, then the next step is to determine if there is systemic or visceral involvement such as the Hennekam syndrome.
  - If not, then it is desirable to exclude patients with disturbed growth, cutaneous manifestations or vascular anomalies, as with the Klippel–Trenaunay, Parkes Weber, Proteus, CLOVE or WILD syndromes (see Chapter 26).
  - Only then should patients be separated into early onset (less than one year old) or late onset (older than one year) disease.
  - Early onset includes Milroy disease and multi-segmental variants.
  - Later onset includes Meige disease and distichiasis lymphoedema.
- Future genetic testing for known and newly discovered mutations and chromosomal defects should allow early recognition to predict primary lymphoedema conditions. It is already becoming clear that some apparently secondary forms may have an underlying primary component.

Secondary lymphoedema

- Secondary lymphoedema is much more common and may affect one or more lymphatic territories.

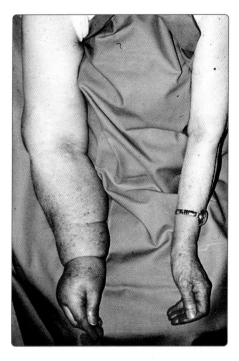

Figure 18.2 Secondary lymphoedema of the right upper limb after treatment for breast cancer.

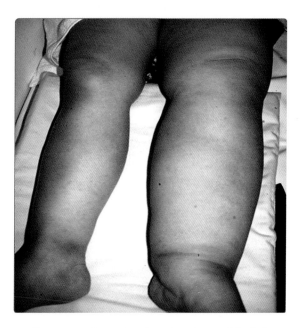

Figure 18.3 Secondary lymphoedema of the left lower limb.

- Its major causes are:
  - surgical excision of lymph nodes
  - surgical or traumatic division of the lymphatics
  - tumours affecting lymph nodes and lymphatics
  - irradiation
  - recurring bacterial infections causing lymphangitis
  - chronic infection such as filariasis
- In *developed nations,* the most common cause is malignancy and its treatment. This ranges from lymph node obstruction due to lymphoma or metastatic cancer, or subsequent to radical lymph node excision and associated radiotherapy (Figures 18.2 and 18.3). The most common sites for lymph node metastases are the axillary nodes for breast cancers or inguinal nodes for lower-body melanoma and other skin cancers. About 30% of patients treated for breast, reproductive and gastro-intestinal system cancers will at some stage develop into variable degrees of lymphoedema, and most present within the first two to three years after surgery or radiotherapy. Following treatment for breast cancer, lymphoedema occurs in about 30% of patients after axillary lymph node clearance, but only in about 5% after sentinel node biopsy.
- In *developing nations,* the most common cause of secondary lymphoedema is filariasis. Mosquito-borne nematode infection with the parasites *Brugia malayi, Brugia timori* or *Wuchereria bancrofti* is the most common cause.
- *Surgical trauma* to lymphatic vessels can cause lymphoedema after varicose vein surgery, peripheral vascular surgery, vein harvesting for coronary artery surgery or burn scar excision. Penetrating or even blunt trauma can interrupt lymphatics to cause localized lymphoedema.

Pathology

- Oedema results if lymphatic transport falls below the capacity to handle the presented load of microvascular filtrate that normally leaks from the blood stream into the interstitium. This consists of excess fluid, plasma proteins, extravascular blood cells and parenchymal cell products, and culminates in excess deposition of ground matrix substances. Stagnation of high-molecular-weight proteins in the interstitium with protein concentrations of 1.0–5.5 mg/mL results in a high oncotic pressure that favours additional fluid accumulation.

- Oedema usually occurs only after lymph outflow has been reduced by 80% or more depending on each individual's lymphatic functional reserve. Those with a low reserve may show oedema after relatively insignificant lymph outflow reduction.
- Fibrosis within regional lymph nodes or around the major lymph collectors for any reason causes increased resistance to lymph flow reducing lymph transport. There are bottlenecks for lymph collectors in the legs at the medial ankle, knee and groin, and in the arm at the elbow and axilla.
- Histological studies show that there is usually only a small volume of stagnant lymph in sub-epidermal lymphatics, and that most tissue fluid accumulates in spaces, in subcutaneous tissues along and around small veins, and superficial and deep to the muscle fascia.[6]
- Excessive fluid accumulation may not be clinically evident in its early stages but may become apparent in later life when the outflow is chronically disrupted.
- Chronic interstitial fluid accumulation leads to valvular incompetence in the remaining outflow tracts with reversal of flow from subcutaneous tissues into the dermal plexus. Lymph vessels then become fibrosed, and fibrinoid thrombi accumulate within their lumen, obliterating many remaining previously functional lymph channels. Spontaneous lympho-venous shunts may form as part of the response, and there are fibrosed shrunken lymph nodes that lose their normal architecture and function.
- Long-term chronic high protein levels in the interstitial fluid initiates an inflammatory reaction, increased macrophage activity and elastic fibre destruction. Fibroblasts migrate into the interstitium and deposit collagen, causing fibrosclerosis. The net effect is to change from the initial pitting oedema to a brawny non-pitting oedema. The overlying skin becomes thickened and can display a peau d'orange (orange skin) appearance. This may present in all or just some of the lymphatic territories, and each territory can change at a different rate or be in a different stage.

- Chronic lymphatic failure may result in change in the protein composition of lymph in affected areas, often with a decrease in alpha-2 globulin levels and increase in the albumin-to-globulin ratio. The outcome is suppressed local immunologic surveillance with increased risk of chronic infection and susceptibility to malignant change.
- Chronic lymphatic failure also leads to reduced tissue oxygen tension, and higher tissue levels of adipogenic factors, eventually manifesting as excessive epifascial fat deposition. Fat further restricts lymph outflow resulting in a progressive deterioration.

Clinical features

History

- Ask about the reason for presentation. This may relate to embarrassment about appearance, functional impairment, restriction in the range of motion of adjacent joints, difficulty in fitting shoes or episodes of lymphangitis.
- Aim to diagnose or exclude cardiac, hepatic or renal causes for oedema, regional tumours that could cause secondary lymphoedema, thyroid dysfunction that may cause myxoedema or venous disease causing high-output lymphoedema. Note that pain generally suggests acute or chronic venous disease or other vascular pathology, as lymphoedema is usually painless.
- Determine if there is a family history of limb swelling and the age of onset if primary lymphoedema is a possible diagnosis. Enquire about past surgery, radiotherapy or trauma in the region if secondary lymphoedema is suspected.

- Note the oedema location which can affect any region, often corresponding to one or more lymphatic territories. Ask about variations in swelling which is most often unilateral and may worsen when the weather is warm, before menstruation, after the limb is dependent for a long time and in the evenings. Venous oedema is more likely than lymphoedema to improve overnight.
- Enquire as to medications such as calcium channel-blockers, prednisolone and non-steroidal anti-inflammatory drugs which can cause leg oedema.

Examination

- Perform a general examination for cardiac and renal disease in particular, and general assessment of height, weight and body mass index. Check thyroid function.
- Examine regional lymph node fields for lymphadenopathy and examine the abdomen for a palpable liver or spleen. Look for features of varicose disease.
- Look for surgical or traumatic scarring.
- Inspect for swelling and confirm by tape measurements of limb circumferences at recorded levels along the limbs comparing the two sides. Clinically manifest oedema usually means a circumference difference of 2 cm or more allowing for limb dominance. Remember that the latent phase of lymphoedema which is difficult to detect clinically without special equipment, can result in symptoms without measured swelling.
- Recommended sites to make measurements are:
  - upper limb:
    - dorsum of the hand
    - wrist
    - 10 cm below the olecranon process
    - 10 cm above the olecranon process
  - lower limb:
    - 2 cm above the medial malleolus
    - 10 cm below the inferior pole of patella
    - 10 cm above the superior pole of patella.
- Note the distribution of oedema. Unilateral oedema can be due to venous or lymphatic disease, while bilateral oedema can be due to systemic or lymphatic disease. The dorsum of the foot is spared with venous disease or lipoedema (see below) but is very much involved in lymphoedema.
- Tenderness is a sign of deep vein thrombosis or lipoedema, whereas lymphoedema is usually non-tender.
- Examine for pitting oedema in the early stages. Press firmly for 30–60 seconds and diagnose pitting oedema if indentation then persists. The pitting test can be applied not only on the dorsum of the hand and foot but also in the mid points of all lymphatic territories. With time, oedema progresses to non-pitting oedema as fibrosis occurs and the subcutaneous fat levels increase.
- Fibrosis can be detected using the Stemmer sign test[*], which is characteristic for lymphoedema but not for other oedemas. A positive Stemmer sign is the inability to pinch the skin on the dorsum of the foot for example at the base of the second toe or hand at the index finger. The Stemmer sign can be used in any lymphatic territory where the pitting test is performed.
- Examine the skin texture. Hyperkeratosis and papillomatosis with brawny induration are characteristic of chronic lymphoedema. Brown haemosiderin deposits on the lower legs and ankles are consistent with venous disease. Reflex sympathetic dystrophy initially leads to warm tender skin with increased sweating. In the late stages of chronic lymphatic failure, the skin becomes thin, shiny and cool, then atrophic and dry with flexion contractures. At this stage, look for skin thickening as peau d'orange, eventual elephantiasis with cobble-stoned plaques and fissuring, ulceration or lymphorrhea (Figure 18.4).
- Look for confounding conditions such as obesity, occult trauma and repeated infection that may complicate the clinical picture.

---

[*] Robert Stemmer described the sign in 1976. It had previously been alluded to by Moritz Kaposi in 1887.

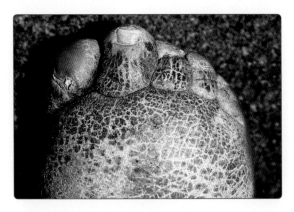

Figure 18.4 Skin changes associated with advances chronic lymphoedema.

Clinical staging

- Lymphoedema has been classified into the following stages:
  - Stage 0 (latent): Lymphatic vessels have sustained some damage which is not yet apparent. Transport capacity is still sufficient and lymphoedema is not clinically detectable.
  - Stage I: There is reversible pitting oedema that decreases when the limb is elevated. The limb is near normal on waking.
  - Stage II: Non-pitting oedema does not decrease when the limb is elevated. Fibrosis has commenced.
  - Stage III: Lymphostatic elephantiasis with a large increase in the size of the limb and hardened skin.
- A functional severity assessment can be used within each stage based on increase in limb volume, assessed as minimal (<20% increase), moderate (20%–40% increase) or severe (>40% increase).

Complications

- The most common complication is infection in stagnant lymph causing cellulitis or lymphangitis which causes further damage to already compromised lymphatic vessels and regional lymph nodes. Bacteria can enter through minute breaches in already damaged skin, but commonly through tinea between the toes. Red inflammatory streaks along lymphatic tracts is diagnostic, associated with systemic malaise,

rigors and fever. If left untreated, infection can lead to septicaemia, skin abscesses, ulceration or tissue necrosis. It needs to be distinguished from acute or chronic lipodermatosclerosis which has no systemic features and no local spreading erythema.
- Patients with chronic lymphoedema for ten years or more have a small risk of developing lymphangiosarcoma (Stewart–Treves syndrome[*]), which commonly presents as a reddish-purple discoloration or nodule that tends to form satellite lesions. It is highly aggressive, requires radical amputation of the involved extremity and has a five-year survival rate of less than 10%.

Differential diagnosis

Lipoedema

- Lipoedema presents as symmetrical bilateral lower limb swelling due to deposition of adipose tissue (Figure 18.5). It is distinct

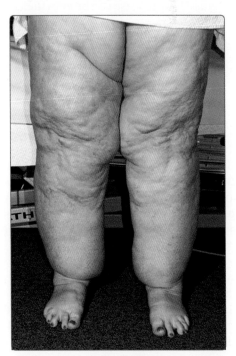

Figure 18.5 Lipoedema.

---

[*] Described by Fred Stewart and Norman Treves from the Memorial Hospital for Cancer and Allied Diseases in New York City in 1948.

from lymphoedema in its early stages and is not a manifestation of obesity. In later stages, excess epifascial fatty tissue interferes with lymphatic drainage to cause secondary lymphoedema or lipo-lymphoedema. Pain due to lipoedema can limit a patient's willingness and ability to wear compression garments which can worsen the lymphatic component and predispose to complications such as infection.

- Lipoedema generally involves the lower limbs between the hips and ankles but not the feet, and occasionally the upper limbs as well. It mostly commences in women after puberty or pregnancy and may affect as many as 10% of post-pubertal females. There is an occasional family history, and it is postulated that it is caused by both genetic and hormonal factors. A hormonal basis is further supported by occasional cases in males associated with liver disease causing high oestrogen levels.
- Progression of disease can be classified as three stages:
  - Stage 1: Smooth skin with increased underlying fat.
  - Stage 2: Indentations and nodules causing 'mattress-like' skin.
  - Stage 3: Large extrusions of skin and subcutaneous fat with subcutaneous fibrosis.
- There may be ankle fat pads only, 'stove-pipe' legs, large buttocks or 'saddle bags'. The distribution respects skin creases so that tissues 'fold' across the ankles over the normal foot. Subcutaneous tissues have a thickened 'doughy' texture with nodularity, and appearances can resemble cellulite. The limb is tender to pressure, bruises easily and shows hyper-flexibility. Varicose veins are present in about 40%.
- The distinction from lymphoedema is made on clinical grounds from the symmetrical distribution and appearance, but they can be difficult to distinguish in more advanced stages.
- Treatment options for lipoedema are limited. An anti-inflammatory diet may be of benefit, but diuretics are ineffective. Past attempts to reduce size by lipectomy or liposuction were not recommended as they risked causing mechanical damage to the lymphatics, but newer techniques are safer and effective. Although long-term low-level compression is unlikely to reverse lipoedema, it may help prevent its worsening and progression to lipo-lymphoedema. Simply giving these patients a 'diagnosis' can have enormous psychological benefit as it can relieve guilt that they are simply fat and should try harder to lose weight.

Cellulite

- Cellulite is a condition of unknown aetiology in which underlying fat deposits give the skin a dimpled lumpy appearance.[7] It is most noticeable on the buttocks and thighs and usually occurs in women after puberty. Histology shows discrete perivascular lymphocitic infiltrates in the dermis with oedematous collagen fibres, reduced elastin and oedematous intercellular matrix. Dermal lymphatic vessels are usually visibly distended, subcutaneous fat cells appear enlarged and adipose tissue septae show a normal structure but some oedema. Interlobular septae are arranged vertically in women but horizontally and diagonally in men, which may allow dermal fat protrusion. No physical or dietary treatment has been shown to be of benefit.

Myxoedema

- Myxoedema from hypothyroidism has a similar appearance to lymphoedema, but the skin is more dry, rough, cool and pale, with coarse hair and hair loss. Oedema is non-pitting due to infiltration with glycosoaminoglycans. It is most common around the pre-tibial area of the legs.

History

- Sculptures on the façade of Queen Hatasu's temple at Deir el-Bahri in Egypt, carved nearly 3500 years ago record her voyage to Somalia and show her being greeted by the Prince and his wife Princess Ati who was clearly suffering from lymphoedema.[8]

- The first account of lymphoedema now attributed to filariasis is found in the Ebers Papyrus written in about 1550 BC. It is speculated that the soldiers of Alexander the Great returning from India spread it to Southern Europe and Northern Africa, that the Crusaders brought it to Western and Northern Europe, and that it was later introduced to the Americas through the slave trade from Africa.
- Aulus Cornelius Celsus (25 BC–50 AD) is credited with first use of the term elephantiasis, followed by the Persian physicians Ali Ben Abbas (930–994) and Avicenna (980–1037). The cause was unknown but its endemic occurrence was well-recognized.
- Otto Wuchereria (1820–1873) and Joseph Bancroft (1836–1894) gave their names to the parasite Wuchereria bancrofti that causes filariasis.
- William Halstead (1852–1922), surgeon at Johns Hopkins Hospital in Baltimore, reported the first cases of surgically-induced lymphoedema.

References

1. Consensus document of the International Society of Lymphology. The diagnosis and treatment of peripheral lymphedema. *2013 Lymphology* 2013;46:1–11. http://www.u.arizona.edu/~witte/2013consensus.pdf

2. Position statement of the National Lymphoedema Network. The diagnosis and treatment of lymphoedema. 2011. http://www.lymphnet.org/pdfDocs/nlntreatment.pdf

3. Lee BB, Antignani PL, Baroncelli TA, Boccardo FM, Brorson H, Campisi C, Damstra RJ et al. IUA-ISVI consensus for diagnosis guideline of chronic lymphedema of the limbs. *Int Angiol* 2015;34:311–32. https://pdfs.semanticscholar.org/3d5f/468d9a281d592 23ca1d2d3e8bc6fe96a5024.pdf

4. Feldman JL. Hereditary lymphoedema. National organization for rare diseases. 2015. https://rarediseases.org/rare-diseases/hereditary-lymphedema/

5. Connell F, Brice G, Mansour S, Mortimer P. Presentation of childhood lymphoedema. *J Lymphoedema* 2009;4:65–72. http://www.woundsinternational.com/media/issues/849/files/content_11171.pdf

6. Olszewski WL, Cwikla JB, Zaleska M, Domaszewska-Szostek A, Gradalski T, Szopinska S. Where do lymph and tissue fluid flow during intermittent pneumatic massage of lower limbs with obstructive lymphoedema? *Phlebolymphology* 2011;18:188–95. http://www.phlebolymphology.org/where-do-lymph-and-tissue-fluid-flow-during-intermittent-pneumatic-massage-of-lower-limbs-with-obstructive-lymphedema/

7. Afonso JPQM, Tucunduva TC, Pinheiro MVB, Bagatin E. Cellulite: A review. *Surg Cosmet Dermatol* 2010;2:214–9. http://www.surgicalcosmetic.org.br/detalhe-artigo/82/Celulite--artigo-de-revisao

8. Hajdu SI. A note from history: Elephantiasis. *Ann Clin Lab Science* 2002;32:207–209. http://citeseerx.ist.psu.edu/viewdoc/download?doi=10.1.1.505.375&rep=rep1&type=pdf

19 Lymphoedema – investigation and treatment

Written with Neil Piller

> This chapter includes recommendations from the Union Internationale de Phlebologie, and position statements from National and International lymphoedema groups.[1-6]

Investigations

- Diagnosis is usually based on clinical assessment. Imaging is rarely needed to diagnose lymphoedema but can be used to confirm the diagnosis and assess its extent and severity.
- Blood tests may be required to help exclude other underlying events or disorders.
- Plain X-rays are performed if there are suspected associated bony abnormalities. CT or MR imaging and ultrasound may be performed to diagnose or exclude regional pathology that might be causing secondary or high-output lymphoedema. They may also be used to examine tissue characteristics.
- Lymphangiography was once the front-line investigation but is now rarely used because of potential adverse effects.
- Lymphoscintigraphy is the standard diagnostic technique to define anatomy and patency, evaluate flow dynamics and functional lymphatic status and determine the severity of obstruction.
- Fluorescence micro-lymphography is less invasive than lymphoscintigraphy and is increasingly being used to demonstrate smaller and more superficial lymphatics and to indicate their functional status.
- Biopsy is occasionally required.

Lymphoscintigraphy

- This technique is relatively non-invasive, involves only a low dose of irradiation and has no known significant adverse effects.[7] However, the technique has not been standardized, with use of various radioisotopes and doses, one or more intra-dermal or subcutaneous injection sites, varying protocols for passive and active physical activity and different imaging times. The technique provides good imaging for both lymphatics and lymph nodes with quantitative and qualitative information relating to lymph transport and the major deep and superficial pathways. Lymphoscintigraphy is particularly helpful to investigate chronic oedema of uncertain origin and to assess clinically diagnosed primary lymphoedema.
- A lymphoscintogram ideally must be 'loaded' following some form of exercise. Filtered Tc99 albumin suspended in saline, is introduced by intradermal injection into the web space between the first and second toes or fingers to create a wheal, and the region is massaged for two minutes immediately after injection. A high-resolution collimator is used to give images at 10, 40 and 160 minutes. The time for radionuclide to arrive at the knees, groin or other areas of interest in the lower limbs or elbows and axillae in the upper limbs is

recorded. Normally whole body images are also obtained. It normally takes about 45 minutes to travel from toes to the inguinal region and about 15 minutes to travel from the fingers to the axilla, but these times vary considerably depending on the many factors described above. Ideally, lymphoscintigraphy is undertaken bilaterally and the sides compared if a unilateral situation is being assessed.

- In the lower limbs, there should be symmetric migration of the radionuclide seen through three to five lymph vessels in the calf and one to two vessels in the thigh. Typically, approximately one to three popliteal lymph nodes and two to ten ilio-inguinal nodes are then seen, and ilio-inguinal nodes should be apparent within one hour for the lower limbs.
- Dermal backflow is the hallmark sign of lymphatic obstruction on lymphoscintigraphy.
  Dermal backflow with a spreading blush rather than linear spread along the limb is diagnostic of obstruction, particularly if seen in the popliteal or inguinal region. Disease is present if inguinal lymph nodes cannot be seen. The examination looks for flow obstruction, collateral lymph vessels, dermal backflow, delayed flow, lymphocoeles, delayed visualization or non-visualization of lymph nodes, a reduced number of lymph nodes, dilated lymphatics, thoracic duct obstruction or leakage. In severe cases, the nucleotide may not leave the injection site, indicating no lymphatic system function.
- Primary lymphoedema cannot be reliably differentiated from secondary lymphoedema on the basis of lymphoscintigraphy alone.

Indocyanine green lymphography (fluorescence microlymphography)

- This demonstrates smaller, more superficial lymphatic vessels. Indocyanine green is injected intradermally and followed up draining lymphatic pathways under fluorescent lighting. It binds to all proteins, especially albumin, and fluouresces green when exposed to 760 nm near infrared light. Its advantages allow for examination of drainage live and from any angle, and it is well suited to intra-operative use. It can give live guidance to lymph drainage direction, pathways, areas of blockage and dermal back-flow, and helps guide techniques involving manual lymphatic drainage. Its limitation is that it cannot be used to observe lymph vessels more than 2 cm deep in subcutaneous tissues.
- Indocyanine green lymphography has allowed a staging scale for lymphoedema to be developed:
  - Stage 0: Many patent lymphatic vessels, no dermal backflow, normal contractility.
  - Stage 1: Many patent lymphatic vessels, minimal patchy dermal backflow, slightly delayed contractility.
  - Stage 2: Moderate patent lymphatic vessels, segmental dermal backflow, moderately delayed contractility.
  - Stage 3: Few patent lymphatic vessels, extensive dermal backflow involving the entire limb, minimal contractility.
  - Stage 4: No patent lymphatic vessels, severe dermal backflow in the entire limb and dorsum extending to the digits (finger/toe sign) and volar (palm/sole sign), no contractility.
  - Stage 5: No patent lymphatic vessels, no dye movement, no contractility.

Lymphangiography

- This invasive investigation is now seldom needed for diagnosis, but is occasionally used for differential diagnosis or to identify precise sites of disease, such as chylous leakage or thoracic duct injury. It can be used to refine a diagnosis prior to surgical or other invasive treatments.

Volume plethysmography

- Volume change due to disease progression or response to treatment can be monitored by measuring water volume displaced by a submerged limb. It is an older but reliable technique although care must be taken to avoid cross-infection between patients. The technique measures total limb volume including fat, muscle, fluids and bone.

Measuring both limbs when investigating unilateral disease allows a controlled comparison.

Bio-impedance spectroscopy

- Bio-impedance spectroscopy can be used to measure water content in tissues. The test is performed by passing a small painless electrical current through the limb to measure the resistance or tissue impedance. Low frequencies only travel in the extracellular fluid and high frequencies travel in both extracellular and intracellular fluid. The higher the water content in interstitial tissue, the lower the impedance. The technique is not as accurate with advanced fibrotic oedema and cannot differentiate lymphoedema from other types of oedema. However, it is an excellent technique to indicate the impact of lymphoedema treatments and is much more accurate than serial measurements of limb circumference. It can provide an indication of total limb fluids or segmental limb fluids. It provides an accurate quantitative measure that is frequently used after breast cancer surgery.

Tissue dielectric constants

- This technique can measure the levels of fluids at specific points in the tissues, normally at specific points within each major lymphatic territory. Fluids at depths of up to 3 cm or more can be detected using various size heads.

Tonometry/indurometry

- These techniques can be used to measure the extent of fibrotic tissue accumulation at specific points within each lymphatic territory. They work by applying a pressure to the tissues, physically or electronically, and measuring the resistance to compression. They can be used in concert with ultrasound.

Biopsy

- Regional lymph node biopsy in a patient with long-standing lymphoedema can aggravate distal swelling and fine needle aspiration biopsy may be preferred. However, sentinel node biopsy in the groin or axilla to stage breast cancer or melanoma, respectively, without removal of normal lymph nodes, is appropriate.
- Skin biopsies are sometimes required to diagnose local complications.

Principles of treatment

- Proactivity to attempt early diagnosis of lymphoedema is critical. Detection of pre-clinical lymphatic failure when there is little or no change in limb volume or circumference is possible with current diagnostic techniques described above. This allows earlier, more conservative and less onerous treatment. Unfortunately, many clinicians still wait until there is clinically detectable increase in size, volume and composition of the affected lymphatic territory, making treatment more intensive, time-consuming and costly.
- The goal is to preserve function, reduce physical and psychologic suffering and prevent skin damage and infection. For secondary lymphoedema, the underlying pathology must also be treated. Other co-existing factors which may add to lymph load should also ideally be dealt with first. These include hypertension management, kidney or liver issues, medications check and thyroid function check.
- For newly presenting patients, treatment should be commenced early before irreversible interstitial fibrosclerotic changes develop. Most patients can be successfully managed by conservative measures although treatment may need to persist throughout their lifetime. Strict compliance is required even though treatment may be uncomfortable and inconvenient.
- In the neonate, initial parental observation alone may be sufficient, as delayed lymphatic development can result in spontaneous improvement. Treatment in children is by intense conservative measures avoiding surgery. Adult patients, and often their partners or carers, should be encouraged to be actively involved in management.

- The intensity and sequencing for treating lymphoedema largely depends on the clinical stage, but also on the patient's age and general health. Generally, there is an early intensive treatment phase followed by a management phase.
  - Stage I is generally adequately managed by exercise, skin care and appropriate compression garments.
  - Stage II requires higher levels of management, usually with addition of manual lymphatic drainage techniques.
  - Stage III requires intensive treatment, often from a range of health professionals under supervision.

General measures

- Aim to target and sequence treatment and be as pro-active as possible.
- Elevate the limb whenever possible. Raise the foot of the bed at night, although straight leg raising can impede popliteal drainage, as with venous disease. Avoid constrictive clothing or bandages or garments which exert a tourniquet effect on the groin, knee area or ankles, or the wrist, elbow or upper arm.
- Aim for a diet which can manage any weight issues. Ideally involve a dietician or nutritionist. Seek advice about the benefits of an anti-inflammatory diet – one richer in omega3 and plant products rather than meat products with high omega6 content.
- Provide education for risk identification and reduction, such as avoiding trauma and treating wounds early. Manage cardiac, renal and other co-morbid conditions.
- Provide genetic counselling for families that include a patient with primary lymphoedema.
- Arrange for rehabilitation if severe lymphoedema impairs daily activities. Provide psychological counselling, pain management and palliative care for advanced disease if required.

Decongestive lymphatic therapy

- Decongestive lymphatic therapy may be required regardless of whether lymphoedema is primary or secondary. It consists of exercise, skin care, manual lymphatic drainage and compression. Trained lymphoedema therapists come from physiotherapy, occupational therapy and nursing professions.

Exercise

- Exercise promotes lymphatic and venous drainage and maintains joint mobility. Exercise machines may help establish a regular program. Hydrotherapy is an excellent means to provide gentle repetitive exercise while applying some external pressure in a graded fashion. Exercise classes are a means for establishing a routine using techniques such as Pilates. Deep breathing promotes lymphatic flow.
- Initially, supervision by a physiotherapist is of benefit. Structured exercise should supplement normal regular activities such as walking. Swimming, cycling and low-impact aerobics are recommended, while heavy lifting exercises should be avoided. Flexibility exercises are advised to maintain joint mobility. Motivation for self-management is essential.

Skin care

- Give advice about preventing skin trauma. Avoid phlebotomy, intravenous catheterization or vaccination in the affected limb.
- Remove keratin debris and surface bacteria. This is particularly important if there is hyperkeratosis, dryness or skin sensitivity. Clean and dry the skin regularly and inspect to detect minor wounds or early infection. Take particular care between the toes and fingers.
- Simple moisturisers such as glycerine prevent skin cracking and dramatically reduce infection risk as they increase the barrier to the external environment. Topical emollients and keratolytics stabilize skin; ammonium lactate 5% lotion decreases scaling and pruritus, while topical urea preparations promote hydration and remove excess keratin.

Manual lymphatic drainage

- Manual lymphatic drainage stimulates lymph transport by moving accumulated fluids, opening collateral lymph pathways and reducing fibrosclerosis. It is most effective when started in the early stages. Introduction immediately after treatment for breast cancer and other tumours may reduce the severity and perhaps the incidence of subsequent secondary lymphoedema.
- Manual lymphatic drainage by massage aims to progressively move fluid from more distal to proximal sites. Various techniques are advocated, but they have several features in common. Ideally, a session should last for about one hour, performed at least daily, for a course of up to three weeks. Manual lymphatic drainage should commence with a deep breathing program to clear the abdominal and thoracic lymphatics and prepare them for fluid delivery from the more distal sites.
- Gentle massage commences above the region of interest then works from proximal to distal to progressively move fluid out of the region. Massage must be gentle to avoid risk of trauma to lymphatics, and is slow, light and rhythmical aided by deep breathing. Excessive pressure stimulates blood flow to cause hyperaemia and further fluid accumulation.
- Manual lymphatic drainage should be avoided if there is infection in the region or if there is occlusive peripheral arterial disease. However, a theoretical risk of promoting metastasis from dormant tumours with secondary lymphoedema is usually far outweighed by the benefits.
- The aim is to teach the patient, partner or carer to perform simple lymphatic drainage, which is a modified form of the professionally performed manual lymphatic drainage. However, not all are sufficiently dexterous or motivated to learn the techniques.
- Manual lymphatic drainage should always be combined with compression if possible, but may be the only option if compression is not feasible, for example with oedema affecting the breast, trunk or genitalia.
- Various massage pads and vibrating devices that may help promote lymph drainage are also available, but patients should seek health professional advice before their use.

Compression

- Principles underlying compression using bandages, stockings, other devices or a pneumatic pump have been discussed in Chapter 11.[4] It is important to realize that chronic lymphoedema requires constant compression, and that if it is discontinued then oedema will rapidly re-appear. The combination of compression and manual lymphatic drainage is considerably more effective than either alone.
- Multiple layers of short-stretch bandages with 50% overlap and 50% stretch to cover the entire limb are used at first. Any part of the limbs can be bandaged including fingers and toes, and compression gloves and socks are also available.
- For severe or stubborn lymphoedema, multi-layer bandages or double stockings increase compression, and wearing garments for 24 hours a day reduces rebound oedema. Multi-layer bandaging is particularly indicated if there are wounds, lymphorrhoea or skin problems. However, they usually need to be applied by an experienced practitioner, for poorly applied bandages can do more harm than good, with the biggest problem being a potential tourniquet effect with a reverse pressure gradient.
- Bandages tend to slip if left for longer than 24 hours, particularly as oedema is controlled, so that prolonged treatment can cause logistical management problems. It is here that Velcro devices with adjustable straps enable patient self-management, thus easing the demand on specialist services and allowing more frequent attention to skin care. This continuing adjustment is very important, for otherwise once some fluid is removed then resultant compression declines and further drainage ceases leading to a sub-optimal result.
- Low stretch elastic garments are then required for long-term use. These may be

below- or above-knee stockings for lower limbs, above-elbow sleeves for upper limbs, bras, compression shorts,or face or neck compression wear, depending on the part affected (Figure 19.1). They should be as tight as can be tolerated, preferably grade III (>40 mm Hg) for the lower limbs. However, there must always be a compression gradient for an optimal outcome.

- Garments need to be measured for size or custom-made, and fitted when oedema is best controlled ensuring that they are comfortable. They should have graduated compression on the affected limb that increases from distal to proximal, but with no tourniquet effect. Two pairs are required, one to wear while the other dries after washing. Compression garments for children must be replaced to allow for growth, usually several times each year for young children and babies.

- Patients should use compression garments continuously during the day. They may be removed at night when the extremity is elevated in bed but should be replaced promptly each morning after the proximal lymphatic territories and collectors are emptied by a gentle slow deep breathing program.

- Intermittent pneumatic compression with a sequential gradient pump is of particular value for elderly patients, those confined to bed or those who have a disability that limits self-management. It is thought to act by reducing capillary filtration and lymph formation rather than by increasing lymph outflow. Recommended pump pressures generally range from 30–60 mm Hg adjusted according to the skin condition and pain tolerance, and each treatment session is usually for one hour. A compression garment or short-stretch bandages should be worn between pump treatments to maintain oedema control. Care must be taken to avoid development of a fibrosclerotic ring above the pump which would exacerbate lymph flow obstruction.

Measuring for compression garments

- These are manufactured in several size combinations which hopefully will cater for

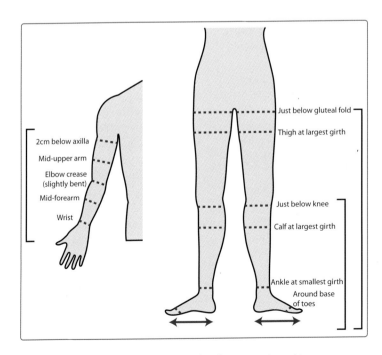

Figure 19.1 Measurements for sleeves and stockings.

most patients. If possible, measure in the morning when the limb is least swollen, and if the limb is swollen then elevate it for a time. Try to measure lower limb garments with the patient standing.

- Measurements to select the best size should be taken by a trained fitter where possible. If the garment is too tight, the patient will be uncomfortable and unlikely to wear it all day. If it is too loose, the patient will spend all day pulling it up.
- If measurements are at the very end of the size scale, there will be minimal stretch left in the garment and it is best to move up to the next size. This will still give the correct compression, but it will be more comfortable and easier to put on.
- If the patient is very elderly or has poor muscle strength, start with a lower compression garment. Once the patient is used to it, you may be able to introduce a higher compression if needed.
- If the patient has poor muscle strength, consider use of two light compression garments, one over the other, as each is easier to put on and take off, leading to better compliance.
- Advise the patient to wear the garment for a couple of hours a day at first, then gradually increase the time as the patient gets accustomed to wearing it.

Pharmacologic therapy

Vaso-active drugs

- The efficacy of pharmacologic therapies is uncertain.
- Benzopyrones including coumarin and flavonoids are believed to bind to accumulated interstitial proteins inducing macrophage phagocytosis and proteolysis so that resulting protein fragments are removed through venous capillaries and lymphatics. Hepatotoxicity has been reported in up to 6% of patients taking coumarin.
- Oral and topical retinoids may help normalize keratinization and decrease inflammatory and fibrotic changes.

Antimicrobials

- A course of antibiotics is required for acute lymph stasis-related cellulitis or lymphangitis with both local and systemic evidence of infection. Long-term prophylaxis is used for recurring episodes of infection. Consider using a beta-lactamase-resistant antibiotic that is effective against gram-positive organisms.
- Fungal infection, which is a common association with lymphoedema, is treated with a topical or systemic antimycotic drug.
- Lymphatic filariasis is treated with anthelmintic agents as well as broad-spectrum antibiotics to counter secondary bacterial infection.

Other drugs and agents

- Diuretics are not effective for treating lymphoedema. They may only have a role for oedema of systemic origin.
- No gene therapy for hereditary lymphoedema is available as yet.

Surgery

- Surgery for lymphoedema in the past has generally been considered as a final option, but practice now is to consider some procedures at an earlier stage.[6]
- Surgical treatment is palliative and not curative, and compliance with life-long compression after surgery is the most important factor for ensuring lasting success.
- Surgery is considered if a multidisciplinary team concludes that there has been steady progression of disease despite maximum conservative treatment over an arbitrary two-year period. However, reconstructive surgery may be considered earlier before fibrotic changes have developed in the lymphatics.
- Treatment of secondary lymphoedema commences with managing its cause.

Lymphatic reconstructive surgery

- Lympho-venous anastomosis by microsurgery is best used in the early stages of lymphoedema prior to development and progression to the fatty fibrous stages where lymph vessels may become fibrotic. Venous–lymphatic anastomosis surgery is most effective for secondary lymphoedema. The capacity for these operations is limited by the small number of centres with sufficient expertise to perform them.

- Surgery may require lymphatic–venous, lymphatic–lymphatic and lymphatic–venous–lymphatic anastomoses. Lymphatic–venous anastomosis may involve an interposition autologous vein graft between lymphatics above and below the lymphatic obstruction. Free lymph node transplant surgery is a controversial procedure with questions being asked about its impact on the node donation site.
- Other physiologic surgical procedures have been used to attempt to promote lymphatic drainage, including omental transposition, buried dermal flaps and entero-mesenteric bridging.

Excisional surgery

- Surgical debulking is required for a limb that is so large that it restricts daily activities and prevents successful conservative management. Debulking is also required if there is significant fibrotic induration or increased frequency or severity of infections.
- Various excisional procedures have been described. The Charles procedure* in the lower limb involves radical excision of affected subcutaneous tissue down to the deep fascia, after which the area is covered with skin grafts taken from the resected specimen. Successful outcomes have been reported, but the operation is rarely performed due to complications, including skin graft breakdown, nerve damage, late skin complications, poor cosmetic result and worsening of foot oedema distal to the operation site.
- Staged excision is now the option of choice. This involves removing only a portion of

skin and subcutaneous tissue, followed by primary closure. After approximately three months, the procedure is repeated on a different area of the extremity. This procedure is safe and reliable and demonstrates the most consistent improvement, with the lowest incidence of complications.

- Liposuction can remove associated fat deposition and has been reported to be effective for secondary upper limb lymphoedema following mastectomy and more recently for lower limb lymphoedema. It is of doubtful benefit for primary lymphoedema because of technical difficulties due to associated subcutaneous fibrosis. Bulk excision is necessary once fibrosis has set in. Redundant skin excision can remove foci of infection.

Outcome of treatment

- Prior to treatment, and at intervals after, documentation includes photography, tape measurements and limb volume by water displacement, ideally obtained in the morning after elevation of the limb in bed overnight.
- Serial measurements by bio-impedance spectroscopy and tissue dielectric constants can provide an objective measure of response.

References

1. Lee BB, Antignani PL, Baroncelli TA, Boccardo FM, Brorson H, Campisi C, Damstra RJ et al. IUA-ISVI consensus for diagnosis guideline of chronic lymphedema of the limbs. *Int Angiol* 2015;34:311–32. https://pdfs.semanticscholar.org/3d5f/468d9a281d592 23ca1d2d3e8bc6fe96a5024.pdf
2. Consensus document of the International Society of Lymphology. The diagnosis and treatment of peripheral lymphedema. *2013 Lymphology* 2013;46:1–11. http://www.u.arizona.edu/~witte/2013consensus.pdf
3. Position statement of the National Lymphoedema Network. The diagnosis and treatment of lymphoedema. 2011. http://www.lymphnet.org/pdfDocs/nlntreatment.pdf
4. Moffatt C, Partsch H, Schuren J, Quéré I, Sneddon M, Flour M, Towers A et al. International lymphoedema framework position document. Compression therapy: A position document on

---

* Richard Charles described an operation for scrotal lymphoedema in 1901. Archibald McIndoe mistakenly attributed a similar operation in the lower limb to Charles in 1950.

compression bandaging. 2012. http://www.soffed.co.uk/lymphorg/wp-content/uploads/2016/03/Compression-bandaging-final.pdf

5. Cormier J, Damstra R, Brorson H, Suami H, Chang D. International lymphoedema framework position document. Surgical intervention: A position document on surgery for lymphoedema. 2012. http://www.soffed.co.uk/lymphorg/wp-content/uploads/2016/03/Surgery-final.pdf

6. Moffatt C, Doherty D, Morgan P. Best practice for the management of lymphoedema. *International Consensus* 2006. http://www.soffed.co.uk/lymphorg/wp-content/uploads/2016/03/Best_practice.pdf

7. Keeley V. The use of lymphoscintigraphy in the management of chronic oedema. *J Lymphoedema* 2006;1:42–57. http://www.journaloflymphoedema.com/media/issues/757/files/content_11075.pdf

20 Haemostasis and fibrinolysis

This chapter incorporates recommendations from an international consensus statement on the prevention and treatment of venous thromboembolism.[1]

Haemostasis

- Haemostasis is the response to stop bleeding following injury to a blood vessel.[2] It involves simultaneous primary haemostasis due to vasoconstriction and adhesion of platelets, and secondary haemostasis by initiation of a coagulation cascade. Both are controlled by blood cells and endothelial cells. Normally, there is a balance between factors that activate haemostasis and inhibitors that prevent excess thrombus propagation to avoid pathological thrombosis or bleeding. Venous thrombo-embolism (VTE) may be manifest as deep vein thrombosis (DVT) and pulmonary embolism (PE).

Primary haemostasis

- The initial stages involve interactions between the vessel wall and platelets resulting in vessel wound closure within a few seconds by a white platelet-rich clot.

The blood vessel wall

- Endothelial cells are normally anti-thrombotic due to negatively charged heparin-like glycosaminoglycans such as heparan sulphate and phospholipids, platelet and coagulation inhibitors and fibrinolysis activators.
- The sub-endothelial layer is normally pro-thrombotic due to collagen, von Willebrand factor and chemicals involved in platelet adhesion. Endothelial trauma also causes exposed tissue to become pro-thrombotic due to secretion of platelet-activating agents and fibrinolysis inhibitors.
- Smooth muscle cells in the media respond to trauma by vasospasm induced by a local sympathetic response, and by release of endothelin and platelet-derived thromboxane A2.

Platelet function

- Platelets are discoid fragments of cytoplasm with no cell nucleus, and are derived from megakaryocytes in the bone marrow. Blood normally contains $150–450 \times 10^9$/L and they circulate for about ten days.
- The platelet membrane produces thromboxane A2, the glycoproteins GPIb/IX/X, GPVI and GPIIb/IIIa and phospholipids, which are cofactors for platelet procoagulant activity through protein kinase C and phospholipase A2.
- The platelet receptor integrin GPIIb/IIIa plays a critical role in mediating interaction with fibrinogen to cause platelet adhesion. It has two components – αIIb (GPIIb) and β3 (GPIIIa) which form a combined receptor for fibrin and von Willebrand factor under ADP control.
- Platelets contain two types of granules:
  - α granules contain adhesive proteins including P-selectin, pro-thrombotic factors including von Willebrand factor, factor VIII, factor V, fibrinogen and fibronectin and proinflammatory factors, including platelet factor IV, platelet-derived growth factor and tumour growth factor-α

- δ granules contain adenosine diphosphate, calcium, serotonin, histamine and epinephrine
- Platelet microparticles appear when haemostasis is activated and with inflammation, malignancy, angiogenesis and immune reactions.[3] Some 80% are derived from platelets and the rest from megakaryocytes. They have surface antigens and participate in cell adhesion, thromboxane-2 production and generation of small amounts of thrombin.
- The von Willebrand factor[*] is a glycoprotein synthesized by endothelial cells, platelets and megakaryocytes. It acts as a carrier protein for factor VIII preventing its proteolytic degradation in plasma, and as an adhesive protein essential for platelet-endothelium adhesion. It is initially synthesised as high molecular weight molecules that are degraded by the metalloprotease ADAMTS13. It is a principal adhesive protein binding to a glycoprotein Ib-IX-V receptor complex on the platelet surface.
- Thromboxane A2 is produced in platelets from prostaglandin H2 under the control of its enzyme thromboxane-A synthase.

Platelet aggregation

- Loss of the endothelial barrier exposes sub-endothelial collagen and von Willebrand factor to the blood stream. This causes circulating platelets to become activated, progressively adhere to sub-endothelial structures and to each other, and aggregate to form a platelet plug. Activated platelets change from a discoid to a spherical shape with pseudopods that increase their active surface area.
- The platelet membrane secretes thromboxane A2 which facilitates platelet aggregation through the glycoprotein complex GP IIb/IIIa. Thromboxane A2 and platelet activating factor bind to receptors on other platelet membranes leading to new platelet recruitment. Von Willebrand factor forms additional links between the platelets' glycoprotein Ib/

IX/V and collagen fibrils and platelet activation exposes binding sites for activated GPIIb/IIIa and fibrinogen to cause platelet aggregation.
- Activated platelet granules secrete agonists, chemotaxins, clotting factors and vasoconstrictors, and these promote platelet aggregation, thrombin generation and vasospasm. Platelet granules activate phospholipase A_2 which increases membrane glycoprotein IIb/IIIa and the ability to bind fibrinogen.
- Interactions of adenosine diphosphate with platelet receptors and thromboxane receptors activate the GP IIb/IIIa receptors. Subsequent binding of fibrinogen and von Willebrand factor to activated GP IIb/IIIa receptors leads to irreversible platelet aggregation and a stable clot, strengthened by circulating fibrinogen (Figure 20.1).
- Prostacyclin inhibits platelet aggregation, and its balance with thromboxane A-2 constrains platelet aggregation to restrict clot extension.
- The final structure of a clot utilizes the platelet's GIIb/IIIa receptor to simultaneously bind fibrinogen, platelets and subendothelial von Willibrand factor.

Secondary haemostasis

- The traditional account of the coagulation cascade involves a dominant extrinsic pathway and a less significant intrinsic pathway which converge to a common pathway to activate factor X. They are now better referred to as the tissue factor and contact activation pathways, respectively. Clotting factors and their inhibitors are shown in Figure 20.2 and listed in Table 20.1; note the long half-life of factors II, IX and X, and short half-life of protein C.

The coagulation cascade

- Most clotting factors and their inhibitors are synthesized in the liver. However, tissue factor is found in extravascular cells, and factors V, XI and XIII are also found in platelets. Factors II, VII, IX and X need

---

[*] Erik Adolf von Willebrand (1870–1949), a physician from Finland.

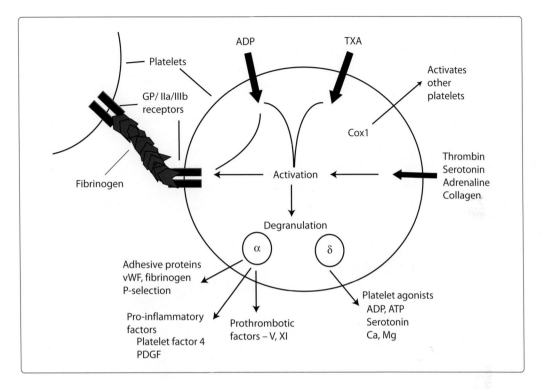

Figure 20.1 Mechanisms for platelet adhesion.

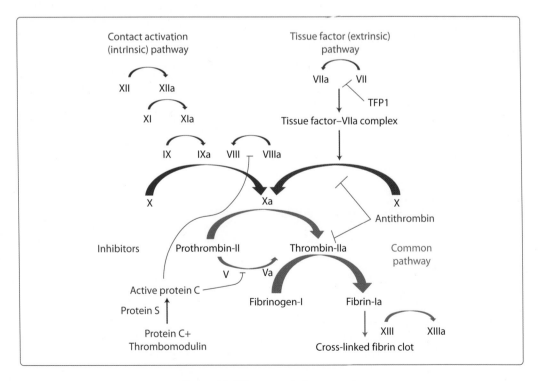

Figure 20.2 The coagulation cascade.

Table 20.1 Coagulation factors and inhibitors

	Factor name	Nature	Function	Half life
Coagulation factors				
FI	Fibrinogen	Glycoprotein	Substrate for clot formation	4 days
FII	Prothrombin	Serine protease	Precursor thrombin	60 hours
FIII	Tissue factor	Cytokine receptor	Initiates clotting	<30 mins.
(FIV)	Calcium	Element	Facilitates binding to phospholipids	–
FV	Proaccelerin, labile factor	Cofactor – not an enzyme	Cofactor for FX-prothrominase complex	12–36 hours
FVII	Proconvertin, stable factor	Serine protease	Activates FIX and FX	5–6 hours
FVIII	Antihaemophilic factor A	Glycoprotein	Cofactor of FIX-tenase complex	8–12 hours
FIX	Antihaemophilic factor B Christmas factor	Serine protease	Activates FX	24 hours
FX	Stuart–Prower factor	Serine protease	Activates prothrombin	40 hours
FXI	Plasma thromboplastin antecedant	Serine protease	Activates FIX	45 hours
FXII	Hageman factor	Serine protease	Activates FIX, FVII and prekallikrein	40–50 hours
FXIII	Fibrin stabilizing factor	Transglutaminase	Cross-links fibrin	8–10 days
	Kininogen and Prekallikrein	Proteins	Cofactors	7 days
Coagulation inhibitors				
	Von Willebrand factor	Glycoprotein	Binds to FVIII, mediates platelet adhesion	9–15 hours
	Antithrombin III	Glycoprotein	Inhibits FIIa and FXa	3–4 days
	Protein C	Serine protease	Inhibits FVa and FVIIIa	6–10 hours
	Protein S	Glycoprotein	Cofactor for protein C	80 hours
	Heparin co-factor II	Protein	Inhibits FIIa	1–2 hours
	Thrombomodulin	Protein	Cofactor – modifies thrombin	8–10 hours

vitamin K to be fully active, as do proteins C and S.

- Control mechanisms exist to localize fibrin formation to the site of injury. Protein C when activated by its cofactor protein S inactivates the cofactors VIIIa and Va. Antithrombin inhibits thrombin and factor Xa as well as FIXa and FXIa. Tissue factor pathway inhibitor and alpha-2-macroglobulin inhibit FXa and thrombin. Other serine protease inhibitors are heparin cofactor II (thrombin inhibitor), protein Z-dependent protease inhibitor (FXa inhibitor) and C1-inhibitor (FXIa inhibitor).
- Although the tissue factor pathway is much stronger than the contact pathway, and they are difficult to distinguish.

Contact activation pathway

- Prekallikrein is converted to kallikrein, and FXII is activated to start this pathway. FXI is formed which when activated produces FIX then FX. FVIII is a cofactor for FIXa which in the presence of calcium and phospholipids, forms the intrinsic tenase complex that converts FX to FXa to initiate clotting.

Tissue factor pathway

- Normal endothelium physically separates extravascular tissue factor from circulating FVII to prevent inappropriate activation of the clotting cascade.[4] Breakage of the endothelial barrier leads to release of tissue factor which activates FVII, which in turn activates FX where the extrinsic and intrinsic pathways converge leading to rapid activation of the clotting cascade.
- Small amounts of tissue factor are also present in blood in microparticles and these levels increase in various diseases such as sepsis and cancer, which may contribute to thrombosis associated with these diseases.

Common pathway

- The prothrombinase complex consists of FXa and FVa bound to phospholipid membranes in the presence of calcium ions. This complex converts prothrombin (FII) to thrombin (FIIa) which then converts fibrinogen to fibrin strands that form the scaffold for the thrombus. FXIII (fibrin stabilizing factor) crosslinks fibrin strands to give strength to the clot.
- The coagulation cascade is now described as having four phases.

Initiation

- Tissue factor released from a damaged vessel binds FVIIa to activate FIX and FX, and FXa binds to FII to form thrombin. However, the amount of thrombin initially generated is not sufficient to form a clot.

Amplification

- Feedback loops bind thrombin with platelets to further activate FV and FVIII. FVIII is a cofactor in the prothrombinase complex and accelerates activation of FII by FXa and of FXa by FIXa.

Propagation

- Accumulated enzyme complexes on platelet surfaces support strong thrombin generation and platelet activation which ensures continuous generation of thrombin and subsequently fibrin to form a sufficiently large clot.

Stabilization

- Thrombin generation leads to activation of the fibrin stabilizing FXIII which links fibrin polymers and provides strength and stability to the clot. FXIIIa begins stabilizing fibrin polymers before a visible thrombus appears as this requires conversion of at least 20% of fibrinogen into fibrin.
- Fibrin clots are attached to collagen types I, II, III, and V in the vessel wall by FXIIIa, a reaction that may prevent the clot from being dislodged from the wall. Thrombin also activates thrombin activatable fibrinolysis inhibitor which protects the clot from fibrinolysis.
- Fibrin forms a mesh of long strands of tough insoluble protein that are bound to platelets. The fibrin clot appears within about 60 seconds and the process is complete within several minutes. Low flow venous clots are red as they contain many erythrocytes while high flow arterial thrombi tend to be white as they contain predominantly platelets.

Coagulation tests

- The coagulation phase can be tested by the activated partial thromboplastin time, prothrombin time and thrombin time. These measure the time elapsed from different points in the activation of the cascade to the generation of fibrin.

Activated partial thromboplastin time (aPPT)

- The aPTT measures the efficacy of both the intrinsic and common coagulation pathways. The test is termed partial due to absence of tissue factor from the reaction mixture. It determines the time to generate fibrin from initiation of the intrinsic pathway by activation of FXII. This requires an external agent which was traditionally kaolin although automated analysers now use micronized silica. It also requires the presence of a phospholipid emulsion that takes the place of platelet factors.

- The normal aPTT is less than 20–35 seconds. The test is abnormal for any of the inherited or acquired factor deficiencies in the intrinsic and common pathways. A prolonged aPTT that cannot be completely returned to normal with addition of normal plasma indicates the presence of a circulating inhibitor of coagulation such as therapeutic heparin or lupus anticoagulant.

Prothrombin time (PT) and International Normalized Ratio (INR)

- The PT measures the integrity of the extrinsic and common pathways. It determines the time to generate fibrin after activation through factors VII, V, X, prothrombin and fibrinogen. Citrated plasma is incubated at 37°C with tissue factor as an activating agent in the presence of calcium, and the time is measured until fibrin filaments are seen.
- The normal prothrombin time is 8–14 seconds. As with aPTT, a prolonged PT may reflect either factor deficiency or a circulating inhibitor of coagulation, and the distinction is again made by repeating the test after mixing with normal plasma.
- The International Normalized Ratio (INR) is where the PT is adjusted by a factor between 0.9 and 3 to standardize the activity of a manufacturer's tissue factor against that set by the World Health Organization.

Thrombin time

- This test measures the time to drive the reaction of fibrinogen to fibrin in the presence of thrombin. Citrated plasma is incubated at 37°C with thrombin and the time is measured to the generation of fibrin filaments. The normal thrombin time is 13–21 seconds. A prolonged TT indicates deficient fibrinogen, abnormal fibrinogen (dysfibrinogenemia) or an inhibitor to the reaction which can be further clarified by measuring the fibrinogen

concentration. The most common acquired inhibitors for this reaction are heparin, direct thrombin inhibitors and fibrin degradation products.

Conditions associated with abnormal PT and aPTT

- If the aPTT is prolonged and the PT (INR) is normal, the problem is localized to the intrinsic pathway (Table 20.2).
- If the aPTT is normal and the PT (INR) is prolonged, the problem lies in the extrinsic pathway.
- If both the aPTT and PT (INR) are prolonged, the problem is in the final common pathway and the thrombin clotting time can be used to assess conversion of fibrinogen to fibrin. If the thrombin time is normal, the problem resides in the common pathway due to abnormalities in factors II, V, or X.

Other investigations for coagulation

- *The ecarin clotting time* can be used to monitor treatment with direct thrombin inhibitors (e.g. argatroban, dabigatran). Ecarin activates prothrombin to intermediate meizothrombin which forms complexes with direct thrombin inhibitors.
- *The dilute Russell viper venom time* is very sensitive to the amount of phospholipid available for the prothrombinase complex and therefore to the presence of antiphospholipid antibodies, especially anti-B2GP1. It uses a 1:1 mixture of patient and control plasma with limited thromboplastic material. It is used for pro-thrombotic screening.
- *FXa activated clotting time* detects procoagulant phospholipids and is sensitive to platelet activation, hypercoagulability and presence of microparticles. It is useful for detection of plasma procoagulant phospholipids.
- *Anti-factor Xa activity* is sometimes used to assess heparin activity when the aPTT is inaccurate due to antiphospholipid antibodies (heparin resistance), if there has been thrombosis despite heparin or for low molecular weight heparin activity when

Table 20.2 Causes of abnormal PT and aPTT

PT	aPTT	
Prolonged	**Normal**	**Inherited**
		Inherited FVII deficiency
		Acquired
		Warfarin treatment
		Acquired FVII deficiency
		Inhibitor of FVII
		Liver disease
Normal	**Prolonged**	**Inherited**
		Deficiencies of factors VIII, IX or XI
		Deficiency of FXII or prekallikrein
		Von Willebrand disease
		Acquired
		Heparin treatment
		Acquired deficiency of factors VIII, IX, XI, XII
		Acquired von Willebrand disease
		Lupus anticoagulant
Prolonged	**Prolonged**	**Inherited**
		Deficiency prothrombin, factors V or X
		Deficiency fibrinogen
		Acquired
		Combined heparin & warfarin treatment
		Liver disease
		Disseminated intravascular coagulation
		Inhibitors of prothrombin, factors V or X
Normal	**Normal**	**Bleeding diathesis**
		Thrombocytopenia
		Mild von Willebrand factor deficiency
		Platelet dysfunction
		Fibrinolytic system disorder
		FXIII deficiency (rare)

dosing is difficult in severe renal disease, obesity or in paediatrics.

- *Thrombo-elastography* gives information about every stage of clot formation and lysis. It measures reaction time to initial fibrin formation, rate of clot formation, strength of clot and clot lysis. It is currently mainly used in bypass surgery.

- *The euglobulin lysis time* measures overall fibrinolysis.
- Specific tests are emerging for the newer direct oral anticoagulants.
- Recommended investigations for possible clotting abnormalities before elective operations are shown in Table 20.3.

Table 20.3 Investigations for clotting abnormalities

Level	Bleeding history	Surgical procedure	Evaluation
I	Negative	Minor	None
II	Negative	Major	Platelet count, aPTT
III	Equivocal	Major	Platelet count, aPTT, PT, TT, FXIII assay, von Willebrand tests
IV	Positive	Minor or major	If negative for above, add FIX and XI assay, α2-antiplasmin, tissue plasminogen activator, platelet aggregation tests

Fibrinolysis

- Fibrinolysis is an enzymatic reaction that breaks down a fibrin clot to limit the extent of thrombosis (Figure 20.3). Tissue plasminogen activator (tPA) and urokinase plasminogen activator (u-PA) released from vascular endothelium act on fibrin-bound plasminogen to produce the enzyme plasmin. Plasmin breaks down the clot into fibrin degradation products (FDPs) that are cleared by other proteases or by the kidney and liver. Tissue plasminogen activator is very slowly released into the blood such that it takes several days after bleeding has stopped for the clot to be broken down, allowing time for wounds to initiate repair. Plasmin activity is regulated to prevent widespread fibrinolysis by plasminogen activator inhibitor, α2 antiplasmin, α2 macroglobulin and thrombin-activatable fibrinolysis inhibitor. D-dimer is a type of FDP that contains the cross-linkage that FXIII had applied to fibrin, and thus indicates the lysis of completed clot. It allows a very sensitive but not specific test which is only useful as a negative test to rule out clotting.

Thrombophilia

- Altered levels of clotting factors or inhibitors can increase the likelihood that VTE

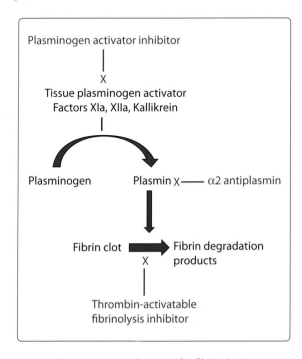

Figure 20.3 Mechanisms for fibrinolysis.

will develop or recur, and this is termed thrombophilia which can be either inherited or acquired.[1,5] Thrombophilia affects approximately 5% of the population although most of these will only develop thrombosis if there is an additional risk factor, and it is found in some 50% of patients who have had spontaneous VTE not provoked by another cause.

Acquired thrombophilia

- Acquired thrombophilia is more common than the hereditary conditions.
- Some acquired conditions causing thrombophilia are as follows:
  - antiphospholipid syndrome
  - hormone treatment
  - myeloproliferative disorders
  - heparin-induced thrombocytopenia
  - JAK2 mutation
  - acquired clotting factor deficiencies
  - dysfibrinogenaemia
  - paroxysmal nocturnal hemoglobinuria
- Predisposing factors for acquired thrombophilia include the following:
  - advanced age
  - major surgery/trauma
  - medical diseases
  - malignancies
  - pregnancy
  - oral contraceptives
  - hormone replacement therapy
  - obesity
  - smoking

Antiphospholipid syndrome

- The antiphospholipid syndrome is an autoimmune disorder characterized by antiphospholipid antibodies, arterial and venous thrombotic events and complications in pregnancy. It was first described in the 1980s after reports of specific antibodies in people with systemic lupus erythematosus and thrombosis. The diagnostic antibodies are lupus anticoagulant and anti-B2-glycoprotein-1, a type of anti-cardiolipin antibody.
- A subset of anti-cardiolipin antibodies bind to apoH which inhibits protein C, some antibodies bind to protein S, decreasing the efficiency of protein C, while other antibodies bind to and activate prothrombin. Antibodies can block phospholipid-dependent steps so as to be procoagulant yet with a prolonged aPTT which is referred to as the *lupus paradox*. Antiphospholipid antibodies are also found in patients with autoimmunity, infections, drug-induced lupus or myeloproliferative, neoplastic and lymphomatous disorders.
- The prevalence of antibodies in healthy people is 1%–5%, but the prevalence of the clinical syndrome is only about five in 100,000. Unlike the congenital thrombophilias which only cause venous thrombo-embolism, antiphospholipid syndrome can also cause arterial thrombosis. Associated findings are thrombocytopenia, heart valve disease, skin ulcers and livedo reticularis or racemosa, renal thrombotic microangiopathy, haemolytic anaemia and cognitive impairment. A clinical diagnosis requires the presence of antibodies plus a history of venous and/or arterial thromboembolic phenomena and/or obstetric problems, namely one or more foetal losses after ten weeks, premature delivery because of severe pre-eclampsia or three or more miscarriages before ten weeks' gestation.
- *Catastrophic antiphospholipid syndrome* is a life-threatening condition found in about 1% of these patients. Precipitating events include infection, surgery, medications and inconsistent anticoagulation. It has a 50% mortality associated with disseminated intravascular coagulation. The diagnosis is based on involvement of at least three organ systems or tissues, presence of antibodies and histological evidence of small vessel occlusion.
- Lupus anticoagulants and anticardiolipin antibodies are not considered hereditary, but they are often included in the thrombophilia panel because besides their prothrombotic risk, they can interfere with many of these tests, in particular clot-based tests that depend on phospholipid.
- Recommended treatment following VTE is with indefinite anticoagulation at an INR of

2–3 if using warfarin, or higher for arterial thrombosis. Recommended management for a pregnant woman with antiphospholipid syndrome and previous VTE is with low-dose aspirin and therapeutic LMWH. Other measures used include statins, chloroquine or B-cell depletion therapy.

Acquired coagulation factor abnormalities

- Acquired decrease of protein C, protein S or antithrombin are much more common than hereditary deficiencies and need to be excluded before diagnosing a hereditary cause. They may be decreased by liver disease, active thrombosis, surgery or disseminated intravascular coagulation. They are low at birth, and protein C can remain below adult reference range throughout adolescence. Pregnancy or oestrogen use decrease protein S and antithrombin. Acute phase reactions decrease free and functional protein S but not total protein S. Heparin or proteinuria decrease antithrombin, whereas vitamin K deficiency or vitamin K antagonist therapy such as warfarin decrease protein C and protein S.

Other acquired disorders

- Myeloproliferative disorders such as polycythemia vera and essential thrombocytosis predispose to thrombosis through hyperviscosity and dysfunctional platelets. Paroxysmal nocturnal haemoglobinuria (see Chapter 17) is a rare condition resulting from acquired alterations in the PIGA gene which plays a role in the prevention of red cell lysis by complement. It increases the risk of venous thrombosis as well as haemolytic anaemia. Cancer, the nephrotic syndrome due to loss of antithrombin in the urine and inflammatory bowel disease predispose to thrombosis.

Hereditary thrombophilias

- The common conditions causing hereditary thrombophilia are autosomal dominant and heterozygous in most patients seen in practice. Factor V Leiden and Pr20210 mutations increase VTE risk over three-fold while proteins C and S and antithrombin deficiencies increase it about six-fold, and the risk of recurrence is higher if the first episode was unprovoked. Heterozygous hereditary thrombophilia does not reduce life expectancy but homozygous inheritance can result in early mortality.
- The most prevalent conditions are listed in Table 20.4. Genetic mutations causing gain of function include thrombophilia due to factor V Leiden and prothrombin gene 20210A. Dual inheritance is not uncommon, the most frequent being mutations for these two genes. Thrombophilia due to abnormal levels of other coagulation proteins include elevated FVIII levels, homocysteinaemia and abnormalities of fibrinolytic proteins. Mutations causing loss of function lead to antithrombin and protein C and protein S deficiency.

Table 20.4 Some causes of hereditary thrombophilia

Condition (heterozygous)	Population prevalence	Prevalence in VTE	Risk of thrombosis	Annual risk to relatives
Factor V Leiden	3%–5%	15%–20%	Moderate	<0.5%
Prothrombin G20210A	2%–3%	4%–5%	Moderate	<0.5%
Hyperhomocysteinaemia	5%	–	–	–
Protein C deficiency	0.3%	2%	Moderate	1%–2%
Protein S deficiency	0.3%	2%	Moderate	1%–2%
Antithrombin deficiency	0.2%	2%	High	0.3% unprovoked 20% provoked
High factor VIII levels	Common	–	Very low	<0.5%

- Except for antithrombin deficiency, VTE in patients with hereditary thrombophilia is most frequently associated with a precipitating factor such as taking an oral contraceptive or hormone replacement therapy, surgery, trauma, medical illness or other reasons for immobilization, pregnancy and post-partum, and cancer and chemotherapy. The more factors present, then the higher is the risk.
- Presentation is usually with lower limb DVT or PE, but hereditary thrombophilia rarely presents as thrombosis at other sites such as in renal, splanchnic, hepato-portal, cerebral or upper limb veins.

Factor V Leiden

- Factor V Leiden is the most common mutation causing thrombophilia, present in some 20% of patients who present with VTE. It only rarely causes arterial thrombosis and has a small risk of causing obstetric complications. It results from replacement of arginine by glutamine in the factor V gene, typically at position 506, denoted as Arg506Gln. This causes activated protein C resistance and failure to inactivate factors Va and VIIIa. Factor V Leiden functions normally with a normal aPTT and PT but cannot be inhibited by protein C. Transmission is autosomal dominant with impaired penetrance. It was identified as a cause of hereditary thrombophilia in 1994, is most common in Caucasian subjects, less common in Latinos and dark-skinned races and rare in Asians. Heterozygous inheritance increases the risk of VTE by some four to eight times, and homozygous inheritance increases risk by up to 80 times.

Prothrombin gene mutation

- Prothrombin G20210A mutation results from replacing guanine with adenine at position 20210 of the DNA of the prothrombin gene. It was identified in 1996 and occurs almost exclusively in Caucasians. It is estimated that most carriers will not develop VTE in their lifetime so that screening in asymptomatic family members of carriers is not usually required.

Hyperhomocysteinaemia

- Hyperhomocysteinaemia is a risk factor for VTE as well as atherosclerosis. Plasma levels >13 μmol/L are common and considered to be a cardiovascular risk while DVT is uncommon and occurs with levels >20 μmol/L. It is not to be confused with the rare disease of homocysteinuria which causes neurologic, vascular and optic complications due to very high plasma levels.
- Homocysteine is an amino acid synthesized from methionine. In part, it is converted back to methionine through the methionine synthase (MTHF) pathway which requires active folate and vitamin B12. The rest is converted into cysteine with vitamin B6 as a co-factor. Homocysteine levels increase with age, smoking, hypothyroidism, renal failure, alcoholism, vitamin B6, B12 or folate deficiency, rheumatoid arthritis and various drugs.
- The most common form of genetic hyperhomocysteinaemia results from production of a thermolabile variant of methylene tetrahydrofolate reductase (MTHFR). Homozygous MTHFR variant is present in over 10% of Caucasians and is a common cause of mildly elevated plasma homocysteine levels in the general population, while heterozygous MTHFR variants are found in up to 40% of Caucasians. Accordingly, it is recommended not to test for MTHFR polymorphism because it is so common and is rarely a cause of VTE.

Antithrombin deficiency

- Antithrombin deficiency was the first cause of hereditary thrombophilia described by Egeberg in 1965. This autosomal dominant condition is rare but carries a high risk of VTE when provoked.

Thrombophilia testing

- Testing for thrombophilias should only be performed if it is anticipated that results will improve or modify management. It is not necessary to screen all patients with a first episode of spontaneous VTE.

- Potential advantages from testing include patient satisfaction from having identified a biologic risk factor underlying a thrombotic event, and an increased likelihood of using prophylaxis in high-risk situations. A woman can be made aware of the risk–benefit ratio associated with the oral contraceptive and hormone replacement therapy to allow more informed decisions, particularly if testing reveals the more significant protein C or S deficiency or antithrombin deficiency that increase VTE risk six-fold.
- Disadvantages from testing are cost, false positive results (2% per test and over 5% cumulative when multiple tests are ordered), spurious results due to inappropriate timing of testing, misinterpretation of results causing unnecessary anxiety, and the possibility of genetic discrimination.
- There are several problems with thrombophilia testing.
  - Doctors are testing too many normal subjects, or inappropriately testing patients with acute VTE or who are being anticoagulated.
  - Results do not affect management of acute VTE.
  - There is no good evidence that testing reduces recurrence rates.
  - A positive result carries psychological implications for the patient.
  - There is a risk of excessive investigation and anticoagulation in future, with patients more likely to report non-specific symptoms such as chest pain.
  - Their doctors are more likely to commence anticoagulation if a diagnosis is indeterminate.
  - There are possible insurance implications since patients must declare all known medical conditions.

National Institute for Health and Clinical Excellence (NICE) guidelines for thrombophilia testing

- Do not test:[6]
  - patients who are being treated by anticoagulation

- patients who have had provoked VTE
- first-degree relatives of people with a history of DVT or PE and thrombophilia
- upper-extremity DVT, central venous catheter-associated DVT, retinal vein thrombosis, arterial thrombosis or pre-eclampsia at term

International consensus statement

- Test for:[1,5]
  - first unprovoked episode of VTE under the age of 60 years
  - first episode of VTE whether unprovoked or provoked under the age of 40 years
  - unprovoked VTE after ceasing anticoagulation
  - pregnant women with a previous VTE event due to minor risk factors
  - recurrent VTE irrespective of the presence of risk factors
  - women with more than two past miscarriages
  - superficial vein thrombosis in the absence of varicose veins
  - VTE in a subject with a family history of VTE in two or more members, or with known protein C or S or antithrombin deficiency
  - VTE at unusual sites such as cerebral venous sinus, mesenteric or hepatic veins
  - warfarin-induced skin necrosis and neonates with purpura fulminans not related to sepsis
- Many women who are about to commence taking the oral contraceptive will wish to be tested to ensure that this is safe. Defensive medicine dictates that many practitioners will test for thrombophilia if there is a suggestive obstetric background, repeated past VTE or family history of VTE, particularly if their patient is scheduled for treatment with a procedure that would not normally be covered by thrombo-prophylaxis, such as endovenous treatment for chronic venous disease.
- The timing for testing in relation to ongoing anticoagulation varies for different factors.
  - Non-clot based genetic assays for protein C resistance to detect factor V Leiden and

factor II mutation can be performed at any time.

- Clotting-based assays such as for proteins C and S may be influenced by the acute phase of thrombosis, pregnancy, oral contraception or by treatment with vitamin K antagonists. Protein C and S deficiency is best assessed at least two months after cessation of vitamin K antagonist treatment.
- Prolonged treatment with heparin slightly decreases the levels of antithrombin. However, a precise diagnosis of anti-thrombin deficiency is mandatory since heterozygous antithrombin sub-type II HBS (heparin binding site) is not associated with an increased risk of VTE so that its detection can prevent the need for anticoagulation.
- Diagnosis of hereditary deficiency of coagulation inhibitors should be only established after ruling out acquired deficiency of these proteins.
- Testing relatives could identify those at risk for future VTE. The annual risk of first VTE in a relative with a strong thrombophilic defect is less than 2%, although this is some 15–20 times the risk for the general community. Surgery, pregnancy and oral contraceptive are common precipitating events. Prophylaxis during pregnancy would then prevent VTE in one of ten subjects.

20.1 Recommended investigations for thrombophilia

- Blood cell count, prothrombin time, and activated thromboplastin time.
- Coagulation inhibitors – levels of antithrombin, protein C, protein S.
- Activated protein C resistance – if positive, Factor V Leiden mutation or genetic study since there are other less common causes of activated protein C resistance.
- Prothrombin G20210A mutation.
- Lupus anticoagulant detection, anti-β2 GP1antibodies.
- Fasting homocysteine (optional).

Bleeding disorders

- Acquired bleeding disorders are more common than inherited causes. Platelet disorders tend to present with petechial rash and epistaxis, whereas clotting factor disorders commonly present with haemarthroses and post-operative bleeding.

Impaired platelet function

- Medications such as aspirin, non-steroidal anti-inflammatory drugs, GpIIbIIIa antagonists such as abciximab, thienopyridine ADP receptor blockers such as clopidogrel and nitrates, and theophylline are relatively common causes of bleeding due to impaired platelet function. Aspirin irreversibly inhibits cyclooxygenase-1 which platelets cannot replenish as they have no nucleus or DNA, and it takes one week to replace the platelets.
- Myeloproliferative disorders can result in clotting from thrombocytosis and hyperviscosity.

Thrombocytopenia

- There are three mechanisms for reduced platelet numbers.
  - Decreased production – bone marrow disorders, liver and kidney disease, or vitamin B12 and folate or other nutritional deficiencies.
  - Increased destruction – drug-induced including heparin-induced thrombocytopenia, immune thrombocytopenia, non-immune thrombotic thrombocytopenia, paroxysmal nocturnal haemaglobinuria, or disseminated intravascular coagulation.
  - Sequestration by the spleen due to splenomegaly.
- The Kasabach–Merritt phenomenon consists of profound sustained thrombocytopoenia, profound hypofibrinogenaemia, consumptive coagulopathy and elevated D-dimer associated with haemangioendothelioma or other vascular tumours (see Chapter 26).

- Clinical presentation is with epistaxis, muco-cutaneous bleeding, petechiae and menorrhagia. The platelet count falls from a normal level of $150-450 \times 10^9/L$ to $<50 \times 10^9/L$ and a fall to $<10 \times 10^9/L$ is dangerous, requiring transfusion, though this is not very helpful in the presence of antibodies, when steroids are more helpful.
- Some patients require treatment with immune-suppressants or thrombopoietin receptor agonists, while splenectomy may be required.

Von Willebrand's disease

- Von Willebrand's disease is the most common inherited coagulation abnormality and has mixed platelet and coagulation defects. Biochemical abnormalities occur in 1:100 of the population, but clinical disease prevalence is just 1:10,000. It is autosomal dominant, with variable penetrance and expression. There are different types according to the degree of impaired factor VIII function.
- It presents with epistaxis and menorrhagia, post-dental extraction bleeding and, rarely, haemarthroses or muscle haematomas. The aPTT is variably prolonged depending on plasma FVIII levels, von Willebrand factor is low and factor VIII coagulant activity is very low in severe forms.
- Patients can be treated with desmopressin (DDAVP) given by intravenous administration of 0.3 μg/kg in 100 mL saline or by the intranasal route, or von Willebrand factor concentrates depending on the type of disease. DDAVP is a modified arginine-vasopressin molecule that has a longer half-life that natural vasopressin, and acts to release von Willebrand factor from endothelial cells and to improve platelet function by activating arginine vasopressin receptors. It is inexpensive, has no transmission risk, and increases factor VIII-VWF levels by four times within 30–60 minutes.

Haemophilia

- Haemophilia A is due to factor VIII deficiency, results from X-linked recessive inheritance and affects 1:5000 live male births. Haemophilia B (Christmas disease) is due to factor IX deficiency, also results from X-linked recessive inheritance and affects 1:30,000 live male births. Haemophilia C is due to factor XI deficiency, occurs equally in both sexes and is mostly found in Ashkenazi Jews. Parahaemophilia is due to insufficient factor V. Acquired haemophilia is associated with cancers, autoimmune disorders and pregnancy.
- It is diagnosed by prolonged aPTT and decreased factor levels, but PT and fibrinogen are normal. Severe disease has less than 1% normal factor VIII levels and patients suffer spontaneous bleeds, moderate disease has 1%–5% levels and does not cause spontaneous bleeding but can cause muscle and joint hematomas after mild trauma or surgery, or bleeding after dental procedures, while mild disease has more than 5% levels and only causes bleeding with severe trauma or after surgery.
- Although factor VIII and IX deficiencies are both X-linked recessive, it is not uncommon for female carriers to need treatment prior to invasive procedures or following trauma. Mild cases are treated with desmopressin as above, moderate severity disease by infusion of clotting factors – 1 unit of factor VIII/kg increases levels by 2%, while serious bleeds requires urgent treatment with 50 units factor VIII/kg to restore normal levels. Prophylaxis for severe haemophilia is with 30 units factor VIII/kg three times weekly.
- Fresh frozen plasma (FFP) from pooled donors contains all factors but only in small quantities so that 1 L FFP would be required to restore 30% factor VIII activity which would be enough for haemostasis but liable to cause fluid overload. Cryoprecipitate formed from FFP has strongly concentrated coagulation factors.

History

- Al-Zahrawi (936–1013), an Arab who has been described as the father of surgery, was the first to describe haemophilia and identify its hereditary nature.
- The Italian biologist and physician Marcello Malpighi (1628–1694) described blood composition, how blood clots and the differences between arterial and venous thrombosis in *De polypo cordis* published in 1666.
- The German pathologist Rudolf Virchow (1821–1902) postulated the interplay of the three processes resulting in venous thrombosis now known as Virchow's triad, in 1856.
- George Gulliver (1804–1882), an anatomist and surgeon working in London, was the first to identify platelets by microscopy.
- Stephen Christmas (1947–1993) was the first patient to be diagnosed with haemophilia B from factor IX deficiency, giving the name to Christmas disease. He was a campaigner for safe transfusion but died from transfusion-acquired AIDS.

References

1. Nicolaides A, Fareed J, Kakkar AK, Comerota AJ, Goldhaber SZ, Hull R, Myers K et al. Prevention and treatment of venous thromboembolism: International consensus statement (Guidelines according to scientific evidence). *Clin Appl Thromb Hemost* 2013;19:116–8. http://europeanvenousforum.org/wp-content/uploads/2015/02/IUA_Guidelines_2013.pdf
2. Gale AJ. Current understanding of hemostasis. *Toxicol Pathol* 2011;39:273–80. http://www.ncbi.nlm.nih.gov/pmc/articles/PMC3126677/
3. Italiano JE, Mairuhu ATA, Flaumenhaf R. Clinical relevance of microparticles from platelets and megakaryocytes. *Curr Opin Hematol* 2011;17:578–84. https://www.ncbi.nlm.nih.gov/pmc/articles/PMC3082287/
4. Mackman N. The role of tissue factor and factor VIIa in hemostasis. *Anesth Analg* 2009;108:1447–52. https://www.ncbi.nlm.nih.gov/pmc/articles/PMC2838713/
5. Stevens SM, Woller SC, Bauer KA, Kasthuri R, Cushman M, Streiff M, Lim W, Douketis JD. Guidance for the evaluation and treatment of hereditary and acquired thrombophilia. *J Thromb Thrombolysis* 2016;41:154–64. http://www.ncbi.nlm.nih.gov/pmc/articles/PMC4715840/
6. NICE guidelines. Venous thromboembolic diseases: The management of venous thromboembolic diseases and the role of thrombophilia. No. 144. 2012. https://www.ncbi.nlm.nih.gov/books/NBK132806/

21 | Anticoagulant, antiplatelet, and thrombolytic agents

Anticoagulant drugs are used to prevent and treat venous thrombo-embolism. Antiplatelet agents are mostly used to inhibit arterial thrombosis, but have a place in managing venous thrombosis. Thrombolytic agents are used to enhance intrinsic fibrinolysis to treat established thrombosis and embolism.

Anticoagulants

- Anticoagulants act at various sites in the clotting cascade (Figure 21.1).[1]

Indirect thrombin inhibitors

- Several compounds with different molecular structures collectively form the heparins, those in clinical use being unfractionated heparin (UFH), low molecular weight heparin (LMWH) and fondaparinux. Heparins are normally stored within secretory granules of mast cells and are released into the circulation at sites of tissue injury to assist immune defence.
- Heparins are indirect anticoagulants as they bind to antithrombin to inactivate factors XIIa, XIa, IXa, Xa and thrombin. They have two separate actions. They contain an active pentasaccharide sequence found on one-third and one-fifth of the chains of UFH and LMWH respectively, and this has a strong electrostatic interaction that binds to antithrombin to activate its anti-FXa activity. Fondaparinux is a synthetic analogue of the naturally occurring pentasaccharide found in heparins and selectively

and irreversibly binds to antithrombin to neutralize FXa. A separate 18-saccharide unit must also bind to thrombin as well as antithrombin to inhibit thrombin, and this effect is proportional to the size of the heparin molecule. Thus, fondoparinux is a pure FXa inhibitor and LMWHs have predominant anti-FXa activity due to less antithrombin effect than UFH. These interactions increase inactivation of thrombin, FXa and other proteases by about 1000 times.

- Comparison of features for the heparins is shown in Table 21.1.[1]

Unfractionated heparin (UFH)

- UFH acts immediately after intravenous injection and within 20–30 minutes after subcutaneous injection of its slowly-absorbed calcium salt calciparine. UFH readily binds to plasma proteins which contributes to its variable anticoagulant response after parenteral administration. If given by subcutaneous injection, doses need to be large enough to overcome its low bioavailability.
- UFH clearance from the circulation is through two independent mechanisms. The initial phase is rapid binding to endothelial cells, macrophages and proteins, where UFH is depolymerized higher molecular weight being cleared more rapidly than lower molecular weight chains. The second phase is a slower renal clearance, resulting in a repeated dose causing

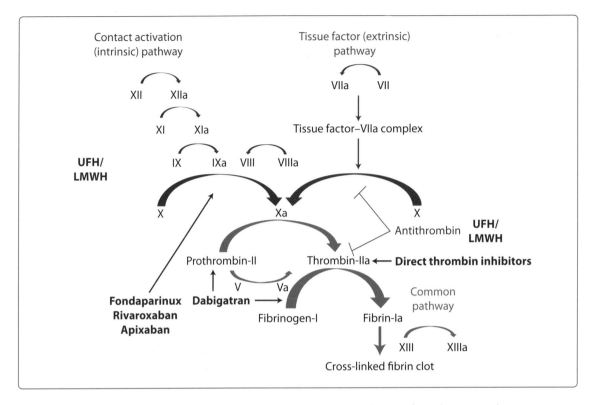

Figure 21.1 Sites of action for anticoagulant drugs other than warfarin shown in red.

Table 21.1 Comparison of heparins

Features	UFH	LMWH	Fondaparinux
Source	Biological	Biological	Synthetic
Molecular weight (Da)	15,000	5,000	1,500
Target	Xa:IIa	Xa > IIa	Xa
Bioavailability (%)	30	90	100
Half-life (hours)	1	4	17
Renal excretion	No	Yes	Yes
Protamine reversal	Complete	Partial	None
Incidence of HIT (%)	<5.0	<1.0	Case reports

a disproportionate increase in the intensity and duration of its anticoagulant effect.

- UFH has a short half-life of no more than 90 minutes so that the anticoagulant effect for intravenous heparin is mostly lost after three to four hours. It does not cross the placental barrier and is not secreted in milk, so it can be safely used during pregnancy and lactation.

- UFH is not very effective at inactivating fibrin-bound thrombin and platelet-bound FXa, sometimes resulting in ongoing propagation despite full heparinization. Conditions that lead to heparin resistance requiring >35,000 u per day to maintain a therapeutic aPTT include antithrombin deficiency, increased heparin clearance, elevated heparin-binding proteins, FVIII or fibrinogen, or fever, thrombosis, sepsis, myocardial infarction, cancer or recent surgery.

- Limitations of UFH include poor bioavailability after subcutaneous injection, a short half-life when administered intravenously requiring continuous intravenous infusion, and a variable response from patient to patient which necessitates frequent coagulation monitoring and a risk of complications. Contraindications to UFH are a history of heparin-induced thrombocytopenia, uncontrolled active bleeding or a known risk of bleeding or circumstances where coagulation tests cannot be performed at appropriate intervals. A significant advantage is its non-renal excretion.

- Reversal of heparin is with protamine, which inactivates the anionic heparin by ionic binding, the resultant complex being broken down by the mononuclear phagocyte system in the spleen, lymph nodes and liver. Protamine can only partially bind the shorter LMWH chains, resulting in about 60% inactivation of FXa activity. If immediate reversal is required, a protamine dose of 1 mg neutralizes 100 U heparin and 60% of 1 mg of LMWH.

21.1 Dosage for unfractionated heparin (UFH)

For treatment of VTE by intravenous UFH infusion:

- Maintain an aPTT of at least 1.5 times control.
- Give an initial bolus of 80 U/kg.
- Start a constant infusion of 18 U/kg.
- Consider lower doses in older patients.
- Check the aPTT or heparin activity level six hours after the bolus to adjust the infusion rate.
- Check the aPTT or heparin activity level every six hours until two successive values are therapeutic.
- Monitor the aPTT or heparin activity level, haematocrit and platelet count every 24 hours.

Low molecular weight heparin (LMWH)

- Unfractionated heparin is modified by isolating fragments of molecular weight less than 9000 daltons to form low molecular weight heparin (LMWH), and this has made its pharmacodynamics more predictable. Several preparations are available, including enoxaparin (Clexane®), dalteparin (Fragmin®), tinzaparin (Innohep®) and nadroparin (Fraxiparine®). They exert their effect by predominantly inhibiting activated FX; the ratio anti-Xa:anti-IIa for LMWH compared to UFH is 4:1. The smaller molecular weight molecules do not bind randomly to plasma proteins, thereby increasing bioavailability compared to UFH to 90% after subcutaneous injection. LMWH is also able to inactivate platelet-bound FXa, shows resistance to inhibition by platelet factor IV and has a decreased effect on platelet function and vascular permeability causing less risk of haemorrhage.

- An increased bioavailability and longer half-life of LMWH allows for outpatient treatment of DVT in most patients. However, in-patient management is required if there is proven or suspected concomitant PE, a significant comorbidity, extensive ilio-femoral DVT, morbid obesity, renal failure or if poor follow-up is expected.

- The onset of action after subcutaneous injection is one to two hours, the peak activity is at three to five hours and the half-life is 12 hours. It is metabolized in the liver and excreted in the urine, and the dose should be reduced if there is renal impairment. It appears that there is no difference in efficacy or risk of complications for once daily compared to twice daily injections, though twice daily dosing gives smoother pharmacokinetics.

- The dose–response is predictable, with peak anti-FXa activity occurring three to five hours after injection so that laboratory monitoring is usually not necessary. Monitoring is an option to adjust dosing in high-risk patients with renal insufficiency, obesity or pregnancy.

- The incidence of heparin-induced thrombocytopenia (HIT) is one-tenth that of UFH, but LMWH should not be administered if there is a past history of HIT or if platelets are observed to drop by more than 30% by day five.

- Protamine completely reverses the anti-FIIa activity of LMWH, but only reverses 60% of anti-FXa activity. If immediate reversal is required within eight hours of LMWH administration, a protamine dose of 1 mg is administered for each 1 mg LMWH, and if bleeding continues, a second dose of 0.5 mg of protamine per 1 mg LMWH can be given. Experience has allowed practitioners to become comfortable with variations in dosage.

21.2 Dosage for low molecular weight heparin

- For prevention of VTE following surgery, enoxaparin 40 mg daily or daltaparin 5000 U daily.
- For treatment of VTE with enoxaparin:
  - Dosage: 1 mg/kg subcutaneous bd or 1.5 mg/kg subcutaneous daily.
  - If using warfarin, initiate warfarin therapy after first dose given.
  - Continue enoxaparin until INR is 2–3 and for a minimum of five days when preceding warfarin.
  - Monitoring by aPTT is not required.
  - Give doses bd and adjust to anti-FXa levels between 0.5 and 1.0 U/mL in the very young and morbidly obese (weight >150 kg or BMI >40 kg/m^2),
  - Reduce dosing with decreased renal function, and avoid enoxaparin if eGFR is <30 – illness and dehydration can cause the eGFR to fall.
- There are considerable variations in recommended dosage regimes with standard guidelines for enoxaparin of 40 mg daily for prophylaxis after orthopaedic surgery, 1.5 mg/kg daily for unstable angina and intermediate dosing commonly used for in-hospital prophylaxis, superficial vein thrombosis and other indications.

Fondaparinux

- Fondaparinux sodium (Arixtra) is a synthetic analogue of the pentasaccharide sequence in the heparins that mediates their interaction with antithrombin. The drug is at least as effective as UFH or LMWH for prevention or treatment of VTE, and in contrast has no inhibitory activity against thrombin and mainly targets FXa, although it also inhibits FIXa.
- Its peak action occurs at two hours, its half-life is about 16–20 hours allowing for sustained antithrombotic activity, and it is excreted by the kidneys with clearance reduced in patients with renal impairment. It does not affect PT or aPTT, nor does it affect platelet function or aggregation. As with LMWH, predictable pharmacokinetics means that monitoring anti-Xa levels is not usually required.
- It does not cause heparin-induced thrombocytopenia because it does not bind to platelet factor IV and therefore cannot make the heparin–platelet factor IV complex that reacts with platelet activating antibodies. There is no antidote, and treatment for over-dosage is with four-factor prothrombin complex concentrate (II, VII, IX and X) if available or three-factor prothrombin complex concentrate (lacks VII).
- Idraparinux is a derivative of fondaparinux with a half-life of 80 hours allowing once weekly dosage, with 100% bioavailability following subcutaneous injection and a linear response with no need for monitoring.,

---

21.3 Dosage for fondaparinux

- Prevention of VTE for major orthopaedic surgery as an alternative to LMWH – fondaparinux 2.5 mg once daily by subcutaneous injection.
- Treatment of VTE – fondaparinux once daily by subcutaneous injection, giving 7.5 mg for a 50–100 kg adult.

Vitamin K antagonists

- Vitamin K antagonists are administered by mouth for prolonged anticoagulation (Figure 21.2). The most widely used vitamin K antagonist is warfarin (Coumadin). Warfarin's mechanism of action is unique among anticoagulants in that instead of binding to active clotting factors to induce anticoagulation, it reduces the total amounts of clotting factors in the circulation.
- Vitamin K undergoes a cycle of changes that allows it to affect the clotting process. Vitamin K is converted to a reduced form of vitamin K hydroquinone by vitamin K reductase. Vitamin K hydroquinone is required for normal function of clotting factors. It is then converted to an oxidized form of vitamin K epoxide involving carboxylase. This is then converted back to vitamin K by vitamin K epoxide reductase.
- Clotting factors II, VII, IX and X and natural anticoagulants protein C and protein S have a series of glutamic acid residues at their amino terminus, and these require carboxylation by vitamin K hydroquinone to allow them to bind to phospholipid surfaces on the vascular endothelium. The responsible enzyme is gamma-glutamyl carboxylase.
- Warfarin acts at two main sites. It inhibits the vitamin K-dependent synthesis of biologically active forms of the calcium-dependent clotting factors II, VII, IX and X and protein C and protein S. It also inhibits vitamin K epoxide reductase to diminish available vitamin K and vitamin K hydroquinone, which restricts the carboxylation activity of gamma glutamyl carboxylase. Stores of previously produced active factors are reduced by inactive factors over several days and the anticoagulant effect then becomes apparent.
- Warfarin has several limitations. It is slow to start to act because its anticoagulant effect depends on clearing the vitamin K-dependent clotting proteins, which takes several days. Plasma protein C has a six-hour half-life, shorter than most other clotting factors, causing a potential procoagulant state in the first days of treatment. In addition, the dose required varies because dietary vitamin K intake differs between patients, so that frequent monitoring is required to ensure a therapeutic effect, which is a burden to the patient and a cost to the health care system.
- Warfarin exhibits full effect within about four hours though therapeutic effect requires the circulating clotting factors to be metabolized over several days, and its half-life is about 40 hours. It is metabolized in the liver and excreted in urine. It is a category D drug in pregnancy and must not be used before about 14 weeks due to it causing nasal and skeletal malformations, but is safe to use during lactation. It is contraindicated if there is known deficiency in any of its target clotting factors, while relative general contraindications include severe liver and kidney disease and patient non-compliance. It is also contraindicated with heparin-induced thrombocytopenia until

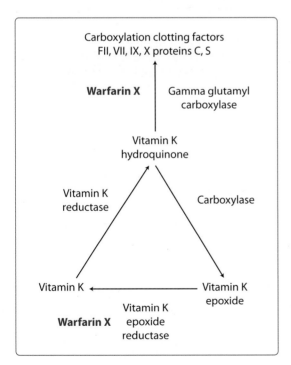

Figure 21.2 Sites of action for warfarin shown in red.

platelet levels return to normal. Antibiotic interactions increase bleeding risk due to alteration of intestinal flora that synthesize vitamin K and inhibition of cytochrome p450 isozymes that metabolize warfarin. The short six-hour half-lives of protein C and FVII can result in unpredictable early effects of warfarin in the first two days, including pro-thrombosis if not covered by other anticoagulants.

- Adverse reactions include the *warfarin necrosis syndrome*, which can occur between the third and seventh day, with pain and redness then tissue necrosis due to extensive thrombosis of venules and capillaries in the subcutaneous fat of the thigh, breast and buttocks in particular. It is uncertain whether necrosis results from hypersensitivity or a direct toxic effect. Another complication is the *purple toe syndrome* which usually occurs one to three months after the start of anticoagulation, with pain and discolouration due to cholesterol emboli from haemorrhagic atheromatous plaques in the aorta.

21.4 Dosage of warfarin

- Begin with 5 mg daily for the first three days.
- Adjust dosage by serial measurements of the International Normalized Ratio (INR) to maintain an INR>2.
- Obtain the first INR on the third day while maintaining cover with other anticoagulation. Continue LMWH for at least five days even if INR is in the therapeutic range due to early FVII depletion before factors II and X have been depleted.
- Lower initial dosing may be warranted for the elderly and patients with underlying comorbidities.

Direct oral anticoagulants (DOACs)

- Evidence is emerging that DOACs are not only as effective as warfarin but safer, particularly with respect to the most feared complication of intracerebral haemorrhage.[2]
- The terminology for the agents has evolved since their introduction in 2010. These new and novel oral anticoagulants were given the acronym NOACs, but as the novelty wore off this was changed to DOAC for direct oral anticoagulant, and this may best reflect both present drugs and future oral anticoagulants that will directly bind to other clotting factors aside from FXa or FIIa.
- The first to be introduced was dabigatran (Pradaxa®), which directly binds to FIIa (thrombin). Subsequently, agents which bind to FXa directly were introduced – rivaroxaban (Xarelto®), then apixaban (Eliquis®) and edoxaban (Savaysa®).
- Advantages over heparin are oral administration with no known risk of heparin-induced thrombocytopenia. Advantages over warfarin include rapid onset of action, eliminating the need for bridging therapy with a parenteral anticoagulant in most situations. Unlike warfarin, they are not affected by dietary vitamin K intake, and have a much lower potential for interactions with other drugs. These features result in a predictable anticoagulant response after fixed-dose administration, so that routine coagulation monitoring is not necessary. Caution is needed for patients with renal impairment as dabigatran is mostly excreted by the kidneys (85%) whereas the FXa inhibitors are excreted in both urine (rivaroxaban 35%, apixaban 25%) and faeces, so that there is less accumulation in patients with renal impairment.
- The reversal agent idarucizumab (Praxbind) which contains antibody fragments is now available to reverse dabigatran. The FXa inhibitor reversal agent andexanet alfa is a 'decoy' protein which is an inactive form of FXa and is at a late stage of development and should soon be able to reverse direct acting FXa antagonist DOACs as well as LMWHs and fondaparinux. Both agents carry a significant pro-thrombotic risk,

and therefore should only be used for life-threatening haemorrhage. Other options for haemorrhage include 3- or 4-factor PCCs, fresh frozen plasma, oral activated charcoal, anti-fibrinolytics such as tranexamic acid and haemodialysis for dabigatran overdose.

- Dabigatran is a pro-drug metabolized to its active form in the liver, active in two hours and with a 14-hour half-life. P-glycoprotein inhibitors such as clarithromycin, amiodarone, verapamil, antifungals and some anti-HIV drugs may raise serum levels.

  Concurrent use of aspirin, Cox2 inhibitors, short and short half-life NSAIDs post operation do not increase bleeding risk.

  Some studies have suggested an increased gastro-intestinal bleed rate and acute coronary syndromes compared with warfarin.

- Rivaroxaban has a peak action at two to four hours and a half-life of five to nine hours. Its use is not recommended during pregnancy or lactation. Strong inducers of CYP3A4 such as rifampicin, phenytoin, carbamazepine, phenobarbital or St John's wort may reduce the plasma concentration and efficacy of rivaroxaban.
- Timing to recommence DOACs after surgery depends on the operation and risk of bleeding.
  - For procedures with immediate and complete haemostasis, commence a DOAC six to eight hours after operation.
  - For procedures with a risk of post-operative bleeding, resume parenteral thrombo-prophylaxis for example with low dose LMWH six to eight hours after operation and change to a DOAC at 48–72 hours when haemostasis is assured.
- To change from warfarin to a DOAC, wait until the INR is <2.5. To change from an DOAC to warfarin, cease the DOAC on day three or four of warfarin providing the INR is >2.0 on the two previous days.
- Comparison of their pharmacodynamics is shown in Table 21.2.

21.5 Dosage of direct oral anticoagulants

- Full anticoagulant dosing:
  - Rivaroxaban – 15 mg twice daily by mouth for 21 days then 20 mg daily.
  - Apixaban –10 mg twice daily by mouth for 7 days then 5 mg twice daily.
  - Dabigatran – 150 mg twice daily after 5–10 days of parenteral anticoagulation.
- Suggested orthopaedic prophylaxis:
  - Rivaroxaban – 10 mg daily for 35 days for hip replacement, and 12 days for knee replacement.
  - Dabigatran – 110 mg one to four hours after surgery, followed by 220 mg once daily for 28–35 days for hip replacement or ten days for knee replacement.
  - Apixaban –2.5 mg twice daily for 35 days for hip replacement or 12 days for knee replacement.

Reasons to avoid DOACs – renal impairment, pregnancy, breastfeeding, mechanical heart valve, erratic compliance, gastro-intestinal bleed risk or body weight <50 kg or >120 kg.

Direct parenteral thrombin inhibitors

- Some directly inhibit thrombin and thrombin generation, including hirudin analogues desirudin and bivalirudin and argatroban derived from the amino acid arginine. They can be used if heparin is contraindicated for example, if a patient develops heparin-induced thrombocytopenia.
- They exert their effect through direct selective reversible binding to the enzymatic catalytic site and anion binding site of thrombin, leading to formation and inhibition of activation of factors V, VIII, XIII, protein C and platelet aggregation.
- Bivalirudin has the shortest half-life, making it a particularly useful agent during procedures. Critically ill patients typically require lower infusion rates than recommended by the manufacturer.

Table 21.2 Pharmacodynamics of DOACs[1]

Features	Dabigatran	Rivaroxaban	Apixaban
Target	Thrombin	Factor Xa	Factor Xa
Prodrug	Yes	No	No
Dosing	Fixed	Fixed	Fixed
Bioavailability (%)	6	80	90
Half-life (hours)	12–17	5–9	12
Renal excretion (%)	80	65	25
Coagulation monitoring	No	No	No
Antidote	Darucizumab	Pending	Pending
Interactions	P-gp inhibitors	Combined P-gp and CYP3A4 inhibitors	Potent 3CYP3A4 inhibitors

Bivalirudin and argatroban are monitored using aPTT with a goal of 1.5–2.5 times control or baseline.

- Danaproid is a mixture of heparin sulfate, dermatan sulfate and chondroitin sulfate and is a direct FXa inhibitor with little cross-reactivity to heparin.
- They are immediately active following parenteral administration, but have a relatively short duration of action. They carry an appreciable risk of causing bleeding and anaphylaxis, and there is no means to reverse their action if bleeding occurs.

Anti-platelet agents

- Anti-platelet agents are mostly used to inhibit arterial thrombosis but can be used to inhibit venous thrombosis (Figure 21.3).

Cyclo-oxygenase (COX) inhibitors

- Aspirin (acetylsalicylic acid) is a non-steroidal anti-inflammatory drug (NSAID) that has several actions which are dose-dependent. Low doses have anti-thrombotic effects, intermediate doses have anti-pyretic and analgesic effects and high doses have anti-inflammatory effects. Although aspirin is mostly used to inhibit arterial thrombosis, aspirin administered in low doses has now also been shown to reduce the incidence of VTE in high-risk patients, and a 50% reduction in the

likelihood of recurrent VTE after six months of anticoagulation has been completed.[4] It may also benefit post-orthopaedic surgery VTE prophylaxis.

- The anti-thrombotic effect results from aspirin blocking the cyclo-oxygenase (COX-1) enzyme to inhibit prostaglandin and thromboxane synthesis. COX-1 is present in most tissues, maintains the normal lining of the stomach and is involved in kidney and platelet function. COX-2 is primarily present at sites of inflammation, and COX-2 inhibitors such as celocoxib and meloxicam seem to have an anti-inflammatory action with less risk of gastro-intestinal bleeding.
- Aspirin in low dose has more effect on platelets than endothelial cells, as cyclooxygenase can only be regenerated by new platelet formation, whereas endothelial cells are nucleated and can re-synthesize the enzyme. As a result, low-dose aspirin inhibits platelet aggregation by blocking thromboxane generation, but has little effect on production of endothelial cell prostacyclin which is a vasodilator and inhibitor of platelet activation. All COX-1 inhibitors can interfere with aspirin's platelet effect if given concurrently, and most NSAIDs, with the possible except of naproxen, may be associated with an increased risk of stroke and heart attack.
- Aspirin overdose symptoms range from tinnitus, nausea and dizziness, to respiratory

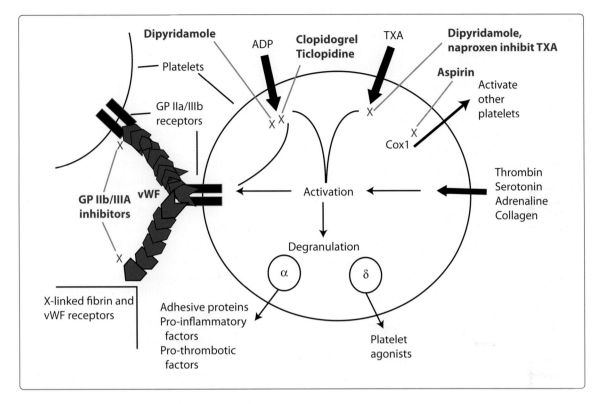

Figure 21.3 Sites of action for ant-platelet agents shown in red.

alkalosis, metabolic acidosis, fitting and coma. It is treated with oral charcoal, intravenous hydration, bicarbonate alkanization and haemodialysis.

Adenosine diphosphate (ADP) receptor inhibitors

- The most commonly prescribed drug of this type is clopidogrel (Plavix), which is used to reduce the risk of arterial thrombosis. The drug specifically and irreversibly inhibits the P2Y12 subtype of ADP receptor, which is important for activation of platelets and cross-linking by fibrin, by blocking activation of the GP IIb/IIIa pathway. This functions as a receptor for linking fibrinogen and vitronectin, and for fibronectin and the von Willebrand factor. Onset of action is slow, so that a loading-dose of 300 mg is usually administered for acute myocardial infarction, whereas the usual dose is 75 mg

daily. As with aspirin, platelet function is only restored by making new platelets, and routine surgery is usually delayed up to a week following cessation of clopidogrel. Clopidogrel is more potent than low-dose aspirin and has an annual gastro-intestinal bleed rate of >2% and cerebral haemorrhage rate of 0.1%. Bleeding risk increases when clopidogrel and aspirin are combined (Co-Plavix).
- The newer more potent P2Y12 inhibitors prasugrel and ticagrelor are associated with more bleeding side-effects but stronger antiplatelet action.

Adenosine uptake inhibitors

- Dipyridamole (Persantin) is used to inhibit thrombosis, particularly for stroke prevention often in association with aspirin. It blocks the phosphodiesterase enzymes that normally break down cyclic adenosine monophosphate (cAMP), and increasing cellular cAMP levels impair platelet aggregation and cause arteriolar smooth muscle relaxation by blocking the platelet response to adenosine diphosphate. This inhibits cellular uptake of adenosine into platelets, red blood cells and endothelial cells.

GP IIb/IIIa antagonists

- GP IIb/IIIa antagonists include abciximab (ReoPro), eptifibatide (Integrilin) and tirofiban hydrochloride (Aggrastat).[5] They are administered intravenously as a bolus followed by infusion. Their action is to prevent platelet aggregation, thrombus formation and distal thromboembolism, while preserving platelet binding to damaged vascular surfaces. They can provide antiplatelet therapy for patients undergoing endovascular interventions.
- Study of a rare bleeding disorder, Glanzmann thrombasthenia, revealed an inherited autosomal recessive GPIIb/IIIa deficiency, where platelets are of normal size and undergo normal activation-related secretion and shape changes, but do not bind fibrinogen and cannot form aggregates. Activation of the GIIb/IIIa complex is the final common pathway for platelet aggregation and for cross-linking of platelets by fibrin. Blocking the platelet's GPIIb/IIIa, fibrinogen and von Willebrand factor receptor sites provides a much stronger action than other antiplatelet medications that block only one of many platelet activators. In addition, GPIIb/IIIa antagonism is able to dissolve platelet-rich clot by disrupting platelet-fibrinogen interactions. Thrombotic thrombocytopenia purpura (TTP) produces antibodies to this same GPIIb/IIIa receptor and is a rare side-effect of usage.

Thrombolytic agents

- Thrombolytic drugs are either used systemically or catheter-directed for PE or extensive proximal DVT, as well as stroke and acute myocardial infarction.[6] PT and aPTT are prolonged due to low fibrinogen concentrations, but anti-FXa is normal.

- Preferred treatment now is with tissue plasminogen activators (tPA) which catalyse plasminogen to plasmin. Commercial agents are alteplase, reteplase and tenecteplase. Other agents that have been used are streptokinase and urokinase.
- *Alteplase* is identical to native tPA. It is fibrin-specific and has a plasma half-life of four to six minutes.
- *Reteplase* is a second-generation recombinant tissue-type plasminogen activator that works more rapidly and may have a lower bleeding risk than alteplase. It does not bind fibrin as tightly as native tPA does so that it can diffuse more freely through the clot rather than bind only to the surface. At high concentrations, reteplase does not compete with plasminogen for fibrin-binding sites, allowing plasminogen at the site of the clot to be transformed into clot-dissolving plasmin. Reteplase does not cause allergic reactions.
- *Tenecteplase* is the latest approved thrombolytic agent. It is produced by recombinant DNA technology and its action is similar to that of alteplase. It has a longer plasma half-life, ranging initially from 20–24 minutes to 130 minutes for final clearance, mostly through liver metabolism. This allows single-bolus administration with decreased bleeding side effects as a consequence of a high fibrin specificity.

21.6 Dosage for thrombolytic agents

- Continuous infusion rather than bolus or pulse-spray infusion for treating DVT. Set infusions at low rates anticipating multiple visits to the interventional suite.
- Typical doses of alteplase by catheter – continuously 0.5–1.0 mg/kg/hour with 40 mg maximum after a bolus of 2–5 mg or by pulse spray – 0.5 mg/mL at 0.2 mL every 30–60 seconds.
- Recommended dosage of alteplase for acute PE – 10 mg intravenous bolus followed by 90 mg infusion over two hours then routine parenteral anticoagulation.

Antifibrinolytics

- Tranexamic acid is a synthetic analogue of the amino acid lysine that acts as an antifibrinolytic agent by reversibly binding lysine receptor sites on plasminogen or plasmin. This prevents plasmin from binding to and degrading fibrin and preserves the framework of fibrin's matrix structure. Tranexamic acid has roughly eight times the antifibrinolytic activity of an older analogue, ε-aminocaproic acid. It is marketed in the USA and Australia in tablet form as Lysteda and in intravenous form as Cyklokapron. It is used following major trauma, dental procedures for haemophiliacs, heavy menstrual bleeding and operations with a high risk of blood loss.

History

- Medicines made from willow and other salicylate-rich plants are referred to in the Ebers Papyrus. Hippocrates referred to the use of salicylic tea to reduce fevers around 400 BC.
- Heparin was discovered by Jay McLean (1890–1957) working as a medical student at Johns Hopkins University under William Henry Howell (1860–1945) in 1916. It was originally isolated from canine liver cells, hence its name. It was elected to define one unit of heparin as the *Howell Unit*, which is an amount approximately equivalent to 0.002 mg of pure heparin and is the quantity required to keep 1 mL of cat's blood fluid for 24 hours at 0°C. It was not introduced into clinical practice until Erik Jorpes (1894–1973), working at the Karolinska Institutet, published his research on the structure of heparin in 1935.
- Warfarin first came to attention when it was found to be produced in spoilt sweet clover to cause a fatal bleeding disease in cattle,

and it is still used as a pesticide. Its structure was revealed by Karl Paul Link (1901–1978) and co-workers in 1940 and subsequently developed at the Wisconsin Alumni Research Foundation from which it gained its name.

- John Vane, Sune Bergström and Bengt Samuelsson were awarded the 1982 Nobel Prize in Physiology or Medicine 'for their discoveries concerning prostaglandins and related biologically active substances' resulting from Vane's discovery in 1971 that aspirin suppressed production of prostaglandins and thromboxanes.

References

1. Alquwaizani M, Buckley L, Adams C, Fanikos J. Anticoagulants: A review of the pharmacology, dosing, and complications. *Curr Emergency Hosp Med Reps* 2013;1:83–97. http://link.springer.com/article/10.1007/s40138-013-0014-6

2. Yeh CH, Fredenburgh JC, Weitz JI. Oral direct FXa inhibitors. *Circ Res* 2012;111:1069–78. http://circres.ahajournals.org/content/111/8/1069

3. Hinojar R, Jimenez-Natcher JJ, Fernandez-Golfin C, Zamorano JL. New oral anticoagulants: A practical guide for physicians. *Eur Heart J – Cardiovasc Pharmacother* 2015;1:134–45. http://ehjcvp.oxfordjournals.org/content/ehjcardpharm/1/2/134.full.pdf

4. Simes J, Becattini C, Agnelli G, Eikelboom JW, Kirby AC, Mister R, Prandoni P, Brighton TA. INSPIRE Study Investigators (International Collaboration of Aspirin Trials for Recurrent Venous Thromboembolism). Aspirin for the prevention of recurrent venous thromboembolism: The INSPIRE collaboration. *Circulation* 2014;130:1062–71. https://www.ncbi.nlm.nih.gov/pubmed/25156992

5. Stangl PA, Lewis S. Review of currently available GP IIb/IIIa inhibitors and their role in peripheral vascular interventions. *Semin Intervent Radiol* 2010;27:412–21. https://www.ncbi.nlm.nih.gov/pmc/articles/PMC3324199/

6. NICE Clinical Guidelines. *Venous Thromboembolic Diseases: Thrombolytic Therapy for DVT. National Clinical Guideline Centre (UK).* 2012; London: Royal College of Physicians No. 144. https://www.ncbi.nlm.nih.gov/books/NBK132803/

22 Venous thrombo-embolism: pathology and clinical features

This chapter incorporates recommendations from an international consensus statement for prevention and treatment of venous thrombo-embolism.[1]

Pathogenesis

- The annual venous thrombo-embolism (VTE) incidence is about 1–2:1000, of which two-thirds are deep vein thrombosis (DVT) and one-third pulmonary embolism (PE).
- Virchow's triad underpins development of venous thrombosis – venous stasis, hypercoagulability and changes in the endothelium (Figure 22.1). Venous thrombosis typically begins by activation of clotting within venous valve sinuses where flow is more stagnant and blood is relatively oxygen-deprived. A thrombus is likely to propagate along a vein, initially partially fixed to the wall with a *free-floating* tail and only subsequently becoming fully adherent to occlude the vein.
- Thrombosis initiates inflammation in the vein wall involving leukocytes, cytokines and tissue factors. P-selectin is produced to cause leukocyte–endothelial adhesion and potentiate the inflammatory response, while P-selectin inhibiting mechanisms facilitate a fibrinolytic response. These release platelet-derived microparticles that further potentiate thrombosis and inflammation, while leukocytes also activate fibrinolysis.

Tissue factors and other mediators initiate a fibrotic reaction, and the balance between fibrinolysis and fibrosis determines the degree of damage to the vein wall and valves. The vein may become partially or completely occluded and valves may lose normal function, leading to post-thrombotic syndrome (see Chapter 15).

- It is necessary to distinguish between thrombosis provoked by one or more precipitating factors, or unprovoked indicating the need to search for an underlying predisposition. Principal clinical provoking factors are surgery, medical diseases, injury and immobilization, pregnancy and long-haul travel, on a background of advancing age, obesity, infection, varicose veins, past VTE and hormone prescription. Unprovoked attacks are likely to result from predisposition due to thrombophilia.

Risk factors

Surgery

- There is a variable risk for VTE after surgery without thrombo-prophylaxis depending on the patient's age and associated risk factors (Table 22.1).[2]
- The increased incidence of VTE during and for up to several weeks after surgery, is related to immobility causing venous stasis, impaired fibrinolysis and effects on coagulation factors, particularly increased thrombin activation and elevated plasminogen activator inhibitors.

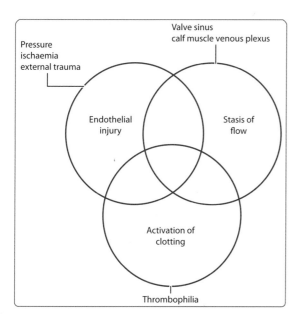

Figure 22.1 Virchow's triad.

Pregnancy

- Pulmonary embolism is the leading cause of maternal mortality in Western countries.[1,3] The prevalence of VTE is approximately 0.3–1:1000 pregnancies, up to 10 times higher than in women not pregnant and not using oral contraception. Factors I, II, VII, VIII, IX and X increase in pregnancy, and there is increased resistance to the anti-thrombotic factors proteins C and S.
- Two-thirds of DVTs occur ante-partum, distributed equally throughout all three trimesters, and 80% are in the left lower limb. In contrast, 40%–60% of pregnancy-related PEs occur at 4–6 weeks post-partum. Risk factors have been defined by the Royal College of Obstetricians and Gynaecologists.[4]

Pre-existing risk factors for VTE in pregnancy

- Previous VTE
- Thrombophilia
- Medical comorbidities
- Age >35 years
- Obesity (BMI $\geq$ 30 kg/m^2)
- Smoking
- Gross varicose veins
- Paraplegia.

Obstetric risk factors for VTE in pregnancy

- Parity $\geq$3
- Current pre-eclampsia
- Caesarean section
- Prolonged labour (>24 hours)
- Mid-cavity or rotational operative delivery
- Stillbirth
- Pre-term birth
- Post-partum haemorrhage.

New onset/transient risk factors for VTE in pregnancy

- Any surgical procedure in pregnancy or puerperium except immediate repair of the perineum

Table 22.1 Approximate risk of VTE without thrombo-prophylaxis

Risk	Patient	Calf DVT (%)	Proximal DVT (%)	Clinical PE (%)
Low	Minor surgery. Patient aged <40 years. No additional risk factors.	2	0.4	0.2
Moderate	Minor surgery, Patient with additional risk factors. Surgery in patient aged 40–60 years. No additional risk factors.	10–20	2–4	1–2
High	Surgery in patient >60 years. Additional risk factors (e.g. prior VTE, cancer).	20–40	4–8	2–4
Highest	Surgery in patient with multiple risk factors (age >40 years, cancer, prior VTE). Lower limb orthopaedic surgery.	40–80	10–20	4–10

- Bone fracture
- Hyperemesis, dehydration
- Ovarian hyperstimulation syndrome
- Assisted reproductive technology
- Immobility
- Current systemic infection
- Long distance travel.

Contraception

- The most widely used form of contraception is the combined oral contraceptive. Other options are progestin-only pills, subcutaneous implants, depot medroxyprogesterone acetate injections and medicated intrauterine devices.[1]
- In addition to providing contraception, the combined oral contraceptive results in control of menorrhagia and dysmenorrhea, and less risk of ovarian cyst and ovarian or endometrial cancers. This is at the expense of a three-fold to fourfold increased risk for VTE, mostly attributed to its oestrogen component through its effect on clotting factors, with increased APC resistance, decreased protein S and increased prothrombin. The risk is highest in the first year of use, especially the first three months, but an increased risk persists until about three months after the contraceptive is discontinued. Progestin-only contraception by the oral route, IUD or implant have no increased VTE risk and can be used in preference to combined oral contraception.
- The combined oral contraceptive contains 20–50 µg of ethinylestradiol and a progestin. There are four generations, determined by the progestin.
  - First generation – norethisterone.
  - Second generation – norgestrel, levonorgestrel.
  - Third generation – desogestrel, gestodene, norgestimate.
  - Fourth generation – drospirenone, a progestin of the spirolactone group.
- The dose of oestrogen was reduced to lessen the risk, but new progestins incorporated to improve efficacy and help acne in third and fourth generation preparations have doubled the risk of VTE compared to second generation compounds. Risk is high with a personal past history or family history of VTE. The risk increases with age and body mass index, and further by smoking, long-haul travel and immobilization. The combined oral contraceptive is absolutely contraindicated by a personal history for VTE, and caution and counselling are required with a strong family history of VTE or known thrombophilia. Progestin-only contraception rather than combined contraception, or thrombophilia testing prior to prescribing the combined oral contraceptive are recommended for women with a family history of severe VTE before the age of 50 in a first-degree relative. Use of the oral contraceptive in a woman with thrombophilia due to heterozygous factor V Leiden increases the risk by some 15–30 times, approaching that for the homozygous condition. However, screening all women for thrombophilia prior to prescribing the oral contraceptive would require about two million screens to prevent one VTE death, as the background annualized risk in this cohort is only about 1:10,000.

Hormone replacement therapy

- Hormone replacement therapy can be used to relieve symptoms of menopause.[1] Risks with oral administration include increased incidence of breast cancer, heart disease, stroke and a twofold to fourfold increased risk of VTE. As a result, treatment should be with the lowest dose that helps and for the shortest time needed, and should be re-evaluated every six months. The oestrogen dose in drugs used for hormone-replacement is generally only 20%–25% of that contained in modern oral contraceptives, but despite their much lower biological potency, their risk of causing VTE is much the same, presumably as a reflection of age.
- If the uterus has not been removed, then treatment is with an oestrogen and progestin, as oestrogen alone can stimulate endometrial growth increasing the risk of uterine cancer; treatment after hysterectomy can be with oestrogen alone. The preparations are different to those used for oral contraception. They are based on conjugated oestrogens,

synthetic conjugated oestrogens, or esterified oestrogens or 17β-oestradiol. Natural plant-derived progesterone creams sold over the counter contain too little progesterone to be effective.

- Oestradiol, when taken orally, is converted to oestrone in the liver, and this releases C-reactive protein and clotting factors, which are associated with heart disease and stroke. Oestradiol directly enters the bloodstream when used trans-dermally as a patch, gel or pessary, avoiding this risk, which is advantageous for women with diabetes, hypertension and other cardiovascular risk factors, and it has not been associated with any increased VTE risk.

Traveller's thrombosis

- There is a threefold to fourfold increased risk of thrombosis with travel by train, bus, plane or car, the increasing risk commencing after more than about four hours of travel.[5] This equates to an absolute risk of VTE for flights greater than four hours of 1:4500–6000, although the risk is at least doubled for subjects with thrombophilia or women taking the contraceptive pill, and considerably higher again with multiple risk factors.

Superficial vein thrombosis

Pathology

- Superficial vein thrombosis (SVT) results from thrombosis causing secondary chemical inflammation, and is usually self-limiting.[6,7] The alternative term superficial thrombophlebitis or simply phlebitis are commonly used, and there is usually a marked inflammatory reaction. However, the frequent response is to commence antibiotic treatment, which should be discouraged, as the pathology is a sterile inflammatory response that should not be confused with infection.
- SVT usually affects the lower limbs and is bilateral in 5%–10%. Lower limb SVT is usually benign and self-limiting, but deep vein thrombosis (DVT) and even pulmonary embolism (PE) can occur, particularly if

saphenous veins are thrombosed. The great saphenous vein (GSV) is involved in 60%–80% of patients and the small saphenous vein (SSV) in 10%–20%, but SVT usually commences in varicose tributaries from these systems. Ultrasound examination is recommended to exclude coexistent DVT, for clinical examination alone does not reliably exclude saphenous vein involvement.

- The strongest risk factors for developing SVT are varicose disease, pregnancy and obesity. SVT in the absence of varicose veins can be due to underlying cancer, vasculitis, collagen disorders or haematological diseases. SVT in the upper limbs is usually a consequence of intravenous catheters, injections used for treatment or drug abuse.
- Recent French studies identified concomitant DVT in 25%–30% of patients with SVT, and a PE in 4%–7% of patients.[7] The risk of sub-clinical PE is even higher if investigated. Below-knee thrombosis is twice as common as above-knee thrombosis, and some 40% of DVTs are not contiguous with the SVTs. The most common association is extension from the above-knee GSV into the femoral vein, whereas SVT confined to the below-knee GSV has a low risk of associated DVT.
- Inflammation usually resolves in about three weeks, and the vein can recanalize in about six to eight weeks, or it becomes a fibrous cord to cure that segment of varicose veins.
- SVT risk resembles calf vein DVT with roughly 20% chance of propagation and 4% chance of PE.

Clinical presentations

- The onset is acute and the vein is a warm red tender cord. The differential diagnosis is for cellulitis or lymphangitis. A frequent problem now is presentation with a thrombosed surface vein after sclerotherapy for varicose veins, which is frequently incorrectly treated with antibiotics as an infection.
- Migratory superficial vein thrombosis associated with cancer is known as

Trousseau's syndrome[*] and has particularly been associated with pancreatic cancer. SVT usually presents in the lower limb, but also occurs in the breast or dorsal vein of the penis after trauma, known as Mondor's disease.[†]

Deep vein thrombosis

Pathology

- Most lower limb DVTs commence in below-knee veins. Approximately 20% of below-knee DVTs spread to above-knee veins, and about 20% of these – or 4% of all patients – progress to cause symptomatic PE. The terms proximal and distal DVT should no longer be used, instead referring to calf, femoro-popliteal or ilio-femoral DVT.[8]
- Thrombosis can occur in other veins, such as the subclavian vein (see Chapter 16). DVT is frequently occult, detected only by investigation with ultrasound, presenting later with the post-thrombotic syndrome (see Chapter 15), or developing a potentially fatal PE. If an ultrasound scan is positive for DVT, then approximately 30% are bilateral. Confirming this does not affect immediate treatment but is of value to assess long-term prognosis for the post-thrombotic syndrome. The cumulative recurrence rate for DVT is about 10% at two years.
- Sudden occlusive ilio-femoral thrombosis can compromise the venous and arterial circulation causing *phlegmasia cerulea alba* (white painful inflammation), then the superficial collateral circulation as well leading to *phlegmasia cerulea dolens* (blue painful inflammation). This is characterized by severe pain, swelling, cyanosis and oedema, with a risk of venous gangrene. It most often affects one or both lower limbs, but rarely occurs in an upper limb. An underlying malignancy is found in 50% of cases, and it can complicate heparin-induced thrombocytopenia.

---

[*] Armand Trousseau (1801–1867), French physician who worked at the Hôtel Dieu in Paris.
[†] Henri Mondor (1885–1962), French professor of clinical surgery in Paris.

Clinical presentations

- The diagnosis cannot be made with confidence from the clinical features alone, whether DVT is in the lower limb or less frequently in the upper limb or other sites. Some 50% of patients with 'classic symptoms' have negative investigations, and as many as 50% of those with image-documented venous thrombosis lack specific symptoms.
- If DVT becomes symptomatic then clinical features include:
  - oedema which is the most specific feature
  - leg pain, present in 50% of patients, but nonspecific
  - warmth and redness or discoloration of the skin over the region
  - pain and tenderness due to DVT does not usually correlate well with the location and extent of the thrombus
- Examination may reveal suggestive signs:
  - swelling
  - calf tenderness
  - distention of surface veins
  - a moderately raised temperature
  - a traditional test has been to elicit discomfort behind the knee on forced dorsiflexion of the foot (Homans' test) but it has such low accuracy for diagnosis for DVT as to be of no value
- The differential diagnosis includes cellulitis, torn calf muscle, ruptured Baker's cyst, sub-fascial haematoma, ruptured plantaris muscle, prolonged limb dependency, lymphangitis or nerve entrapment.

Pulmonary embolism

- Some 25% of PEs present with sudden death, most often within 30 minutes of onset of symptoms. PE is responsible for 10% of in-hospital deaths, and many of these are preventable with prophylaxis.

Pathology

- Thrombus may break away from veins to pass through the right atrium and ventricle to occlude pulmonary arteries as a PE. Approximately 10%–20% of lower limbs DVTs lead to PE, and PE is proportionately more common in older people. PE is most likely in the early stages of thrombosis when clot is less adherent. However, approximately one-third of patients with PE confirmed by investigation have no evidence of lower limb DVT from ultrasound study. Autopsy studies show thrombus in pelvic veins in most cases, and many of these could have been diagnosed by magnetic resonance venography.

- Embolism can also be due to air, tumour, fat or amniotic fluid of venous origin. It can be detected during sclerotherapy for chronic venous disease, particularly if foamed sclerosant is used.

Clinical presentations

- Presentation may be silent and only detected by investigations, symptomatic without compromising the circulation, catastrophic causing cardiogenic shock or with sudden death. Some 10% of symptomatic PEs are fatal. Symptoms include sudden onset dyspnoea, deep then pleuritic chest pain and a cough with blood-streaked sputum. The severity of symptoms and general disability relates to the size of the thrombus and of the arteries occluded. Resolution in those who survive is usually complete, but persistence of diffuse occlusion can lead to subsequent pulmonary hypertension in less than 5%.

Paradoxical embolism

- A patent foramen ovale (PFO) is present in approximately 30% of the population. Paradoxical embolism occurs if an embolus passes from the right to left atrium through to the arterial circulation, frequently to the brain causing stroke. This would not normally happen unless the right atrial pressure exceeds the left, as during a Valsalva manoeuvre or with pulmonary hypertension. The PFO increases in size with advancing age, from a mean of 3 mm in the first decade to 6 mm in the tenth decade. Paradoxical embolism is usually isolated, but it can be associated with PE if this causes the pulmonary artery pressure to rise increasing the pressure gradient between the atria.

- Transcranial Doppler (TCD) detects small emboli during sclerotherapy using foamed sclerosant. Some 12 sclerotherapy-related strokes have been reported. TCD bubble studies are used to look for PFOs in conditions such as cryptogenic strokes.

History

- The earliest known cases of deep vein thrombosis were described by the Indian physician Sushruta in his book *Sushruta Samhita*, thought to be written by 300 BC.
- Perhaps the first well documented case of venous thrombosis is depicted in an illustrated manuscript preserved at the Bibliothèque nationale de France regarding a 20-year-old man, Raoul, who was cured of infected ulceration after praying at the church of Saint Denis in 1271.
- Wilhelm Fabry, also known as Hildanus (1560–1634), and referred to as the father of German surgery, described phlegmasia cerulea dolens.
- Gerard van Swieten (1700–1772), a Dutch–Austrian physician, reported in 1776 that injurious substances introduced into the veins of dogs 'rendered the blood grumous, through which grume flowing through the veins from a smaller to a larger capacity pass to the right ventricle and thence to the lungs'.
- A public health recommendation was issued in the late 1700s to encourage women to breast feed as a means to prevent DVT, as it was thought to result from milk building up in the leg.
- René Laennec (1781–1826), a French physician who invented the stethoscope, first described the pathologic features of haemorrhagic pulmonary infarction in a treatise on diseases of the heart and lung published in 1819.
- Jean Cruveilhier (1791–1874), a French pathologist, in his book entitled *Anatomie pathologique du corps humain* hypothesized that the cause of all disease was phlebitis and detailed the pathologic anatomy of pulmonary apoplexy.
- Rudolph Virchow (1821–1902), German pathologist, finally described the current understanding that 'a venous thrombus can

break loose from its origin, travel through the blood stream, and involve the vessels of other organs'.

References

1. Nicolaides A, Fareed J, Kakkar AK, Comerota AJ, Goldhaber SZ, Hull R, Myers K et al. Prevention and treatment of venous thromboembolism: International Consensus Statement (Guidelines according to scientific evidence). *Clin Appl Thromb Hemost.* 2013;19:116–8. http://europeanvenousforum.org/wp-content/uploads/2015/02/IUA_Guidelines_2013.pdf

2. Agnelli G. Prevention of venous thromboembolism in surgical patients. *Circulation* 2004;14;110(24 Suppl 1):IV4–12. http://circ.ahajournals.org/content/110/24_suppl_1/IV-4

3. Biron-Andreani C. Venous thromboembolic disease and pregnancy: Prevention and treatment. *Phlebolymphology* 2010;17:77–86. http://www.phlebolymphology.org/venous-thromboembolic-disease-and-pregnancy-prevention-and-treatment/

4. Royal College of Obstetricians and Gynaecologists. Reducing the risk of venous thromboembolism during pregnancy and the puerperium. Green-top Guideline No. 37a. 2015. https://www.rcog.org.uk/globalassets/documents/guidelines/gtg-37a.pdf

5. Johnston RV, Hudson MF, on behalf of the Aerospace Medical Association Air Transport Medicine Committee. Travelers' thrombosis. *Aviat Space Environ Med* 2014; 85:191–4. https://www.asma.org/asma/media/asma/Travel-Publications/Medical%20Guidelines/Travelers-Thrombosis.pdf

6. Kalodiki E, Stvrtinova V, Allegra C, Andreozzi G, Antignani PL, Avram R, Brkljacic B et al. Superficial vein thrombosis: A consensus statement. *Int Angiol.* 2012;31:203–16. http://www.minervamedica.it/en/journals/international-angiology/article.php?cod=R34Y2012N03A0203&acquista=1

7. Gillet J-L. Management of superficial vein thrombosis of the lower limbs: Update and current recommendations. *Phlebolymphology* 2015;22:82–9. http://www.phlebolymphology.org/management-of-superficial-vein-thrombosis-of-the-lower-limbs-update-and-current-recommendations/

8. de Maeseneer MG, Bochanen N, van Rooijen G, Neglén P. Analysis of 1,338 patients with acute lower limb deep venous thrombosis (dvt) supports the inadequacy of the term "proximal DVT". *Eur J Vasc Endovasc Surg.* 2016;51:415–20. https://www.ncbi.nlm.nih.gov/pubmed/26777542

23 | Venous thrombo-embolism: diagnosis

This chapter incorporates recommendations from an international consensus statement for prevention and treatment of venous thrombo-embolism.[1]

Clinical scores can help determine probability of deep vein thrombosis (DVT) and pulmonary embolism (PE). Diagnostic procedures for VTE include D-dimer blood tests, ultrasound, isotope studies and computed tomographic angiography. Many practitioners proceed directly to imaging where the possibility of VTE is high.

Wells scores

- Clinical assessment for the probability of DVT and PE can be calculated from the Wells scores. Computer or smartphone apps now allow simple calculation of the scores, which help choose the most appropriate investigations and provide medico-legal protection.[2,3]

Risk prediction for DVT

- Each of the following clinical features scores one point.
  - Active cancer – treatment within the last 6 months or palliative
  - Calf swelling ≥ 3 cm compared to asymptomatic calf measured 10 cm below tibial tuberosity
  - Swollen unilateral non-varicose superficial veins in the symptomatic limb
  - Unilateral pitting oedema in the symptomatic limb
  - Previous documented DVT
  - Swelling of the whole leg
  - Localized tenderness along the deep venous system
  - Paralysis, paresis or recent cast immobilization of lower extremities
  - Recently bedridden for ≥3 days, or major surgery requiring regional or general anaesthetic in the past 12 weeks
  - If an alternative diagnosis is at least as likely, then two points are deducted
- The possible range is from −2 to +9. Patients with a Wells scores of two or more have a 30% chance of having a DVT, whereas those with a lower score have a 5% chance.

Risk prediction for PE

- Wells scores for PE are calculated from the following criteria.
  - Clinical signs and symptoms of DVT
    – Yes + 3
  - PE is primary diagnosis OR equally likely
    – Yes + 3
  - Heart rate >100 – Yes + 1.5
  - Immobilization >3 days OR surgery in previous 4 weeks – Yes + 1.5
  - Previous, objectively diagnosed PE or DVT
    – Yes + 1.5
  - Haemoptysis – Yes + 1
  - Malignancy, treatment within 6 months or palliative – Yes + 1
- Traditional score.
  - Score >6.0 – High probability
  - Score 2.0–6.0 – Moderate probability
  - Score <2.0 – Low probability
- Alternative interpretation.
  - Score >4 – PE likely: consider diagnostic imaging.
  - Score ≤4 – PE unlikely: consider D-dimer to rule out PE.

D-dimer test

- D-dimer is a simple, rapid and cost-effective blood test to exclude VTE in low-probability patients.[4] D-dimers are fibrin degradation products that include cross-linkage from the action of FXIII. Levels can become elevated if coagulation and fibrinolysis have been activated, but can also be due to many other conditions. The D-dimer assay depends on a monoclonal antibody binding to the D-dimer fragment.
- D-dimer has about 95% sensitivity and high negative predictive value so that it can be used to select patients who do not warrant further investigation. However, it has only 50% specificity so that a positive test does not diagnose DVT as there may be other causes for elevation. It is a good screening test to exclude VTE in low- to medium-probability patients, although high-probability patients go directly to more definitive investigations.
- The reference value for D-dimer is ideally established by the performing laboratory. However, the upper limit of a normal D-dimer is normally given as 500 ng/mL, while evidence now suggests that this can be raised by 100 ng/mL for each decade over 50 years old.
- False-positive readings can be due to liver disease, high rheumatoid factor, inflammation, malignancy, trauma, pregnancy, recent surgery and advanced age. However, D-dimer levels are not affected by body mass index, oestrogen use, family history of PE, recent trauma, travel or prior VTE under treatment. The D-dimer level in individuals with factor XIII deficiency remains low even in the presence of a large thrombus owing to an impaired crosslink formation.
- False-negative readings can occur if the sample is taken too early after thrombus formation, if testing is delayed for several days or if the patient has been anticoagulated. The D-dimer is of little use after open or endovenous intervention, firstly because it is likely to be positive for about a week post-procedure and secondly because these patients are no longer at low risk for VTE so that a D-dimer test would be inappropriate.

Venous thrombosis: ultrasound

- This is the most widely accepted investigation to detect venous thrombosis.[5,6] The sensitivity for ultrasound is >95% for above-knee thrombosis and >85% for below-knee thrombosis for scans where adequate imaging is obtained. Principles of ultrasound are discussed in Chapter 4.

Select transducers

- Both deep and superficial veins are best imaged with a medium- to high-frequency linear array transducer. A lower-frequency curved array transducer may be required to scan an obese or oedematous limb, deep veins in the thigh, particularly the femoral vein at the adductor hiatus, or peroneal veins. Curved or phased array transducers are required if the examination involves the inferior vena cava and iliac, pelvic or ovarian veins.

Prepare the patient

- Ask the patient for a history of deep vein thrombosis and to indicate the site of pain. Check whether iliac veins are to be scanned, particularly if there is a history of pain or swelling in the thigh, recent pregnancy or past iliac DVT. Consider fasting the patient prior to the examination if iliac veins are to be scanned. Alter patient positioning to access veins with the least discomfort if pain is severe. Ask to be informed if the area being compressed is particularly painful as this may indicate sites for thrombosis.

Normal vein characteristics

- Compressible with transducer pressure.
- Thin-walled.
- Larger than the corresponding artery.
- Smooth interior lumen.
- Echo-free lumen.

- Augment with distal compression causing full colour filling of the lumen.
- Phasic flow with respiration and cessation of flow with the Valsalva manoeuvre in upper thigh veins.
- Increase of the common femoral vein diameter by 15–20% with the Valsalva manoeuvre.

23.1 Age of thrombus

- Acute thrombus:
  - Loss of compressibility
  - Thrombus with low echogenicity
  - Increased vein diameter
  - Free-floating thrombus
  - No flow on distal augmentation or the Valsalva manoeuvre.
- Subacute thrombus:
  - Lost or partial compressibility
  - Increased thrombus echogenicity
  - Reduced vein diameter
  - Thrombus adherent to wall
  - Recanalization.
- Chronic thrombus:
  - Partial compressibility
  - Moderate to marked thrombus echogenicity
  - Reduced vein diameter – it may be atrophied
  - Collateral flow in the region
  - Recanalization
  - Thick vein wall.

Thrombosis: direct evidence

- Inability to compress the vein. Thrombus prevents the vein closing with compression. The vein can be part compressed with partially occlusive thrombus, but is incompressible with fully occlusive thrombus.
- Intraluminal clot. Fresh clot is echolucent while old thrombus is increasingly echogenic. This feature is highly dependent on image quality and instrument settings.
- Absent flow in the vein. There is no flow with occlusive thrombosis and only peripheral flow around a central non-occlusive thrombus. This is an important indicator for iliac DVT, where it is often not possible to test for compressibility.
- Diameter of the vein. The diameter increases from the bulk of the thrombus in the acute phase. It then gradually shrinks to become smaller than normal in the chronic phase.
- Thickening of the vein wall. The wall thickness gradually increases with time.

Thrombosis: indirect evidence

- Loss of phasic flow with respiration or little or no response to the Valsalva manoeuvre in the common femoral vein suggests proximal obstruction. However, normal spectral Doppler cannot exclude DVT since there may be only partial thrombosis in the proximal veins.
- Loss of change of diameter with the Valsalva manoeuvre. No change in the CFV diameter suggests proximal occlusive thrombosis.
- Minimal flow augmentation after calf compression. This suggests occlusion between the examination and augmentation sites.
- Increased diameter and flow in superficial veins. They enlarge if they are acting as collaterals.
- Large deep veins may be seen adjacent to the thrombosed vein acting as collaterals.

Techniques

B-mode

- Locate veins and map their course. Centre each vein with B-mode in transverse to assess whether it can be compressed or contains visible thrombus. Confirm thrombus in longitudinal (Figure 23.1). Use pressure from the transducer or counter-pressure from the other hand to assess compressibility. Examine at 2–3 cm intervals down the limb for compressibility and flow. Measure thrombus extent and location from an anatomical landmark. Classify the age of thrombus.

23.2 Tips for ultrasound detection of venous thrombosis

- Deep veins always accompany their corresponding arteries and this helps to correctly identify deep veins rather than collaterals, particularly if chronic thrombosis has caused a vein to atrophy.
- The age of thrombus can be difficult to define.
- Colour Doppler can obscure partial thrombus if colour gain and echo/write priority are set too high.
- Veins to be studied can be obscured by overlying ulceration.
- It can be difficult to compress veins at deep sites or if there is pain from thrombus.
- Low flow within a partially recanalized vein can be difficult to detect.

Colour Doppler

- Distinguish veins from arteries and identify collaterals. Examine with colour Doppler in longitudinal and transverse to determine whether the vein is patent, partially or fully occluded and whether thrombus is fixed or free-floating. Assess from restriction of venous flow if partially occlusive (Figure 23.2) or loss of venous flow compared to adjacent arterial flow if fully occlusive (Figure 23.3).

Spectral Doppler

- Use spectral Doppler in longitudinal to help distinguish the vein from the artery. Examine for phasicity with normal respiration and cessation of flow with the Valsalva manoeuvre; reduced or absent phasicity indicates occlusion proximal to the test site. Confirm whether or not there is flow at the site of thrombosis. The sample volume does not need to be steered absolutely parallel to the vein wall.

Scanning

Groin veins

- Lay the patient supine with the affected leg externally rotated and examine for the femoral and proximal great saphenous veins through the femoral triangle. Scan distally to identify the sapheno-femoral junction and the confluence of the femoral and deep femoral veins.

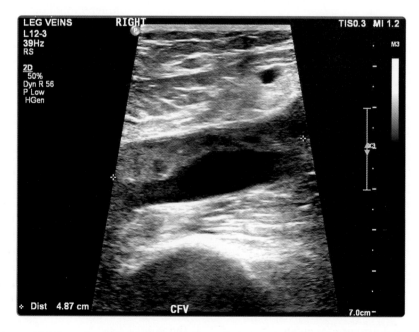

Figure 23.1 B-mode ultrasound of partially occlusive common femoral vein thrombosis.

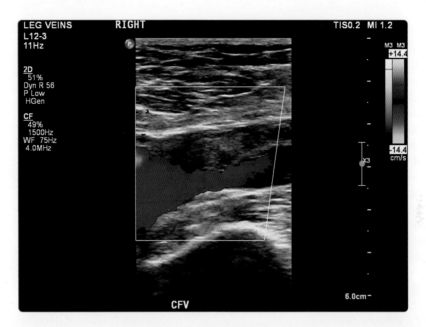

Figure 23.2 Duplex ultrasound showing flow around partially occlusive common femoral vein thrombosis.

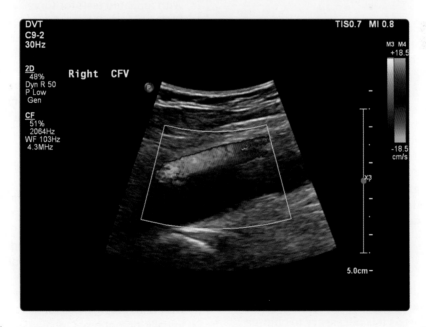

Figure 23.3 Duplex ultrasound showing no flow in the common femoral vein due to thrombosis.

Thigh veins

- Continue with the patient laying supine and the limb externally rotated to examine the femoral and great saphenous veins from an antero-medial approach. Image quality may deteriorate when you reach the adductor hiatus. Straighten the leg and use an anterior approach through the vastus medialis muscle as the vein is further from the transducer but the image is improved.

Posterior veins

- Turn the patient prone or in lateral decubitus position with the knee slightly flexed and use posterior windows. Identify the single or paired popliteal vein, which is usually superficial to the popliteal artery. In the mid-popliteal region, note the several communications including the small saphenous vein, medial and lateral gastrocnemius veins and soleal sinuses. Extra force may be needed to compress the distal popliteal vein. Examine the gastrocnemius veins to as far down into the gastrocnemius muscles as possible. Soleal sinuses are situated lower and deeper in the calf than the gastrocnemius veins and are frequently only visible if distended with thrombus. Within the popliteal fossa, check for the presence and integrity of a Baker's cyst.

Calf veins

- A preferred method to view calf veins is to sit the patient on the side of the bed facing the sonographer with the foot on the sonographers knee to allow calf muscles to drop away and better fill veins. Scan from the medial or posteromedial aspect for the posterior tibial and peroneal veins. The peroneal veins can also be seen through a posterior or anterolateral window. The below-knee great saphenous vein can be seen through a medial window. Anterior tibial vein thrombosis is so rare that many consider that it is not worth scanning these veins.

Abdominal veins

- Scan with the patient laying supine. If iliac veins need to be examined then it is best to do this last as it is necessary to change to the lower-frequency curved or phased array transducer for deeper penetration. It is difficult to compress abdominal veins. Image the inferior vena cava from an anterior approach through the rectus abdominis muscles to the right of the midline, superior to the umbilicus and at the umbilical level. It can be viewed with the patient in left lateral decubitus and a coronal (flank) window if the patient is gassy or obese. Image from an oblique approach to separate the iliac veins and arteries. When technically difficult, the iliac veins can also be imaged with the patient in a lateral decubitus position.

Superficial tributaries

- At all levels, scan for superficial vein thrombosis (Figure 23.4).

23.3 Tips for ultrasound scanning for deep vein thrombosis

- Do not compress the vein any more than necessary if there has been recent thrombosis for fear of detaching thrombus to cause PE.
- With repeated tests for surveillance after DVT, ensure that levels for the extent of thrombus for each test are taken from the same bone, surface or confluence landmarks.
- Enlarged lymph nodes in the groin can be confused with a mass of thrombus, but they can be distinguished since lymph nodes are closed-ended.
- It can be difficult to compress the distal femoral vein by imaging through the antero-medial window. If so, place your free hand behind the thigh and push the limb into the transducer rather than trying to compress the vein through the anterior muscles.
- Remember that the femoral and popliteal veins may be duplicated and both veins need to be assessed.
- Adjacent arteries and nerves can be confused with veins during ultrasound examinations.
- Initially, do not press too hard since the normal vein collapses very easily making it difficult to find.
- The gastrocnemius veins and soleal sinuses are common sites for thrombosis. They are always paired and often contain stagnant blood that may resemble fresh thrombus.

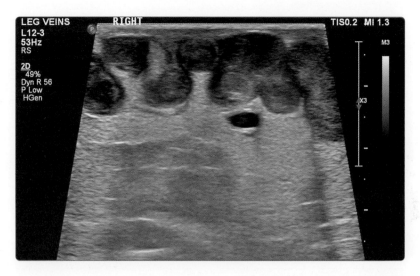

Figure 23.4 B-mode ultrasound of superficial venous thrombosis of varices in the leg.

Venous thrombosis: computed tomography

- CT venography shows thrombus as a complete or partial filling defect. Other signs are upstream venous dilatation compared with the normal contralateral side, perivenous soft-tissue swelling from oedema, contrast highlighting of vasa vasorum of the venous wall and contrast in collateral veins.[7]

Pulmonary embolism: ventilation/perfusion scan

- The ventilation/perfusion (V/Q) lung scan has been a traditional investigation to indicate whether there is a probability that a PE is present, although it has largely been replaced by computed tomographic pulmonary angiography. Medical isotopes are used to evaluate whether air reaches all parts of the lungs and how well blood flows in the pulmonary circulation. Findings are matched with a chest X-ray, as lung disease increases the chance of an indeterminate scan.
- The ventilation phase involves inhaling a gaseous radionuclide such as xenon or technetium through a mask, and the perfusion phase involves intravenous injection of radioactive technetium macro-aggregated albumin (Tc99 m-MAA) (Figure 23.5). A gamma camera acquires images for both phases.

23.4 Results of V/Q scans

- Normal: no perfusion deficit.
- Low probability (<20%): perfusion deficit with matched ventilation deficit.
- Intermediate probability (20%–80%): perfusion deficit that corresponds to parenchymal deficit on chest X-ray.
- High probability (>80%): multiple segmental perfusion deficits with normal ventilation.

Pulmonary embolism: computed tomographic pulmonary angiography

- Diagnostic criteria for acute PE by a computed tomographic (CT) pulmonary angiogram (Figure 23.6) are:[8]
  - Failure of contrast material to fill the entire lumen of an artery leaving a central filling defect
  - Partial filling defect surrounded by contrast material on a cross-sectional image

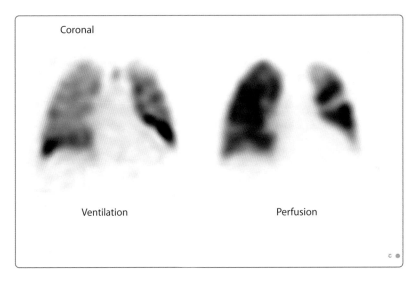

Figure 23.5 V/Q scan showing unmatched perfusion defect in the left mid-zone.

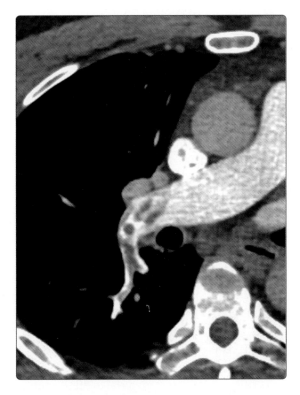

Figure 23.6 CT pulmonary angiogram showing multiple filling defects in the right main pulmonary artery extending into the right lower lobar artery.

- Contrast material between the central filling defect and the artery wall on an in-plane, longitudinal image
- A peripheral intraluminal filling defect that forms an acute angle with the artery wall
- Maximal venous enhancement occurs in less than one minute after the start of intravenous contrast injection and modern scan times are under ten seconds. Even with the best technique, a small number of studies are suboptimal particularly for sub-segmental PE.

Diagnostic pathways

Superficial vein thrombosis

- SVT is usually easily recognized by clinical examination.[9] However, ultrasound examination for both superficial and deep veins of both legs is required in all patients to show the extent and site of superficial thrombosis and the possible presence of associated DVT (Figure 23.7). The extent of thrombus demonstrated by ultrasound is usually considerably greater than is clinically apparent. Serial studies are recommended if the initial ultrasound scan shows SVT in the great or small saphenous veins

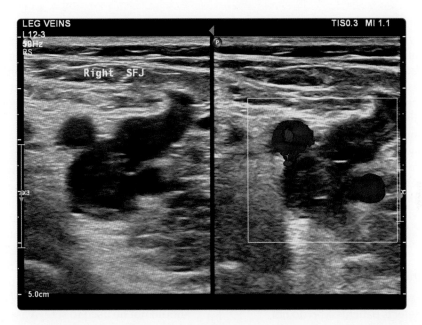

Figure 23.7 B-mode and Doppler ultrasound of superficial venous thrombosis of the great saphenous vein extending to the sapheno-femoral junction and completely occluding the common femoral vein.

to ensure that the process is not progressing and to ensure resolution.

Deep vein thrombosis

- Clinical diagnosis of DVT is unreliable.[8,10,11] Investigation in the past by venography and indirect techniques have now been replaced by the D-dimer blood test, ultrasound and CT venography in selected patients. The aim is to detect patients with DVT who will benefit from prompt commencement of anticoagulation but to avoid the dangers of bleeding from unnecessary anticoagulation in those who do not have a DVT.
- D-dimer is used to select patients who do not warrant further investigation by ultrasound. The D-dimer test should be reserved for patients with suspected DVT and should not be used to screen high-risk subjects. Patients who have had a prior DVT frequently present with residual manifestations of previous episodes or an apparently new episode, and many will have a persistently elevated D-dimer from the first presentation, limiting its predictive value in this group.

- A positive D-dimer test may lead to anticoagulation being commenced pending confirmation of DVT by an ultrasound scan at the next convenient time. However, this practice is dangerous, since the occasional patient with a strong clinical diagnosis and positive D-dimer test will in fact have bleeding into the leg from a muscle tear rather than a DVT, and anticoagulation then can cause persistent bleeding resulting in compartment syndrome. Anticoagulation can usually wait overnight for suspected DVT, although it is usually started immediately pending investigation for PE.
- Ultrasound is the investigation most often used to determine the presence, site and extent of thrombus. The yield is about 30% for leg pain or swelling suspected due to DVT and 20% for DVT as a suspected source of PE. A positive ultrasound scan then determines whether to commence or continue anticoagulation unless contra-indicated, and indicates the site and extent of disease, which has implications for long-term prognosis. If the initial scan clearly excludes DVT, then conversion to a positive scan is extremely

unlikely. Ultrasound also provides an opportunity to make a differential diagnosis in most patients. The accuracy with ultrasound for ilio-caval thrombosis is considerably less, and if there is clinical suspicion of proximal DVT, then contrast-enhanced CT venography is an effective investigation.

- There is concern regarding the expense associated with too many negative ultrasound examinations. Some units save time and cost by restricting ultrasound examination to above-knee veins, but most now routinely scan all veins below the inguinal ligament.

23.5 Diagnostic pathway for DVT

- Clinical diagnosis of DVT is unreliable.
- D-dimer selects patients who do not warrant further investigation, and is reserved for patients with suspected DVT and not used to screen high-risk asymptomatic subjects.
- A positive D-dimer test requires confirmation of DVT by an ultrasound scan as soon as convenient.
- A positive ultrasound scan then determines whether to commence or continue anticoagulation unless contra-indicated.
- Ultrasound also provides an opportunity to make a differential diagnosis.
- Contrast-enhanced CT venography may be required for ilio-caval thrombosis.
- Surveillance after a confirmed DVT can be by weekly scans until it is shown that the thrombus is not propagating.

- Surveillance after a confirmed DVT can be by weekly scans until it is shown that the thrombus is not propagating, as well as a scan for future reference at completion of anticoagulation. There is debate as to whether also scanning the contralateral asymptomatic limb is cost-effective, but an unrecognized contralateral thrombus may prove to be even larger than on the symptomatic side and should be documented at the first scan to allow follow-up if present and to assess

future risk of a post-thrombotic syndrome. Bilateral ultrasound scanning is warranted for in-patients, particularly after operation, and those with bilateral symptoms, systemic illness, probable PE, cancer, trauma or pro-thrombotic states.

Pulmonary embolism

- Clinical diagnosis of PE is unreliable.[8,10–12] A chest X-ray and ECG will be performed but give normal or non-specific findings, with sinus tachycardia as the most common finding. The D-dimer test, ventilation/perfusion (V/Q) lung scan and CTPA are now the investigations used for diagnosis.
- D-dimer is used to exclude PE in low-probability patients. As with DVT studies, it should not be used to screen asymptomatic patients. The PERC rule (Pulmonary Embolism Rule Out Criteria) was developed to avoid performing any investigations including D-dimer studies on so-called 'no-risk patients'. A patient who answers yes to all following nine criteria can be cleared of the need for investigation. If a low-risk patient does not pass the PERC rule, then a D-dimer is ordered.
- PERC:
  - Low risk by Gestalt or other criteria.
  - Age <50 years.
  - Pulse <100.
  - O_2 saturation on room air >94%.
  - No unilateral leg swelling.
  - No haemoptysis.
  - No recent trauma or surgery.
  - No previous VTE.
  - No oral hormone use.
- The diagnosis of PE is ruled out by a negative D-dimer test in some 50% of patients aged less than 50 years but in only about 5% of patients 80 years of age and older, although the efficacy of the test is improved by setting a higher threshold level in older patients – 500 ug/L + 100 ug/L for each decade over 50.
- Residual DVT is lacking in many patients with PE, either because the entire thrombus has already detached to pass to the lungs

or thrombus is in veins not studied by ultrasound. The sensitivity for detecting PE from a lower limb ultrasound study is no more than 40% so that this is not a cost-effective predictive investigation, although it is usually performed for prognostic reasons if a PE is confirmed.

- The V/Q scan determines whether there is disturbed airflow and circulation through the lungs. A high-probability lung scan shows a segmental perfusion defect with a normal ventilation scan. The V/Q scan can only provide a low, moderate or sometimes high probability of PE, although the accuracy is considerably improved if it is restricted only to patients who have a normal chest X-ray.

- Current techniques for CT pulmonary angiography have very high sensitivity and specificity for detecting even very small PEs. In addition, they provide the opportunity to make a differential diagnosis in most patients. However, recurrent emboli may be difficult to differentiate from residual emboli, which may be present in up to 50% of patients. Contrast-enhanced CT carries a risk of an allergic reaction and nephrotoxicity. Newer techniques such as positron emission tomography, magnetic resonance imaging and even lung surface ultrasound are being evaluated.[8] There is concern as to potential over-use of CT scanning because of patient risk and excessive costs.

23.6 Diagnostic pathway for PE

- Clinical diagnosis of PE is unreliable.
- D-dimer is used to exclude PE in low-probability patients.
- Lower limb ultrasound is not an effective predictive investigation for PE.
- The V/Q scan can only provide a low, moderate or occasional high probability of PE.
- CT pulmonary angiography has a very high sensitivity and specificity for detecting even small PEs.
- CT also provides an opportunity to make a differential diagnosis.

Strategies for underlying causes

Pregnancy

- D-dimer levels increase during pregnancy, rendering this test difficult to evaluate after the first trimester.[13] However, pregnancy has a five- to ten-times increased VTE risk so that no pregnant woman with suspected DVT or PE can be in the low-probability range and should not be investigated by D-dimer but should undergo imaging.

- For suspected PE in a pregnant woman, perform a lower limb ultrasound first, for if positive then there is no need for further investigations before commencing treatment. If the chest examination and X-Ray are normal, a half-dose V/Q scan can be performed first, and a positive result then avoids the need for a full V/Q scan so as to cause minimal foetal risk, as the rate of an indeterminate V/Q scan in pregnant women is only 20% compared to the usual 70% rate for all patients. If the chest examination or X-Ray are abnormal, V/Q is likely to be indeterminate, and low-dose CTPA is better. Place an indwelling urinary catheter for 24 hours post V/Q scan to reduce foetal exposure to radioactive urine.

- The foetal radiation exposure is very low with both modalities, though less with CTPA. However, the maternal breast exposure from CT is relatively high, as breasts are more radio-sensitive in pregnancy and lactation so that this may slightly increase the lifelong risk of breast or lung cancer, while there are theoretical concerns regarding iodine and the developing foetal thyroid. For CTPA in pregnancy, it is advised to use a bismuth shield and automated exposure controls to minimize the absorbed radiation dose to the breasts, and breathing strategies to limit the number of inadequate studies.

Malignancy

- Cancer associated with VTE is usually known to be present so that screening for undiagnosed cancer is not often required. However, a general history and examination, including rectal and pelvic examination, are indicated, and routine age-appropriate cancer screening such as chest X-ray, mammography and breast ultrasound, and blood tests for prostate specific antigens are performed. CT and endoscopy are performed to search for an occult malignancy when indicated.

References

1. Nicolaides A, Fareed J, Kakkar AK, Comerota AJ, Goldhaber SZ, Hull R, Myers K et al. Prevention and treatment of venous thromboembolism: International Consensus Statement (Guidelines according to scientific evidence). *Clin Appl Thromb Hemost* 2013;19:116–8. http://europeanvenousforum.org/wp-content/uploads/2015/02/IUA_Guidelines_2013.pdf

2. Wells' criteria for deep vein thrombosis. MedCalc. https://www.mdcalc.com/wells-criteria-dvt

3. Wells' criteria for pulmonary embolism. MedCalc. https://www.mdcalc.com/wells-criteria-pulmonary-embolism

4. Kabrhel C, Courtney DM, Camargo CA, Plewa MC, Nordenholz KE, Moore CL, Richman PB, Smithline HA, Beam DM, Kline JA. Factors associated with positive D-dimer results in patients evaluated for pulmonary embolism. *Acad Emerg Med* 2010; 17: 589–97. https://www.ncbi.nlm.nih.gov/pubmed/20624138

5. Myers KA, Clough A. *Practical Vascular Ultrasound. An Illustrated Guide.* 2014, CRC Press. https://www.crcpress.com/Practical-Vascular-Ultrasound-An-Illustrated-Guide/Myers-Clough/p/book/9781444181180

6. Zygmunt J, Pichot O, Dauplaise T. *Practical Phlebology: Venous Ultrasound.* 2013; CRC Press. https://www.crcpress.com/Practical-Phlebology-Venous-Ultrasound/Zygmunt-Pichot-Dauplaise/p/book/9781853159480

7. Ghaye B, Szapiro D, Willems V, Dondelinger RF. Pitfalls in CT venography of lower limbs and abdominal veins. *Am J Roentgenol* 2002;178:1465–71. http://www.ajronline.org/doi/full/10.2214/ajr.178.6.1781465

8. Dronkers CEA, Klok FA, Huisman MV. Current and future perspectives in imaging of venous thromboembolism. *J Thromb Haemost* 2016;14:1696–710. http://onlinelibrary.wiley.com/doi/10.1111/jth.13403/full

9. Kalodiki E, Stvrtinova V, Allegra C, Andreozzi G, Antignani PL, Avram R, Brkljacic B et al. Superficial vein thrombosis: a consensus statement. *Int Angiol* 2012;31:203–16. http://www.minervamedica.it/en/journals/international-angiology/article.php?cod=R34Y2012N03A0203&acquista=1

10. Huisman MV, Klok FA. Diagnostic management of acute deep vein thrombosis and pulmonary embolism. *J Thromb Haemost* 2013;11:412–22. http://onlinelibrary.wiley.com/doi/10.1111/jth.12124/full

11. Le Gal G, Righini M. Controversies in the diagnosis of venous thromboembolism. *J Thromb Haemost* 2015;13:S259–65. http://onlinelibrary.wiley.com/doi/10.1111/jth.12937/full

12. Da Costa Rodrigues J, Alzuphar S, Combescure C, Le Gal G, Perrier A. Diagnostic characteristics of lower limb venous compression ultrasonography in suspected pulmonary embolism: a meta-analysis. *J Thromb Haemost* 2016;14:1765–72. https://www.ncbi.nlm.nih.gov/pubmed/27377039

13. Sadro CT, Dubinsky TJ. CT in pregnancy: Risks and benefits. Applied Radiology 2013 October: 6–16. http://appliedradiology.com/articles/ct-in-pregnancy-risks-and-benefits

24 Venous thrombo-embolism: prevention

This chapter incorporates guidelines from an Australian and New Zealand working party on the management and prevention of venous thrombo-embolism, and an international consensus statement.[1,2]

Prevention of venous thrombo-embolism (VTE) involves mechanical measures to prevent stasis and anticoagulation to limit thrombosis.

Assessment for VTE risk

There are several different quantitative scoring systems hospital use to assess VTE risk. An example is the Caprini Score which has been validated prospectively in surgical patients.

Caprini score

- The Caprini score provides an objective measure for VTE risk which in turn determines level of prophylaxis.[3]
- **Add 1 point** for each of the following statements that apply now or within the past month:
  - Age 41–60 years _____
  - Minor surgery (less than 45 minutes) is planned _____
  - Past major surgery (more than 45 minutes) within the last month _____
  - Visible varicose veins _____
  - A history of inflammatory bowel disease (e.g. Crohn's disease or ulcerative colitis) _____
  - Swollen legs (current) _____
  - Overweight or obese (body mass index above 25) _____
  - Heart attack _____
  - Congestive heart failure _____
  - Serious infection (e.g. pneumonia) _____
  - Lung disease (e.g. emphysema or COPD) _____
  - On bed rest or restricted mobility, including a removable leg brace for less than 72 hours _____
  - Other risk factors – BMI above 40, smoking, diabetes requiring insulin, chemotherapy, blood transfusions, and length of surgery over 2 hours (1 point each) _____
- **For women only: add 1 point** for each of the following statements that apply:
  - Current use of birth control or hormone replacement therapy (HRT) _____
  - Pregnant or had a baby within the last month _____
  - History of unexplained stillborn infant, recurrent spontaneous abortion (more than 3), premature birth with toxemia or growth restricted infant _____
- **Add 2 points** for each of the following statements that apply:
  - Age 61–74 years _____
  - Current or past malignancies (excluding skin cancer, but not melanoma) _____
  - Planned major surgery lasting longer than 45 minutes (including laparoscopic and arthroscopic) _____
  - Non-removable plaster cast or mould that has kept you from moving your leg within the last month _____
  - Tube in blood vessel in neck or chest that delivers blood or medicine directly to heart within the last month (also called central venous access, PICC line or port) _____

- Confined to a bed for 72 hours or more _____
- **Add 3 points** for each of the following statements that apply:
  - Age 75 or over _____
  - History of blood clots, either deep vein thrombosis (DVT) or pulmonary embolism (PE) _____
  - Family history of blood clots (thrombosis) _____
  - Personal or family history of positive blood test indicating an increased risk of blood clotting _____
- **Add 5 points** for each of the following statements that apply now or within the past month:
  - Elective hip or knee joint replacement surgery _____
  - Broken hip, pelvis or leg _____
  - Serious trauma (e.g. multiple broken bones due to a fall or car accident) _____
  - Spinal cord injury resulting in paralysis _____
  - Experienced a stroke in the last month _____

Total score

- 0 – very low risk.
- 1–2 – low risk: early ambulation + compression stockings.
- 3–4 – moderate risk: early ambulation + compression stockings or anticoagulant.
- ≥5 – high risk: early ambulation + compression stockings + anticoagulant.

Mechanical measures

- Graduated compression stockings (GCS) effectively reduce the risk of venous thrombo-embolism (VTE) for most patients immobilized in hospital.[4] However, an increased risk of skin damage with breaks, ulcers, blisters or necrosis may outweigh these effects in severely immobilized patients, for example, after stroke.
- Compression stockings and bandaging have been discussed in Chapter 11. GCS reduce the risk of DVT after surgery by about 50%.[2] Knee-high stockings are as effective as thigh-high or pantihose garments for routine prophylaxis and are better accepted by patients. Below-knee compression is also an effective means to reduce the risk of traveller's thrombosis. Thrombo-embolic deterrent (TED) stockings used in hospitals have weak compression and are not truly graduated, and are intended for use in immobilized patients and not for ambulatory use like GCS.
- A review regarding GCS[5] concluded that there is:
  - High-quality evidence to support their use for chronic venous disease, especially patients with ulcers.
  - Low- to moderate-quality evidence for a prophylactic effect against deep vein thrombosis in medically ill patients.
  - Low-quality evidence for a prophylactic effect against deep vein thrombosis in general surgical and orthopaedic patients, but insufficient evidence to support their use during pregnancy.
  - No evidence to support their use for the prevention or treatment of the post-thrombotic syndrome. However, two studies have supported their use to prevent the post-thrombotic syndrome.[6,7]
- A randomized controlled trial of over 2000 patients treated world-wide in 64 centres within one week of acute stroke, found that thigh-length GCS did not reduce occurrence of symptomatic or asymptomatic proximal DVT, and that skin complications with breaks, ulcers, blisters or skin necrosis were significantly more common in those assigned to wearing stockings.[8]
- Intermittent pneumatic compression (IPC) using a sequential compression device with an air pump and inflatable sleeve is widely used to simulate muscle pumping and improve venous circulation in the limbs during and for a time after surgery. They reduce the incidence of asymptomatic DVT after surgery from 25% to under 10%.[2] The devices differ as to patient comfort and medical staff satisfaction. Electrical calf

muscle stimulation has also been widely used to activate calf muscle pumping. Early ambulation is encouraged.

- Manufacturing features for commercial devices have various variable and fixed features that determine the total venous volume expelled per hour, such as applied pressure, cycle rate, pressure rise time and refill time, which determine the peak velocity and pulse volume.

Anticoagulation

- Anticoagulation is the primary means to prevent and treat deep vein thrombosis (DVT) and pulmonary embolism (PE). Prevention requires a balance between reducing the risk of VTE against the risk of bleeding from anticoagulation. Anticoagulants limit extension of a thrombus and reduce the risk of detachment to cause embolism but do not reduce the size of an existing thrombus and have not been shown to lessen the risk of developing the post-thrombotic syndrome. Prolonged anticoagulation is usually required to limit the risk of recurrent DVT or PE, although these benefits must be balanced against the dangers from anticoagulation causing significant bleeding. Newer oral agents are addressing the inconvenience of treatment by injections and the need for repeated blood tests to monitor dosage. Drug inter-actions are less common with the new oral agents. Anticoagulant drugs are described in Chapter 21.

Surgical patients

- Without thrombo-prophylaxis, the inci-dence of silent DVT in patients who undergo general surgery is about 25%, and this rises to some 50% in high-risk patients, while the risk of clinical PE is about 2%.[1] Prevention relies on combined physical methods to reduce venous stasis and anticoagulation. These have mark-edly reduced the incidence of VTE, but there is still a risk, and compliance with recommendations for prevention is far from universal. Anticoagulation for non-surgical thrombo-prophylaxis can be extrapolated from the recommendations for surgery.

- Risk relates to the extent of surgery. Recommendations below
    - Major surgery – any intra-abdominal operation and all other operations lasting for more than 45 minutes.
    - Minor surgery – operations other than intra-abdominal procedures and lasting for less than 45 minutes.

Choice of anticoagulant

- Recommended anticoagulation for general surgery is with unfractionated heparin (UFH) or low molecular weight heparin (LMWH). Prophylaxis with direct oral anti-coagulants (DOAC) has only been approved in Australia for hip and knee replacement surgery.
- LMWHs are preferred to UFH due to there being no need for monitoring and lower incidence of heparin-induced thrombo-cytopenia. However, UFH infusion is still preferred in high-risk situations where precise thrombo-regulation is desired, such as cardiothoracic surgery.
- Subcutaneous calciparine is ideal for patients in renal failure.
- Fondaparinux has been studied for hip surgery in some countries and found to have less risk of causing heparin-induced thrombocytopenia and no increased risk of bleeding.
- Vitamin K antagonists have also been used for orthopaedic surgery but are not active until at least five days post-operation.
- DOACs are increasingly being preferred due to convenience for prolonged post-operative prophylaxis.
- There is now evidence that aspirin has some venous antithrombotic effect. It has been accepted by some groups for orthopaedic surgery, but as yet there is little evidence to support its use for routine non-orthopaedic operative prophylaxis.

24.1 Risk stratification for VTE with surgery

- High-risk
  - Major general surgery, age 40–60 years and cancer or history of DVT/PE or other VTE risk factors.[1,2]
  - Major general surgery, age >60 years.
  - Major orthopaedic surgery.
- Moderate-risk
  - Minor surgery, age 40–60 years and history of DVT/PE or other VTE risk factors.
  - Minor surgery, age >60 years.
  - Major general surgery, age 40–60 years without other VTE risk factors.
- Low-risk
  - Minor surgery, age 40–60 years and no other VTE risk factors.
  - Major general surgery, age <40 years and no other risk factors.
  - Guidelines for pharmacological and mechanical prophylaxis in surgical patients according to the extent of the operation taking into account possible contraindications to prophylactic measures are summarized in Table 24.1.[1,2]
- Contraindications to anticoagulant prophylaxis include active bleeding or a high risk of bleeding, thrombocytopenia (platelet count $<50 \times 10^9$/L), history of gastrointestinal bleeding, severe hepatic disease, adverse reaction to heparin, on current anticoagulation, high falls risk and palliative management.
- Contraindications to mechanical prophylaxis include severe peripheral arterial disease, recent skin graft, severe peripheral neuropathy and severe leg deformity.
- VTE risk factors include thrombophilia, oestrogen therapy, pregnancy or puerperium, immobility, active inflammation, strong family history of VTE and/or obesity.

Prophylactic anticoagulation regimes

- The optimal duration for prophylaxis has still to be determined.[1,2] It has been five to seven days in most studies, but the risk is known to continue for longer. Extending prophylaxis from one week to one month considerably reduces incidence of asymptomatic DVT by 50%–70%. Extended pharmacological prophylaxis beyond seven days should be considered if patients develop post-operative complications such as infection. Patients undergoing

Table 24.1 Guidelines for thrombo-embolism prophylaxis

Nature of surgery	Safe for anticoagulant prophylaxis	Safe for mechanical prophylaxis
High risk		
Hip joint replacement or fracture surgery	YES – Anticoagulation for 28–35 days	YES – Apply IPC and/or GCS
Knee joint replacement. Major trauma	YES – Anticoagulation for 5–10 days	YES – Apply GCS and /or IPC
Other surgery with prior VTE or cancer	YES – Anticoagulation for 5–10 days	YES – Apply GCS and /or IPC
Major surgery age >40 years	YES – Anticoagulation for 5–10 days	YES – Apply GCS and /or IPC
Lower risk		
All other surgery with risk factor	YES – Consider anticoagulation	YES – Consider GCS
All other surgery with no risk factor	YES – No anticoagulation	YES – Consider GCS

abdominal or pelvic surgery for cancer and who do not present contraindications to extended prophylaxis should receive LMWH for up to one month after operation.

- Major orthopaedic surgery such as hip joint replacement or hip fracture surgery carry a high risk of VTE, and the risk persists for up to five weeks after operation. Anticoagulant prophylaxis in Australia is approved for five weeks following hip replacement and two weeks following knee replacement. However, there is also an appreciable risk of bleeding complicating the extensive dissection required. LMWH, fondaparinux, vitamin K antagonists or DOACs are all highly effective, but mechanical prophylaxis alone is an alternative if there is concern about bleeding until it is safe to resume anticoagulation.

- Routine prophylaxis is not recommended for diagnostic arthroscopy, unless other risk factors are present, but may be indicated for arthroscopy with ligament reconstruction.

- Timing for ceasing anticoagulation before surgery and recommencing it afterwards depends on the drug half-life and VTE risk. In general, cease LMWH or DOACs 24 hours before and intravenous UFH two hours before operation, and consider restarting as soon as four hours after operation providing haemostasis is secure if there is a high thrombotic but low bleeding risk.

24.2 Anticoagulant dosing for thromboprophylaxis

- Subcutaneous UFH – 5000 U bd or tds.
- LMWH – enoxaparin 40 mg daily or daltaparin 5000 U daily.
- Fondaparinux – 2.5 mg daily as an alternative for major orthopaedic surgery.

- DOAC – rivaroxaban 10 mg orally once daily, apixaban 2.5 mg bd, dabigatran 110 mg four hours post-operation then 220 mg daily.

Pregnancy

- Salient recommendations from the Royal College of Obstetricians and Gynaecologists in 2015 for reducing the risk of venous thrombo-embolism during pregnancy and the puerperium are summarized as follows.[9]

All pregnant women

- Based on the number of risk factors present during pregnancy and listed in Chapter 22, subsection 'New onset/transient risk factors for VTE in pregnancy', excluding previous VTE and thrombophilia:
  - Two risk factors – LMWH for at least ten days post-partum.
  - Three – LMWH from 28 weeks to six weeks post-partum.
  - Four or more – LMWH throughout the pregnancy to six weeks post-partum.

- For admissions related to hyperemesis gravidarum or ovarian hyper-stimulation – consider LMWH.
- At risk for pre-eclampsia – low-dose aspirin throughout pregnancy from the second trimester.

Previous VTE

- If having treatment with long-term oral anticoagulation, change to LMWH as soon as pregnancy is confirmed, ideally within two weeks of the missed period and before the sixth week of pregnancy.
- If not on long-term anticoagulation, start LMWH as soon as there is a positive pregnancy test.
- Original VTE provoked by major surgery with recovery and no other risk factors – withhold LMWH until 28 weeks but with close surveillance.

- Unprovoked or all non-surgically provoked including oestrogen therapy – prophylactic dose LMWH throughout pregnancy and post-partum.

Associated thrombophilia

- Previous single or recurrent VTE associated with thrombophilia due to antithrombin deficiency or the antiphospholipid syndrome – full-dose LMWH throughout the pregnancy and for six weeks post-partum or until returned to oral anticoagulation.
- Previous VTE associated with other hereditary thrombophilias – low-dose thromboprophylaxis.
- No history of VTE and heterozygous for factor V Leiden or the prothrombin 20210A mutation and a positive family history for VTE – LMWH through pregnancy and for six weeks post-partum.
- No prior history of VTE and heterozygous for factor V Leiden or the prothrombin 20210A mutation and no family history for VTE – clinical vigilance through pregnancy and LMWH for six weeks post-partum.
- All other thrombophilias and no prior VTE and a positive family history for VTE – clinical vigilance through pregnancy and LMWH post-partum.
- All other thrombophilias and no prior VTE with no positive family history for VTE – clinical vigilance rather than pharmacologic prophylaxis through pregnancy and post-partum.

During and after labour and delivery

- Vaginal bleeding or once labour begins – do not inject further LMWH until assessed.
- Avoid epidural anaesthesia if possible until at least 12 hours after the previous dose of LMWH.
- Do not give LMWH for four hours after spinal anaesthesia or after an epidural catheter has been removed.
- Elective Caesarean section – thromboprophylactic dose of LMWH on the day prior to delivery, omit the morning dose and perform the operation that morning, and

resume LMWH as soon as possible after delivery provided there is no postpartum haemorrhage and regional analgesia has not been used. Consider LMWH for ten days after elective Caesarean section if there are any additional risk factors.

Traveller's thrombosis

- A Cochrane review concluded that 'There is high-quality evidence that airline passengers ... can expect a substantial reduction in the incidence of symptomless DVT, and low-quality evidence that leg oedema is reduced if they wear compression stockings. ... There is moderate-quality evidence that superficial vein thrombosis may be reduced if passengers wear compression stockings. We cannot assess the effect of wearing stockings on death, pulmonary embolism or symptomatic DVT because no such events occurred in these trials'.[10]

Inferior vena cava filter

- Inferior vena cava (IVC) filters form a mechanical barrier to flow of emboli larger than 4 mm and were developed to attempt to prevent PE. Benefit from a reduced incidence of PE must be balanced against an increased risk of new or further DVT.
- Indications have broadened with the introduction of temporary removable filters. The decision whether to use a temporary or permanent filter depends on the likely time that the patient is at risk of PE or has a contraindication to anticoagulation. They should be removed if at all possible when the risk is averted, as complications such as DVT and migration intraperitoneally or into the duodenum are well documented.
- Several different filter configurations have been used, including the Greenfield filter which has the longest follow-up, with patency rates greater than 95% and recurrent embolism rates of less than 5%. The conical shape allows central filling with emboli while allowing blood on the periphery to

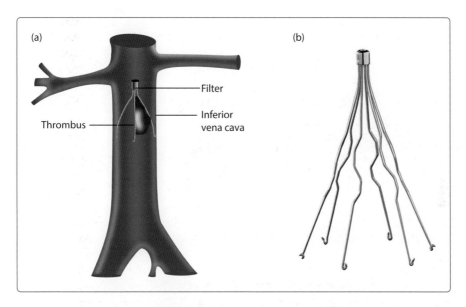

Figure 24.1 Greenfield inferior vena cava filter. The filter is placed just below the renal veins. Its conical shape traps thrombus but allows forward flow.

flow freely (Figure 24.1). The filter collects emboli centrally, though small ones continue to pass. They do not 'overflow' because the captured clot is continually subject to fibrinolysis.

- Regardless of the type of filter chosen, the technique for insertion is similar. Percutaneous approach is through either the common femoral or internal jugular vein. A guide wire and catheter are inserted and a venogram is performed to identify the renal veins and measure the diameter of the IVC to ensure the vein is not too big for the filter. Correct filter placement is infra-renal fixation with central filter extension to the level of the renal veins, though placement in the suprarenal IVC or superior vena cava may be required, according to the site of thrombosis.

Indications for IVC filter

- PE or proximal DVT with contraindications to anticoagulation.[2]
- Recurrent acute PE despite therapeutic anticoagulation.
- Acute PE and poor cardiopulmonary reserve.

Contraindications to IVC filter

- Coagulopathy.
- Total IVC thrombosis.
- Sepsis.
- Caval diameter <15 mm.

IVC filter and anticoagulation

- An IVC filter should not be used routinely as an adjunct to anticoagulation.
- Patients receiving an IVC filter due to a contraindication to anticoagulation should be restarted on anticoagulation whenever the contraindication no longer exists.

References

1. The Australia and New Zealand working party on the management and prevention of venous thromboembolism. Prevention of venous thromboembolism. 4th edn. 2014. http://www.surgeons.org/media/19372/VTE_Guidelines.pdf
2. Nicolaides A, Fareed J, Kakkar AK, Comerota AJ, Goldhaber SZ, Hull R, Myers K et al. Prevention and treatment of venous thromboembolism: International consensus statement (Guidelines according to scientific evidence). *Clin Appl Thromb Hemost.* 2013;19:116–8. http://cat.sagepub.com/content/19/2/116.full.pdf+html

3. Sachdeva A, Dalton M, Amaragiri SV, Lees T. Graduated compression stockings for prevention of deep vein thrombosis. *Cochrane Library* 2014. http://onlinelibrary.wiley.com/doi/10.1002/14651858.CD001484.pub3/full

4. Caprini JA. North Shore University Health System. 2013. http://venousdisease.com/documents/caprini-dvt-risk-assessment.pdf

5. Lim CS, Davies AH. Graduated compression stockings. *Canad Med Assoc J* 2014;186:E391–8. http://www.cmaj.ca/content/186/10/E391

6. Brandjes DP, Büller HR, Heijboer H, Huisman MV, de Rijk M, Jagt H, ten Cate JW. Randomised trial of effect of compression stockings in patients with symptomatic proximal-vein thrombosis. *Lancet.* 1997;349:759–62. https://www.ncbi.nlm.nih.gov/pubmed/9074574

7. Prandoni P, Lensing AW, Prins MH, Frulla M, Marchiori A, Bernardi E, Tormene D, Mosena L, Pagnan A, Girolami A. Below-knee elastic compression stockings to prevent the post-thrombotic syndrome: A randomized, controlled trial. *Ann Intern Med.* 2004;141:249–56. https://www.ncbi.nlm.nih.gov/pubmed/15313740

8. Dennis M, Sandercock PA, Reid J, Graham C, Murray G, Venables G, Rudd A, Bowler G. Effectiveness of thigh-length graduated compression stockings to reduce the risk of deep vein thrombosis after stroke (CLOTS trial 1): A multicentre, randomised controlled trial. *Lancet* 2009;373:1958–65. https://www.ncbi.nlm.nih.gov/pubmed/19477503

9. Royal College of Obstetricians and Gynaecologists. Reducing the risk of venous thromboembolism during pregnancy and the puerperium. Green-top Guideline No. 37a. 2015. https://www.rcog.org.uk/globalassets/documents/guidelines/gtg-37a.pdf

10. Clarke MJ, Broderick C, Hopewell S, Juszczak E, Eisinga A. Compression stockings for preventing deep vein thrombosis in airline passengers. *Cochrane Database System Rev* 2016;(9):Art. No.: CD004002. doi: 10. 1002/14651858.CD004002.pub3. http://www.cochrane.org/CD004002/PVD_compression-stockings-preventing-deep-vein-thrombosis-dvt-airline-passengers

25 Venous thrombo-embolism – treatment

This chapter incorporates guidelines from an Australian and New Zealand working party on the management and prevention of venous thrombo-embolism and an international consensus statement.[1,2]

Treatment for venous thrombo-embolism (VTE) aims to reduce symptoms from superficial vein thrombosis (SVT) and deep vein thrombosis (DVT), avoid the risk of death from pulmonary embolism (PE), and attempt to avoid or restrict the post-thrombotic syndrome.

Treatment options
- Treatment of VTE may involve:
  - Graduated compression stockings or bandages
  - Anticoagulation to limit thrombosis
  - Thrombolysis to remove thrombus
  - Interventional procedures to remove thrombus

Superficial vein thrombosis

- Supportive measures should be instituted for all patients diagnosed with lower limb SVT, with compression bandages or stockings, pain management and extremity elevation whenever possible.
- For patients with SVT not related to endo-venous treatment who are at increased risk for DVT, anticoagulation with DOACs, fondaparinux, LMWH, UFH or vitamin K antagonists are all effective.[3] The CALISTO trial showed that having excluded high-risk SVT, 45 days of intermediate-dose fondaparinux reduced the already low 3%

propagation risk to 1.5%.[4] It is recommended that:
- Low-risk SVT can be managed with NSAIDs, mobilization and ultrasound follow-up.
- Higher-risk SVT, and SVT affecting longer segments or close to the SFJ, SPJ or perforators should probably receive full anticoagulation with serial ultrasound follow-up.
- Patients who present with SVT after endovenous treatment do not require anticoagulation as risk of progression to DVT is very small.
- If thrombus extends into the deep venous system, the patient is treated with standard protocols for DVT. Traditional treatment for saphenous vein thrombosis approaching the junction has been with surgical liga-tion, but studies have not shown any benefit for surgical treatment compared to anti-coagulation alone, and show that the risk of VTE and complications is higher with surgery.[5]

Deep vein thrombosis and pulmonary embolism

- Anticoagulants are used to treat VTE unless contraindicated. Patients with acute DVT require compression bandages or stockings to reduce inflammation and consequent pain, as well as to lessen the risk of thrombus extension by increasing flow in patent veins. Early ambulation is associated with improved blood flow and reduced thrombus extension, with no increased risk of provoking a PE.

Anticoagulation

- The anticoagulants available and dosing options are described in Chapter 21.
- Treatment is essentially the same for SVT, DVT and PE. Traditional treatment has been to commence with subcutaneous LMWH, subcutaneous fixed-dose UFH or intravenous UFH. UFH is continued with warfarin for at least five days and until the INR is >2 for 24 hours. Long-term treatment with subcutaneous LMWH is more effective and is advised with severe ongoing comorbidity such as malignancy and during pregnancy.
- Warfarin is not started when patients require thrombolysis, surgery or have co-morbidities that predispose to major bleeding.

  Use of warfarin is decreasing as it is being replaced by a DOAC from the start due to warfarin's slow onset and long half life, the time many patients spend outside the therapeutic range, multiple drug and food interactions and the inconvenient monitoring that is necessary.
- Because DOACs are therapeutic in two hours they are an alternative to LMWH, or likewise can be initiated later when the LMWH dose would have become due.
- All patients with proven VTE should receive anticoagulation for at least three months, except perhaps for SVT and small calf vein thromboses. This is sufficient for a patient with a major provoking risk factor that has been removed. Prolonged anticoagulation may be appropriate for a patient with an unprovoked VTE but the decision is based on the balance between benefit, risk of bleeding and patient preference, and should be regularly reviewed. Indefinite anticoagulation is appropriate for a patient with more than one episode of VTE.
- Serial ultrasound examinations, although useful to exclude early propagation, may reach a stable state after a few months at which point further imaging is pointless. Return of a D-dimer test to normal indicates that recurrence is considerably less likely if treatment is then ceased. A study found that a normal D-dimer at one month after anticoagulation withdrawal indicated a 4.4% risk of recurrence per year, and that a persistently normal study at three months had a 2.9% risk, whereas an abnormal result at three months predicted a 27% recurrence rate.[6] It is recommended to measure D-dimer at the time of cessation and at one and three months later, and to discuss restarting anticoagulation if the test again becomes abnormal.

Complications of anticoagulation

- When commencing anticoagulants, explain to patients that they will bruise more easily. Warn against contact sports and to report epistaxis, haematuria, bleeding per rectum, severe headaches or unexplained pain.

Haemorrhage

- Risk Prediction for bleeding from anticoagulation can be determined from scores such as the HAS-BLED score. Each scores one point.

Hypertension	Uncontrolled, >160 mm Hg systolic
Abnormal renal function	Dialysis, transplant, creatinine >2.6 mg/dL or >200 µmol/L
Abnormal liver disease	Cirrhosis, bilirubin >2 × normal, AST/ALT/AP >3 × normal)
Stroke history	
Bleeding	Prior major bleeding or predisposition to bleeding
Labile INR	Unstable or high
Elderly	Age ≥65
Drug or alcohol usage	Antiplatelet agents, NSAIDs.

- Serious bleeding is defined as intracranial, requiring hospitalization, haemoglobin decrease >2 g/L and/or transfusion.
  - 0–1 points – low risk (<1 serious bleeds per 100 patient years).
  - 2 points – moderate risk (2 serious bleeds per 100 patient years).
  - 2–4 points – high risk (>3 serious bleeds per 100 patient years).
  - 5 points – very high risk (>10 serious bleeds per 100 patient years).
- Other contraindications to anticoagulation include concurrent surgery or lumbar puncture.

Warfarin

- Risk factors for bleeding on warfarin include age, history of gastrointestinal bleeding within the past 18 months, alcohol-related illness, chronic renal failure, female sex, malignancy and non-white ethnicity. The risk of a major bleed is about 1% per year, of intracranial haemorrhage 0.6% per year and fatal bleed 0.3% per year.
- The risk of bleeding with warfarin is not directly related to the INR level and is affected by other factors such as drug interactions and pre-existing disorders that predispose to bleeding.
- Over-dosage with minor bleeding is treated with oral vitamin K 1–2.5 mg once only, which can correct the INR in 24 hours, or with more urgent intravenous vitamin K 1 mg which takes 6–8 hours but is no more effective at 24 hours.
- More serious bleeding requires infusion of prothrombin complex concentrates (PCC) which contain vitamin K-dependent coagulation factors as well as proteins C and S. These are either three factors (factors II, V, IX) or four factors (FVII as well). A dose of 25–50 IU/kg in 40 ml drops the INR dramatically in under two hours. This volume carries less risk of fluid overload than alternative use of 1000 mL of fresh frozen plasma administered as a blood group specific product, which takes about six hours to act. The plasminogen inhibitor tranexamic acid 15–30 mg/kg may also be used intravenously.

Other anticoagulants

- Treatment of major haemorrhage associated with LMWH is similar to heparin, but the half-life for these is longer and protamine, if used, only reverses 60% of the drug's effects.
- Dabigatran can be removed by haemodialysis, and idarucizumab (Praxbind) is a dabigatran-reversal agent that has become available.
- Direct Factor Xa inhibitors may be treated with prothrombin complex concentrates (PCC) 25–50 IU/kg, and for life-threatening situations consider intravenous tranexamic acid 15–30 mg/kg.

Heparin-induced thrombocytopenia (HIT)

Pathology

- Type 1 HIT is non-immune temporary thrombocytopenia due to enhanced heparin-induced platelet aggregation and splenic sequestration. It is benign and occurs in about 2% of patients. Thrombocytopenia is mild and its onset is early, usually during the first two days after commencement of heparin. The patients' platelet counts seldom drop below 80×10^9/L. Thrombocytopenia resolves spontaneously within a few days even with continuation of heparin and the patients remain asymptomatic.
- Type II HIT is due to an immune reaction against heparin (Figure 25.1).[7] Surgical patients have double the risk for Type II HIT, particularly after cardiac surgery with an incidence of about 4%. It is named for associated low platelet counts but is manifest as venous or arterial thrombosis or areas of skin necrosis. The incidence is at least 1% with heparin treatment for more than four days. Any patient can be affected, and the risk is ten times more likely with UHF compared to LMWH, while there is little risk with DOACs.
- The principal antigen is a complex of heparin and platelet factor 4 which is present in platelet α-granules. This generates heparin-PF4 IgG antibodies

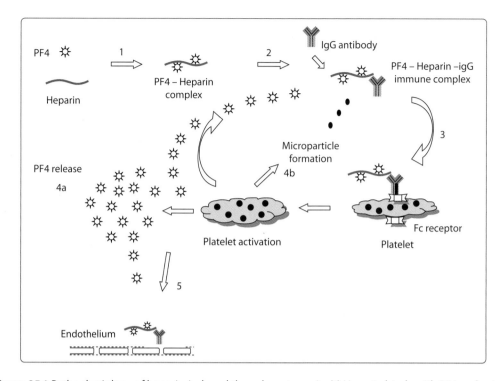

Figure 25.1 Pathophysiology of heparin-induced thrombocytopenia. (1) Heparin binds with PF4 and acts as immunogens. (2) IgG antibody produced, forms PF4–heparin–IgG multimolecular complex. (3) The complex then binds through Fc receptor to platelets and activates them. (4a) activated platelet releases additional PF4 and (4b) prothrombotic microparticles. (5) Immune complex interacts with endothelial cells and promotes immune mediated endothelial damage – a HIT. (Adapted from Ahmed I, Majeed A, Powell R. *Postgrad Med J* 2007;83:575–82. https://www.ncbi.nlm.nih.gov/pmc/articles/PMC2600013/)

causing cross-links between platelets and massive acceleration of platelet activation. The antigen–antibody complexes interact with monocytes and endothelial cells to produce tissue factor, further contributing to activation of the coagulation cascade and thrombin generation. At this point it is called heparin-induced thrombocytopenia and thrombosis (HITT).

- Antibody-coated platelets are cleared by the macrophage system magnifying the thrombocytopenia due to sequestration. Thrombocytopenia refers to a drop of >50% in the patient's platelet count from its baseline and below 100×10^9/L. Thrombocytopenia is moderately severe and its onset is usually delayed until day 5–10 of heparin administration, but its onset can occur earlier if there has been prior exposure to heparin or delayed for up to three weeks well after heparin treatment has been stopped. The platelet count drops gradually to a mean of 50×10^9/L, returning to normal in around a week, though antibodies may take three months to disappear. Thrombocytopenia seldom causes significant bleeding.

Diagnosis

- HIT antibodies can be demonstrated by functional tests and by immunoassays. Functional tests include heparin-induced platelet aggregation and the serotonin release assay. Immunoassays use immuno-enzymatic tests (ELISA) to detect the HIT antibody. However, if HIT is clinically suspected, then treatment should not be withheld pending laboratory results.
- The onset of new thrombosis or extension of pre-existing thrombosis further strengthens the clinical suspicion of HIT. The diagnosis

requires a combination of pre-test probability from clinical assessment and a positive test for platelet-activating antibodies, or is inferred from a strong-positive antigen test result. However, the diagnosis is finally confirmed by demonstrating heparin-dependent platelet-activating antibodies in only about 10% of patients clinically suspected to have HIT. Some patients have the HIT antibody without developing the clinical syndrome.

Prevention

- Limit courses of heparin to less than five days if possible.
- Use LMWH in place of UHF for thrombo-prophylaxis in high-risk patients.
- Monitor the platelet count at least every other day between days 4 and 14 of heparin exposure or until heparin is discontinued.
- Take care not to automatically initiate heparin if a patient is re-admitted for a thrombotic event.

Treatment

- Immediately cease all forms of heparin.
- Send blood samples for laboratory confirmation.
- Monitor carefully for thrombotic event.
- Monitor platelet count until recovery.
- Initiate alternative anticoagulation using non-heparin anticoagulants that do not cross-react with HIT antibodies until warfarin can safely be commenced.
- Drugs that can be safely used are the direct thrombin inhibitor argatroban 2 mg/kg/minute, the heparinoid danaparoid 2500 U intravenous then 400 U per hour (despite being a heparinoid it seldom cross reacts) or the parenteral FX inhibitor fondaparinux 7.5 mg subcutaneous once daily, with adjustments according to weight.
- Theoretically the DOACs should be safe in HITT, but there is little data.
- Do not use warfarin until the platelet count has recovered to avoid the risk of warfarin necrosis due to micro-thrombosis.
- Do not give prophylactic platelet transfusion as it could exacerbate the hypercoagulable state.

- Continue alternative anticoagulation for at least 2–3 months to prevent recurrence.

Thrombolysis and endovascular intervention

- Thrombolytic agents are described in Chapter 15.[2,8-10] They can be used to supplement the natural fibrinolytic process. Thrombolytics can be administered by systemic intravenous infusion, but regional catheter infusion is more effective with less risk of systemic and, in particular, intracranial bleeding. Percutaneous trans-catheter thrombolysis for DVT can be combined with mechanical thrombectomy and correction of venous stenosis or occlusion by angioplasty with stenting if required. The goals are to reduce the severity and duration of lower limb symptoms, prevent PE, diminish the risk of recurrent venous thrombosis and limit or prevent venous valve damage and the post-thrombotic syndrome.
- Particular indications for intervention include symptomatic inferior vena cava thrombosis that responds poorly to anticoagulation alone, phlegmasia cerulea dolens and symptomatic ilio-femoral or rarely femoro-popliteal DVT in patients with a low risk of bleeding. Absolute contraindications are common and include active internal bleeding or disseminated intravascular coagulation, a cerebrovascular event, trauma or recent neurosurgery.
- Continuous infusion rather than bolus or pulse-spray infusion is usually recommended for treating DVT. Low doses have been found to be as effective as higher doses with fewer complications. Typical treatments can involve several visits to the interventional suite over several days. Treatment might release clot fragments as pulmonary emboli, but an inferior vena cava filter is usually not required because ongoing lysis minimizes any damage they may cause.
- Percutaneous mechanical thrombectomy has been developed to shorten treatment time and avoid expensive management in intensive care during thrombolysis. The techniques may not completely remove thrombus but effectively

debulk clot to minimize the dose and time required for thrombolysis. They are categorized as rotational, rheolytic or ultrasound-enhanced, and are most commonly inserted into the ipsilateral popliteal vein.

- Rotational devices employ a high-velocity rotating wire or other device to macerate thrombus. These have a potential to damage endothelium, but it is not known whether this increases risk of re-thrombosis. Rheolytic devices aspirate thrombus into a catheter where it is fragmented by a high-pressure saline jet containing a thrombolytic drug. This carries a theoretical risk of haemolysis that could cause systemic complications. Ultrasound-enhanced devices emit high-frequency, low-energy ultrasound energy which induces cavitational stresses on the fibrin component of thrombus, exposing plasminogen receptor sites, which enhances contact with thrombolytic agents within target thrombus. Although they avoid tissue and blood cell damage, they require longer thrombolytic infusion times than the other techniques.
- Clearance of thrombus frequently discloses an underlying venous stenosis that can be readily controlled by balloon dilatation with intravascular stents (see Chapter 15). Patients are then managed with long-term anticoagulation.
- Meta-analysis shows technical success in more than 80% with a low incidence of PE or systemic events, although bleeding leads to a need for transfusion in some 10% of patients. It was previously considered that thrombolysis for DVT should commence within ten days after onset, but limited results for these techniques suggest little if any difference of outcome for treatment commenced, much later.

Recommendations from National Institute for Health and Clinical Excellence (NICE) guidelines and an international consensus group

- There is reduction in the incidence of the post-thrombotic syndrome (PTS) when thrombolysis is used compared to anticoagulation alone. Pharmaco-mechanical thrombolysis is recommended in preference to either catheter-directed thrombolysis or percutaneous mechanical thrombectomy alone.[2,9]
- For patients with PE, thrombolysis should be performed if PE is massive and considered if PE is sub-massive, provided there are no risk factors for bleeding, but is not recommended for patients with lower risk PE patients, who are best treated by anticoagulation alone.
- Devices have been designed for percutaneous endovascular access to the pulmonary arteries to allow clot to be macerated and simultaneously aspirated from smaller vessels. Open surgical pulmonary embolectomy is having a very limited renaissance. These procedures are only considered for life-threatening PE following unsuccessful thrombolysis and for patients with sub-massive PE who are at increased risk for bleeding with thrombolysis.
- Thrombolysis is likely to increase initial costs of material and length of stay, as well as the cost of treating major bleeding, but is likely to decrease the cost of treating PTS, making intervention more cost-effective.

25.1 Consider catheter-directed thrombolysis for severe iliofemoral DVT or massive PE with

- Symptoms of less than 14 days' duration
- Good functional status
- Life expectancy of one year or more
- Low risk of bleeding

Surgical thrombectomy

- Open surgical thrombectomy has been largely replaced by endovenous techniques, but is still occasionally required for patients with massive swelling and phlegmasia cerulea dolens where there is a contraindication to fibrinolysis or if it is considered that the clot is too extensive to be dealt with by endovascular techniques.

- It is necessary to precisely define the location and extent of thrombosis before operation. Exposure is through the common femoral vein; a Fogarty catheter is passed through the clot and the balloon is inflated and withdrawn along with the clot. Care must be taken to avoid dislodging the clot or breaking it into small fragments, and a temporary inferior vena cava filter is frequently used to reduce the risk of PE. Venography is mandatory since back-bleeding alone does not confirm clot clearance, as this can be through patent tributaries. Venous valves usually prevent retrograde passage but the limb can be tightly wrapped with an Esmarch bandage to force clot extrusion. After thrombus has been removed, an arteriovenous fistula is made between the saphenous and femoral veins to maintain patency by increasing flow velocity through the treated vein.
- Anticoagulation is initiated before surgery and continued for 6–12 months, compression stockings are required long term, and the fistula is closed at about six months. Best results are achieved within the first seven days after thrombosis, and the re-thrombosis rate is about 10%.

History

- Friedrich Trendelenburg (1844–1924) performed an operation to remove an embolus from the pulmonary artery by thoracotomy in two patients in 1872, but neither survived. Martin Kirschner (1879–1942) performed the first successful pulmonary embolectomy in 1924.
- The surgeon John Hunter (1728–1793) advocated ligation of the deep vein after thrombosis, and John Homans (1877–1954) of Boston performed proximal ligation of the femoral veins to prevent pulmonary embolism in 1934.

References

1. Fletcher J, MacLellan D, Baker R, Chong B, Fisher C, Flanagan D et al. The Australia and New Zealand working party on the management and prevention of venous thromboembolism. *Prevention of Venous Thromboembolism*. Fourth edition. 2014. Health education and Management Innovations. http://www.surgeons.org/media/19372/VTE_Guidelines.pdf

2. Nicolaides A, Fareed J, Kakkar AK, Comerota AJ, Goldhaber SZ, Hull R, Myers K et al. Prevention and treatment of venous thromboembolism: international consensus statement (Guidelines according to scientific evidence). *Clin Appl Thromb Hemost* 2013;19:116–8. http://cat.sagepub.com/content/19/2/116.full.pdf+html

3. Di Nisio M, Wichers IM, Middeldorp S. Treatment for superficial thrombophlebitis of the leg. *Cochrane Database Syst Rev* 2013;30;4:CD004982. http://www.cochrane.org/CD004982/PVD_treatment-for-superficial-thrombophlebitis-of-the-leg

4. Leizorovicz A, Becker F, Buchmüller A, Quéré I, Prandoni P, Decousus H, for the CALISTO Study Group. Clinical relevance of symptomatic superficial-vein thrombosis extension: Lessons from the CALISTO study. *Blood* 2013;122:1724–9. http://www.bloodjournal.org/content/122/10/1724?sso-checked=true

5. Gillet J-L. Management of superficial vein thrombosis of the lower limbs: update and current recommendations. *Phlebolymphology* 2015;22:82. http://www.phlebolymphology.org/management-of-superficial-vein-thrombosis-of-the-lower-limbs-update-and-current-recommendations/

6. Palareti G, Cosmi B, Legnani C, Antonucci E, De Micheli V, Ghirarduzzi A et al. on behalf of the DULCIS (D-dimer and ULtrasonography in Combination Italian Study) Investigators. D-dimer to guide the duration of anticoagulation in patients with venous thromboembolism: a management study. *Blood* 2014;124:196–203. http://www.bloodjournal.org/content/124/2/196

7. Ahmed I, Majeed A, Powell R. Heparin-induced thrombocytopenia: diagnosis and management update. *Postgrad Med J* 2007;83:575–82. https://www.ncbi.nlm.nih.gov/pmc/articles/PMC2600013/

8. Morrison HL. Catheter-directed thrombolysis for acute limb ischemia. *Semin Intervent Radiol* 2006;23:258–69. https://www.ncbi.nlm.nih.gov/pmc/articles/PMC3036379/

9. *NICE Clinical Guidelines. Venous Thromboembolic Diseases: Thrombolytic Therapy for DVT*. National Clinical Guideline Centre (UK).No. 144: 2012; London: Royal College of Physicians. https://www.ncbi.nlm.nih.gov/books/NBK132803/

10. Karthikesalingam A, Young EL, Hinchliffe RJ, Loftus IM, Thompson MM, Holt PJE. A systematic review of percutaneous mechanical thrombectomy in the treatment of deep venous thrombosis. *Eur J Vasc Endovasc Surg* 2011;41:554–65. http://www.sciencedirect.com/science/article/pii/S1078588411000165

Vascular tumours and congenital vascular malformations

This chapter includes recommendations and classifications from the International Society for the Study of Vascular Anomalies and the International Union of Angiology.[1-4]

It is necessary to distinguish vascular tumours from congenital vascular malformations, as their pathology, natural history, and management are different.

Nature of vascular tumours and malformations

- In general, vascular tumours are endothelial neoplasms characterized by cellular proliferation and growth that are usually 'self-limited' and develop after birth, whereas vascular malformations are 'self-perpetuating' embryonic tissue remnants that are always present at birth. Most benign vascular tumours undergo spontaneous regression, whereas most malformations never regress, often grow over time and can be exacerbated by treatment. In contrast to vascular tumours, several malformations are known to have a strong hereditary component. However, as will be discussed, the uncommon congenital haemangiomas may not involute, while the naevus simplex malformation can disappear in childhood.
- Diagnosis can usually be made from the history and their appearance. Investigation is reserved for patients who require

intervention. A plain X-ray has limited value, but can show bone abnormalities or phleboliths. Ultrasound is used to evaluate vascularity and determine the types of vessels present. Magnetic resonance imaging (MRI) is used to further characterize the appearance and to determine the extent of larger lesions in relation to their soft tissue components, although MRI usually requires sedation for young children. Computed tomography (CT) is helpful when urgent imaging is required because it is fast and usually does not require sedation. CT provides excellent definition for blood vessels, but it does carry the risks of irradiation and lacks the soft tissue resolution of MR.
- Treatment is usually expectant for benign tumours as they are likely to spontaneously regress, and also for vascular malformations.

Classification of vascular tumours

- The International Society for the Study of Vascular Anomalies (ISSVA) have classified vascular tumours.[1]

Benign vascular tumours

- Infantile haemangioma
- Congenital haemangioma
- Rapidly involuting congenital haemangioma (RICH)
- Non-involuting congenital haemangioma (NICH)

- Partially involuting congenital haemangioma (PICH)
- Tufted angioma
- Spindle-cell haemangioma
- Epithelioid haemangioma
- Pyogenic granuloma (lobular capillary haemangioma)

Locally aggressive or borderline vascular tumours

- Kaposiform haemangioendothelioma
- Retiform haemangioendothelioma
- Papillary intralymphatic angioendothelioma (Dabska tumour)
- Composite haemangioendothelioma
- Kaposi sarcoma

Malignant vascular tumours

- Angiosarcoma
- Epithelioid haemangioendothelioma

Benign vascular tumours

Infantile haemangioma

- Infantile haemangiomas are the most common vascular tumours, affecting 4%–10% of all infants and children. They occur in approximately 10% of Caucasians but are uncommon in dark-skinned children, are three to five times more likely to affect females than males and are more likely to develop in premature babies. Probably more than 50% occur on the head and neck area.
- Focal haemangiomas can be superficial, also called capillary haemangioma, capillary naevus, strawberry haemangioma or strawberry naevus.
- It was previously thought that haemangiomas were derived by angiogenesis from endothelial cells, but it is now considered that they develop from stem cells that remain in an immature arrested state.[7-9] Whether these represent environmental disturbance of normal post-natal stem cells or genetic alterations has still to be determined. Growth factors and blood and connective tissue cells are all involved in a complex process. This potentially allows new avenues for treatment.

- Infantile haemangiomas are further classified[1]:
  Pattern
  - Focal
  - Multifocal
  - Segmental
  - Indeterminate
  Types
  - Superficial
  - Deep
  - Mixed (superficial + deep)
  - Infantile haemangioma with minimal or arrested growth (IHMAG)[5]
- Infantile haemangiomas are mainly composed of proliferating endothelial cells and pericytes and appear as a bluish soft to firm lesion. Segmental haemangiomas are more serious than focal haemangiomas and occur at a younger age, grow up to ten times larger and are more unsightly.

Natural history

- Most haemangiomas are self-limited, although many leave behind a mark at the lesion site. They typically pass through three stages (Figures 26.1–26.4). Proliferation occurs in the first year, usually with a variable growth rate to about 80% of maximum size in the first three months, with cessation by about five months, although some keep growing for up to 18 months. An involuting phase lasts from one to five years. Continued

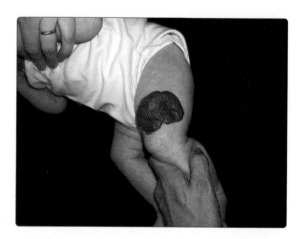

Figure 26.1 Haemangioma involving dermis at six months.

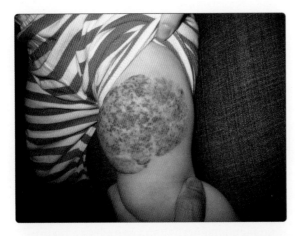

Figure 26.2 Haemangioma showing partial regression.

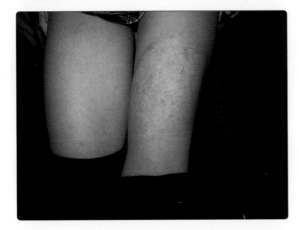

Figure 26.3 Haemangioma has fully regressed but leaving residual skin damage, in particular loss of elasticity that allows some degree of protrusion of the subcutaneous fat.

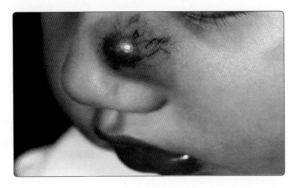

Figure 26.4 Haemangioma involving dermis (red) and subcutaneous tissue (bluish swelling).

involution and regression can take as long as 10 years. The maturing lesion usually has a lighter greyish colour and becomes softer to the touch. After involution, all colour usually disappears leaving no more than an atrophic patch with some telangiectases.

Congenital haemangiomas

- Congenital haemangiomas are considerably less common. They are generally present and fully grown at birth.
  - Rapidly-involuting congenital haemangiomas (RICH) usually involute within about two years.
  - Non-involuting congenital haemangiomas (NICH) are less common and remain without involution into adulthood.
    - They may be partially-involuting (PICH).
- They are composed of capillary lobules associated with large extralobular veins, arteries and lymphatics. Congenital haemangiomas demonstrate relatively high flow, so that a vascular malformation may need to be excluded by imaging. A lobulated soft tissue mass is typical of a haemangioma, whereas dilated vascular channels with feeding arteries or draining veins are characteristic of a malformation.

Other benign vascular tumours

Tufted angioma

- Tufted angiomas are rare benign vascular tumours of young children that only rarely involute (Figure 26.5). Most occur on the upper body localized to the skin and only rarely involving subcutaneous tissues. A lesion is usually a solitary dull red, reddish-brown or purple patch or plaque with a depressed centre. It slowly enlarges over the first few years and then remains stationary with only occasional partial regression. The lesion can become painful and rarely causes the Kasabach–Merritt syndrome (see p. 311). Diagnosis is confirmed by distinctive histology.

Spindle cell haemangioma

- These present as slow-growing solitary or multiple nodules in the skin and subcutaneous

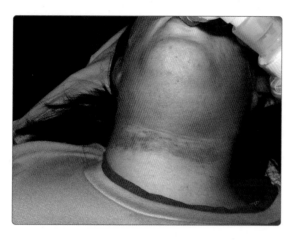

Figure 26.5 Tufted haemangioma with red-brown active edge and some resolution more centrally.

tissues, usually in the distal extremities and usually affecting young to middle-aged adults. Superficial lesions appear blue and may contain phleboliths.[6] They can be associated with the Mafucci or Klippel–Trenaunay syndromes (see pp. 306–307). Diagnosis is confirmed by distinctive histology. They have a tendency to expand and usually require wide surgical excision.

Epithelioid haemangioma

- This condition appears as clustered small translucent brown or red nodules around the ear or in the hairline, and lesions may also involve the inside of the mouth or genitals.[6] These can be asymptomatic, itchy or painful. Patients are commonly young adults but it can affect children. It is particularly common in Japan. Histology shows specific features with thick-walled small blood vessels lined with swollen endothelial cells and surrounded by lymphocytes and eosinophils. Some cases resolve without treatment. Surgical excision may be required with a margin sufficient to prevent local recurrence.

Pyogenic granuloma – lobular capillary haemangioma

- This relatively common lesion usually first appears as a small pinhead-sized red, brownish-red or blue–black spot that grows rapidly over a period of a few days to weeks up to 5 cm

diameter when they develop a raspberry-like appearance.[6] They bleed easily and may ulcerate. Rarely, multiple lesions can develop. A lesion may appear at a site of past trauma or infection and can occur at any age. Histology shows a lobular collection of blood vessels within inflamed tissue, and is required to exclude other conditions such as malignancies. Treatment is usually with curettage and cauterization.

Association with other lesions

- PHACE – posterior fossa anomaly, segmental facial haemangioma (which can be misdiagnosed as Sturge–Weber syndrome – see p. 307), arterial anomalies, cardiovascular anomalies, eye anomalies, sternal clefting and/or supraumbilical raphe. Any infant with a large segmental infantile haemangioma of the face or neck should be investigated for PHACE syndrome, particularly prior to commencement of treatment with propranolol.
- LUMBAR – lower body haemangioma, urogenital anomalies, ulceration, myelopathy, bony deformities, anorectal malformations, arterial anomalies and renal anomalies.
- PELVIS – perineal haemangioma with external genital malformations, lipomyelomeningocoele, vesico-renal abnormalities or imperforate anus.
- Diffuse neonatal haemangiomatosis consists of generalized 0.2–2 cm benign haemangiomas in the skin, or internal lesions especially in the liver, lungs, gastro-intestinal tract or central nervous system. The onset is in the first few months, and it regresses through childhood but may be fatal if there is extensive visceral involvement.

Investigations

- Most lesions can be diagnosed from the patient's history and clinical examination. Investigation commences with ultrasound. B-mode shows a discrete solid mass with low to variable internal echogenicity. Spectral and colour Doppler show increased vascularity with arterial and venous waveforms and mean peak systolic velocity of approximately 15 cm/s. In contrast, arterio-venous malformations show low resistance arterial waveforms and high venous flow in the region, although shunting is sometimes seen in haemangiomas in the growing phase. Serial scans can assess the natural history or response to treatment. MRI is occasionally required to determine the extent of the lesion. Conventional angiography is no longer indicated.

Treatment

- Most haemangiomas resolve without serious long-term complications and require only expectant management, but about 20% become clinically significant, depending on their nature and site so as to require treatment. The disfiguring nature of facial lesions may prompt parents to seek intervention early rather than wait for involution. Other indications for intervention include aggressive growth, proximity to vital structures such as the airway or the eye, visceral involvement, complications such as ulceration and bleeding or even high-output cardiac failure. Treatment is required for NICH after a period of observation to exclude RICH as they do not involute.
- Topical or systemic beta blocker drugs have replaced corticosteroids as the treatment of choice for infantile haemangiomas. They are thought to act by suppressing the signalling pathways of vascular endothelial growth factor and signal transducer and activator of transcription 3 (STAT3). Propranolol is used and is most effective when started during the growth phase in infants. Dosage must be determined on an individual basis, by treating doctors. A response is seen within 24–48 hours, and treatment should be continued for at least six months or until the baby reaches one year of age. Rebound growth can occur on cessation and gradual weaning may be required. Side-effects include hypoglycaemia, bradycardia and hypotension, and it is recommended to closely monitor for cardiovascular effects and blood sugar when starting propranolol. More cardio-selective beta blockers like atenolol are also being evaluated for treatment. Topical timolol has been prescribed for smaller and superficial lesions or when propranolol is contraindicated. Some residual skin changes such as scarring and telangiectasia may remain. Treatment is not always effective.
- Surgical resection and reconstruction is occasionally required if there is a threatening complication or if it is considered that the cosmetic result will be superior to the anticipated outcome after involution, and if it does not endanger an important adjacent structure such as the eye or facial nerve. Surgery may be required after involution to reconstruct a residual scar.
- Surgical resection should be deferred if possible until late childhood when the lesion has matured and the anaesthetic risk to the child is least. However, excision is performed at an earlier age for impending complications or as the child becomes old enough to be aware of the appearance if surgery is considered to be inevitable. Ulceration, when it occurs in haemangiomas, is painful and slow to heal without treatment. Healing can be accelerated and pain relief achieved with appropriate occlusive dressings and topical antibiotics. Pulsed dye laser will also accelerate healing and reduce pain. It is valuable near body orifices where occlusive dressings cannot be attached. Surgical excision of an ulcerated haemangioma, if possible with simple closure, can also be a satisfactory treatment as it gives immediate pain relief, with correction of the long-term scarring consequences of ulceration. Surgery is also indicated in rare cases where deep ulceration risks serious haemorrhage.

Locally aggressive and borderline vascular tumours

Kaposiform haemangioendothelioma

- These are rare vascular tumours that usually occur in the first year or two of life. After a period of growth, lesions usually slowly regress but do not completely disappear. They typically occur on the trunk or proximal extremities as deep purple or red lesions with an adjacent bruise-like appearance. Histology shows both vascular and lymphatic components. They do not metastasise but can involve regional lymph nodes as well as local infiltration. Imaging shows an ill-defined infiltrative lesion with numerous feeding and draining vessels. Larger lesions are associated with platelet trapping (the Kasabach–Merritt phenomenon) which can lead to life-threatening thrombocytopaenia. Treatment is either with steroid and vincristine or, more recently, rapamycin. Surgical excision is rarely possible.

Retiform haemangioendothelioma

- Haemangioendotheliomas are a reactive vaso-proliferation that may present throughout the body occurring at any age. Histology shows thin-walled vessels containing thrombi, solid areas of spindle cells and plump endothelial cells.

Papillary intralymphatic angioendothelioma (Dabska tumour)

- This usually appears in early childhood in either sex but can affect adults too. Surface lesions are usually located on the hands and legs. Advanced cases can become malignant. Treatment involves steroids, chemotherapy, radiotherapy or surgery.

Kaposi sarcoma

- Kaposi sarcoma is due to herpes virus 8 and presents as nonpruritic painless flat or nodular pigmented lesions on the skin or mucosa of the head and neck. It is mainly found in patients with AIDS. It is composed of large endothelial cells surrounded by spindle-shaped cells. Lesions are usually purple in Caucasians and nearly black in people with darker pigmented skin. While skin lesions are mainly a cosmetic concern, oral or aero-digestive tract tumours can cause pain, bleeding or obstruction. Radiation and chemotherapy are helpful but often complicated in this group of patients.

Interferon and intra-lesional vinblastine, cryotherapy and laser excision can be used.

Fabry disease – angiokeratoma corporis diffusum

- This is a rare X-linked genetic lysosomal storage disease due to alpha-galactosidase A deficiency. Glycosphingolipid accumulates in lysosomes of most organs, especially vascular endothelium, causing total body pain, renal, cardiac and ocular effects, with varicose veins, lymphoedema and angiokeratomas of the lower body.

Malignant vascular tumours

Epithelioid haemangioendothelioma

- This is a rare, slowly progressive, distinct pathological vascular tumour that can occur at any age and anywhere in the body, most often affecting bones.

Angiosarcoma

- Angiosarcoma is a rare aggressive neoplasm with a very bad prognosis. It is more common in females and the average age of onset is about four years. Imaging shows an aggressive heterogeneous mass with contrast pooling, usually with multiple liver metastases.

Congenital vascular malformations – classification

- Congenital vascular malformations are distinguished by their embryonic stage of development (see Chapter 1), tissue types and vascular flow. Their classification was previously developed from the Hamburg conference[*2-4] and recently by the International Society for the Study of Vascular Anomalies (ISSVA)[†1]

---

* This classification arose from an international workshop in Hamburg, Germany in 1988.
† This classification was updated at a meeting in Melbourne, Australia in 2014.

Hamburg classification of malformations

- This emphasized the importance of their relation to development in the embryo as well as the tissue type.
  - Extratruncular malformations arise from mesodermal angioblasts in the early reticular stage of embryonic blood vessel development before vascular trunks appear. Primitive cells retain a potential to continue to proliferate and infiltrate after birth, and have a capacity to regrow after therapeutic interventions.
  - Truncular malformations arise at a later stage when vascular trunk development is completed. Abnormal cells have lost the potential to proliferate so that there is little risk of recurrence after treatment.
  - Combinations can occur.
- Each can be further subdivided.
  - Extratruncular
    - Infiltrating and diffuse
    - Limited and localized
  - Truncular
    - Obstruction or stenosis
    - Aplasia, hypoplasia, hyperplasia
    - Stenosis, membrane, congenital spur
    - Dilatation
    - Localised aneurysm
    - Diffuse ectasia
- Morphology allows classification as:
  - Simple malformations
  - Combined malformations
  - Malformations of major named vessels (truncular)
  - Malformations associated with other anomalies

ISSVA classification of vascular malformations

- This classification replaced the Hamburg classification for the ISSVA and is now the classification used by most vascular anomalies multidisciplinary teams worldwide.
- Simple malformations are classified by the predominant tissue as:
  - Capillary malformations (CM)
  - Venous malformations (VM)
  - Lymphatic malformations (LM)
  - Arterio-venous malformations (AVM)
  - Arterio-venous fistula (AVF)
- Combined malformations are two or more combinations of any of the above.
- Capillary, venous and lymphatic malformations are 'low-flow', whereas malformations with an arterial component are 'high-flow'.

Pathology and clinical features

Capillary malformations (CM)

- CM are classified as:[1]
  - Cutaneous and/or mucosal CM ('port-wine' stain)
    - CM with bone and/or soft tissue overgrowth
    - CM with CNS and/or ocular anomalies (Sturge-Weber syndrome)
    - CM of CM-AVM
    - CM of MICCAP (microcephaly-capillary malformation)
    - CM of MCAP (megalencephaly-capillary malformation-polymicrogyria)
  - Hereditary haemorrhagic telangiectasia
  - Cutis marmorata telangiectatica congenita
  - Naevus simplex/salmon patch/'angel kiss', 'stork bite'
- Capillary malformations (CM) are present at birth and appear as pink to red macules on the skin and mucosa (Figures 26.6 and 26.7). Superficial lesions are more pink

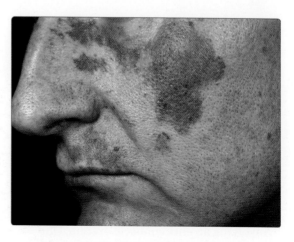

Figure 26.6 Capillary malformation on face.

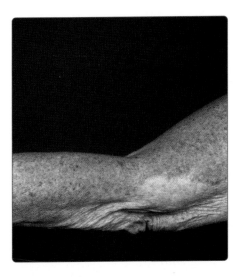

Figure 26.7 Capillary malformation in an adult on the arm showing early hypertrophy and blue nodule formation that would require more deeply penetrating laser.

and deeper lesions more blue, and they darken and thicken over time, sometimes associated with soft tissue or bone overgrowth producing deformity. Most persist throughout life, but occasional variants on the head and face can lighten and even disappear, usually before five years of age. Thicker ones become keratotic later in life.
- Histology shows dilated capillaries and post-capillary venules, while those with soft tissue or bone overgrowth contain deep lobular aggregates of larger vessels.

Venous malformations (VM)

- VM are classified as:[1]
  - Sporadic VM
  - Familial VM cutaneo-mucosal (VMCM)
  - Blue rubber bleb naevus (Bean) syndrome VM
  - Glomuvenous malformation (GVM)
  - Cerebral cavernous malformation (CCM)
- VM are the most common form of malformation. They can affect any tissue or organ and may be focal, multifocal or diffuse, the latter typically involving an entire muscle or limb. One classification refers to 94% sporadic venous

malformations (VM), 5% dominantly inherited glomuvenous malformations (GVM) and 1% dominantly inherited cutaneo-mucosal venous malformations (VMCM).[10]
- Superficial VM present as a blue skin discoloration or as a small soft blue subcutaneous mass that fills when emptied with pressure or elevation, or with increased venous pressure as with dependency or the Valsalva manoeuvre (Figures 26.8 and 26.9). Lesions are commonly single and situated on the face, trunk or limbs. Superficial lesions can cause extensive disfigurement. The size of a growing lesion can lead to problems such as exophthalmia and obstructive symptoms in the respiratory

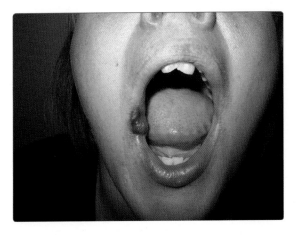

Figure 26.8 Venous malformation at the corner of the mouth that responds well to long pulsed 1064 nm laser.

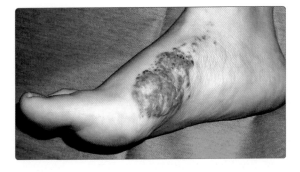

Figure 26.9 Venous malformation of the foot.

and digestive tracts, while deeper lesions that involve muscle or bone can eventually lead to a loss of musculoskeletal function and even pathologic fractures.

- Histology shows a network of thin-walled veins with little or no smooth muscle in the media. VM may be evident at birth, but deeper lesions often present later in life. VM can increase in size with trauma or incomplete surgical excision.
- The anatomical location can be further classified as:
  - Intra-dermal forming superficial telangiectatic and/or venulectatic lesions
  - Subcutaneous presenting with nodules
  - Intra-muscular, intra-articular or deep within other organs
- Local intravascular coagulation (LIC) occurs in many patients with VM. Mild LIC is associated with elevated D-dimer and normal fibrinogen levels, and can result in venous thrombi which often calcify to form phleboliths. Severe LIC is usually associated with extensive VM and produces elevated D-dimer and low fibrinogen levels, which can decompensate into disseminated intravascular coagulopathy, for example during surgery. Typical treatment would be with low molecular weight heparin. Further, D-dimer can help differentiate VM from other vascular anomalies with normal D-dimer levels.

D-dimer and fibrinogen measurements should be a routine investigation for every patient with a significant VM.

Blue rubber bleb syndrome

- This consists of multiple cutaneous, musculoskeletal and gastrointestinal tract VM, the latter responsible for chronic bleeding and anaemia. It occurs in either sex, is present at birth or develops within the first years of life and progresses over time. Lesions are soft and easy to compress, dark blue, about 5 mm in size and situated on the trunk and extremities. Genetic studies are able to distinguish this syndrome from VMCM and other conditions.

Glomo-venous malformations

- In the past, these were incorrectly termed glomangiomas but they are not tumours. They are distinct from glomus tumours which are a tight collection of glomus cells usually found under the nail, (Figure 26.10).
- Malformations form single or multifocal nodular lesions in the skin, sometimes with a cobblestone appearance. They are less compressible and do not empty on elevation. Their histology is necessary for definite diagnosis, and includes rounded 'glomus' cells corresponding to modified immature smooth muscle cells in the vein walls. Although always present at birth, they usually become clinically apparent only later in life. In around 50% of cases they are autosomal dominantly inherited.

Bockenheimer syndrome

- This consists of diffuse phlebectasias affecting the extremities and trunk.

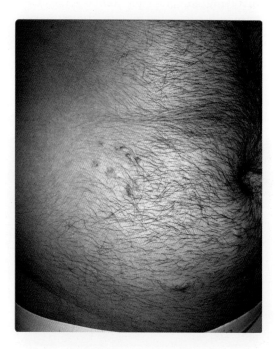

Figure 26.10 Glomuvenous malformation on the abdomen presenting as blue blebs, clinically indistinguishable from a venous malformation, with histology required for diagnosis.

Lymphatic malformations (LM)

- LM are classified as:[1]
  - Common (cystic) LM – macrocystic, microcystic or mixed cystic
  - Generalized lymphatic anomaly (GLA)
  - LM in Gorham-Stout disease
  - Channel type LM
  - Primary lymphoedema
- LM are present at birth and occur mainly on the face, neck and axilla but can occur anywhere in the body (Figure 26.11). They consist of dilated lymphatic channels or cysts lined by endothelial cells of lymphatic origin, in the past referred to as cystic hygromas. They are classified as macrocystic, microcystic or mixed cystic, largely dependent on ultrasound and radiographic features and whether they can be aspirated or sclerosed. Lesions range from small sponge-like blemishes to large bulky masses that cause severe disfigurement. Overlying skin may appear normal or show bluish discoloration. Microcystic lesions are not uncommon involving skin and subcutaneous tissues or mouth, including tongue. The primary lesion is a tiny clear vesicle. Hyperkeratotic changes are common on the skin. It is important to understand the changes visible on the skin represent the 'tip of the iceberg'

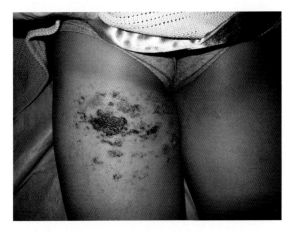

Figure 26.11 Lymphatic malformation of the microcystic type involving the skin. Note both clear and bloodstained vesicles, some showing fluid levels.

overlying honeycomb-like changes in the dermis and subcutaneous tissues.
- Bleeding into a lesion can cause multiple tiny dark-red vesicles, often showing fluid levels. Sudden increase in size is usually associated with bleeding into a cyst, but can also be due to secondary infection. Facial lesions can cause ophthalmologic symptoms, dental problems or a compromised airway. LMs can involve underlying bone and deeper soft tissues, with a risk of pathological fracture. They can also affect thoracic and abdominal viscera and produce chylous pleural effusion or ascites. Primary lymphoedema is a truncular subtype of LM.

Arterio-venous malformations (AVM)

- AVM are classified as:[1]
  - Sporadic
  - In hereditary haemorrhagic telangiectasia
  - In CM-AVM
- AVM are potentially the most aggressive type of malformation and, fortunately, the least common. They have been shown to have increased expression of growth factors responsible for endothelial cell turnover and increased expression of matrix metalloproteinases that can favour their growth. Individual lesions may progress from a quiescent to a more aggressive state, trauma can exacerbate the lesions and rapid growth may be seen during puberty. They can occur almost anywhere in the body, can be single or multiple, and can be limited or very extensive. They have less parenchymal tissue than a high-flow haemangioma. They are the most difficult malformation to treat due to the risk of inducing arterial ischaemia or provoking proliferation of the nidus if only the afferent vessels are closed.
- AVMs are composed of abnormal arteries, veins and capillaries with connections causing arteriovenous shunting, and there are feeding and draining vessels (Figure 26.12). They can be distinguished as three types:
  - Type I – arterial to venous fistulae: at most, three separate arteries shunt to a single draining vein.

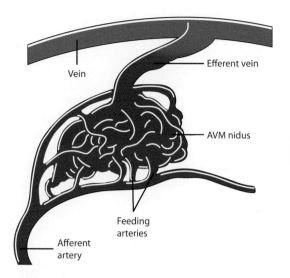

Figure 26.12 Diagrammatic representation of the components of an arterio-venous malformation.

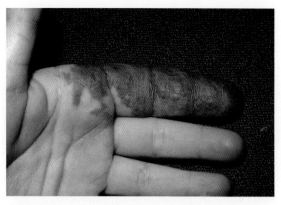

Figure 26.13 Arterio-venous malformation of a finger.

- Type II – arteriolar to venous fistulae: multiple arterioles shunt into a single draining vein.
- Type III – arteriolar to venular fistulae: there are multiple shunts between arterioles and venules, small or large and ectatic.
- Presenting symptoms are varied, with cosmetic disturbance due to skin changes or tissue hypertrophy, pain and complications from ulceration and infection. The appearance in neonates is with a macular pink or red stain resembling a CM or vascular tumour. As the child grows older, a lesion becomes painful and warm progressing to a pulsatile mass, and palpation shows a thrill and auscultation reveals a bruit. Soft tissue and bony hypertrophy result in the affected region becoming larger and warmer than the contralateral side. Severe changes of chronic venous hypertension can lead to venous ulceration or haemorrhage. Repeated thrombosis in the lesion can cause intolerable pain or embolism. Involvement of bone can cause pain. Haemorrhage or a space-occupying mass in a lesion in the central nervous system or other organs can lead to catastrophic presentations. Large lesions can cause shunt-related high-output cardiac failure.

- Dermatological manifestations commence with a stellate lesion with pale patches due to a cutaneous ischaemic steal phenomenon (Figure 26.13). Larger AVMs present with a reticulate appearance with dilated tortuous draining veins. There may be circumscribed pigmented violaceous or dusky lesions. Chronic changes lead to scarring, ulceration and pigmentation.

Combined malformations

- Combined vascular malformations associate any two or three vascular malformations in one lesion. Some malformations combine a cutaneous CM and an underlying VM, denoted as CVM, LM or AVM, or a VM with an LM.

Malformations of major named vessels

- These truncular malformations affect veins, arteries or lymphatics of large calibre vessels (see Chapter 1). They consist of anomalies in their origin, course, number, length or diameter, to cause aplasia, hypoplasia, ectasia or aneurysm formation. Congenital arteriovenous fistulae and persistence of embryonic vessels are also included in this group.

Vascular malformations associated with other anomalies

- Vascular malformations may be associated with anomalies of soft tissue, bone or viscera. These mostly constitute eponymous syndromes.

Klippel–Trenaunay syndrome (KTS)*

- KTS is predominantly a lymphatic anomaly with abnormal venous anatomy, capillary malformations and bony overgrowth (Figure 26.14). Limb hypertrophy occurs in about 70% of patients. The limb is longer and greater in circumference than the healthy limb and often involves the digits. Cutaneous lesions of CM are apparent at birth, while venous varicosities and limb hypertrophy may not be apparent until later.
- A cutaneous CM appears as a flat blue or purplish 'port-wine stain', usually confined to a relatively small area of the lateral surface of the limb and having a geographic border. They often develop dark blue small blebs related to the coexisting lymphatic component. They can involve the entire limb in about 20% and sometimes one side of the entire body. The stain may be confluent or randomly distributed. Additional intra-abdominal or pelvic involvement can affect the genito-urinary tract and large intestine, with visible extension to the abdominal and thoracic wall.

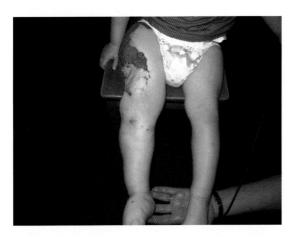

Figure 26.14 Klippel–Trenaunay syndrome. Note dark geographic capillary malformation with blue–black blebs (lymphatic component), an enlarged limb and scar from previous skin graft surgery to deal with leakage from lymphatic blebs.

- The anomalous lateral vein, which typically starts at the foot and extends upwards to drain into the femoral or pelvic veins (see Chapter 2), is a fairly constant feature. There is occasional deep vein occlusion by membrane, agenesis or atresia, venous avalvulia or venous aneurysms. Thrombosis and pulmonary embolism are a significant risk.
- A LM may cause superficial lymphatic vesicles, often complicated by warts, superficial infections or paronychia.
- Some 95% of patients have disease that involves just one lower limb, but pathology can also affect the pelvis, abdomen and thorax. Disease can be bilateral, a few have KTS in an upper limb, and if both upper and lower limbs are affected then it is usually on the same side. There is no racial or sex predilection. Most cases are sporadic, although familial cases have been reported.
- Klippel–Trenaunay syndrome, along with most sporadic LMs and some VMs, is now thought to be caused by a somatic mutation in the gene PIK3CA, and is now thought of as part of a continuum of overgrowth conditions, known as PI3Kinase-Related Overgrowth Spectrum (PROS).

Parkes Weber Syndrome (PWS)†

- This combines CM with arterio-venous fistulae and limb overgrowth. The diagnosis of PWS is made from arteriovenous shunting due to AVM combined with CM. Clinical aspects are similar to KTS, with naevi that are often large and faint pink, but sometimes bright red, limb overgrowth and dilated superficial veins, but it is the AVM that distinguishes PWS from KTS. Compared to KTS, it more frequently affects the upper limbs, less frequently has an abnormal lateral vein and there is no LM component.
- Most cases are sporadic, although familial cases have been reported. Parkes Weber Syndrome is now thought to be synonymous

---

* Maurice Klippel and Paul Trenaunay, French physicians – described in 1900.

† Frederick Parkes Weber (1863–1962) was an English dermatologist who described the Parkes Weber syndrome in several papers up to 1907.

with the AVMs which occur in CM–AVM syndrome, both of which are now thought to be due to an inherited mutation in the gene RASA1.

Sturge–Weber syndrome*

- The Sturge–Weber syndrome has unilateral or bilateral facial and leptomeningeal CM, ocular anomalies, with or without bone and soft tissue overgrowth. Only 5% of children with facial CM have the Sturge–Weber syndrome, and the diagnosis requires MRI evidence of neurologic disorder as well as the CM. These can cause neurologic disabilities, such as seizures and hemiplegia, as well as retardation, and progressive soft tissue and skeletal hypertrophy can develop beneath the malformation. Choroidal anomalies necessitate regular ophthalmologic evaluation. Limbs are occasionally enlarged, with skin changes.

Proteus syndrome

- The condition, also known as elephant man disease, has CM and VM with or without LM, and asymmetric somatic hemihypertrophy and macrodactyly. It is a very rare mosaic genetic disorder characterized by abnormal growth of bones and blood vessels, and various skin lesions including lipomas, epidermal naevi and café-au-lait macules. The condition is usually not evident until late infancy or early childhood. Overgrowth of different body parts is progressive. It resembles KTS but is differentiated by skull changes, naevi, soft tissue masses and plantar hyperplasia.

Maffucci syndrome

- The patient has superficial and deep VM with or without spindle cell haemangiomas, exostoses and enchondromas, especially of the hands and feet, short stature and risk of chondrosarcomas. It presents before five years of age and is possibly an autosomal mutation.

---

* William Sturge (1850–1919), is an English physician and archaeologist who was personal physician to Queen Victoria.

CLOVES syndrome

- This has LM, VM and CM with or without AVM, together with lipomatous overgrowth and spinal and skeletal anomalies causing scoliosis.

Solomon syndrome

- There are epidermal naevi, intracranial AVM, developmental abnormalities of the skin, eyes, nervous, skeletal, cardiovascular and urogenital systems, dysplasia, lipomatous masses and intestinal hamartomatous polyps.

Servelle–Martorell angiodysplasia

- This is characterized by venous or rarely arterial malformations with bony and soft tissue limb abnormalities. Superficial venous ectasia, deep venous hypoplasia, lack of valves or aneurysmal dilation, intra-osseous vascular malformations causing bone hypoplasia with shortening of the limb, intra-osseous vascular ectasias leading to joint destruction and soft tissue limb hypertrophy are all possible features.

Bannayan–Riley–Ruvalcaba syndrome

- There are AVM and VM with lipomatous overgrowth, together with macrocephaly. The presence of CM indicates a possibility of associated central nervous system defects such as microcephaly, ectopic meninges, lipomeningocele, AVM of the spinal cord and other spinal cord abnormalities.

Beckwith–Wiedemann syndrome

- CM of the face with organomegaly cause a large tongue, enlarged abdominal viscera and cardiomegaly. It affects either sex and is inherited. There is a risk of developing a renal or hepatic neoplasm.

Cobb syndrome

- This is a high-flow vascular malformation in the thoraco-lumbar spinal cord medulla causing compression, together with an overlying vascular lesion in the same dermatome. It occurs in either sex, lesions are visible at birth and neurologic complications develop by early adulthood.

Bloom syndrome

- This autosomal recessive inherited disease affects Ashkenazy Jews. It causes short stature, solar telangiectases and butterfly rash on the face, café-au-lait spots, decreased immunity, lung infections, lymphoma and gastro-intestinal malignancy.

Genetic basis

- Many of these malformations have been shown to be associated with gene mutations (Table 26.1).

Investigations

- Baseline D-dimer and fibrinogen levels are recommended for all patients with extensive extratruncular malformations to check for thrombosis and local intravascular coagulation. D-dimer is typically raised for VMs (25% of VMs have D-dimer permanently >1 mg/L) rather than for other malformations. For instance, D-dimer would be expected to be raised in KTS but normal in Parkes Weber syndrome which can be misdiagnosed as KTS.
- Measurement of haemoglobin and platelet counts is recommended to exclude chronic blood loss, particularly from malformations involving the GI tract. Concurrent thrombophilia should be excluded.
- Ultrasound is the first imaging investigation and is frequently all that is required if treatment is to be expectant. However, it does not provide a good three-dimensional picture and has limited ability to adequately show deeper structures or lesions adjacent to bone. Nearby arteries have the usual high-resistance flow signals, unless an AVM is present which will lower resistance with arterialization of venous waveforms.
- X-rays can show phleboliths that are characteristic of VMs, and can also demonstrate any bone involvement by the malformation. MRI is the most useful investigation for obtaining anatomical information, with the best

resolution of soft tissue anatomy. MRI and ultrasound give complementary information about flow. CT can be used where MRI is not possible, and CT angiography can be helpful in high flow lesions.
- Angiography is reserved for AVM being considered for treatment. Venous malformations are not typically visualized on transarterial or transvenous angiography, and if needed are usually imaged by direct percutaneous injection under ultrasound and fluoroscopic control, often as part of treatment.
- Radionucleotide lymphoscintigraphy shows truncular lymphatic malformations causing primary lymphoedema.
- A short course of anticoagulation with low molecular weight heparin is warranted to anticipate the risk of thrombosis during diagnostic or therapeutic intervention.
- Whole-body blood pool scintigraphy using radioisotope tagged erythrocytes is very useful in selected patients to assess the vascularity of malformations, if multiple malformations are present, and to follow up after treatment by sclerotherapy.
- Biopsy can be useful for differentiating AVM from non-involuting congenital hemangiomas which persist indefinitely.
- LM stain positive for D2-40 (podoplanin) which is a marker of lymphatic endothelial cells. Infantile haemangiomas are distinguished from other vascular lesions by staining for Glut1.

Ultrasound

- Scan all affected areas with a high-frequency probe. Use the initial scan to help diagnose the type of lesion and its extent, and serial scans to assess the natural history or response to treatment.[4,11]
- Determine whether the lesion is a haemangioma or a malformation. B-mode shows predominantly soft tissue if it is a haemangioma and vascular channels or lymphatic cysts with little soft tissue if it is a malformation. Examine to see if it is compressible and whether it contains thrombus.

Table 26.1 Causal genes of vascular anomalies (Adapted from ISSVA classification)

Capillary malformations (CM)	Genes
Cutaneous and/or mucosal CM ('port-wine' stain)	GNAQ
CM with CNS and/or ocular anomalies (Sturge–Weber syndrome)	GNAQ
Capillary + arterio-venous malformations (CM + AVM)	**Genes**
CM of CM-AVM	RASA1
Hereditary haemorrhagic telangiectasia – HHT1	ENG
Hereditary haemorrhagic telangiectasia – HHT2	ACVRL1
Juvenile polyposis haemorrhagic telangiectasia	SMAD4
Lymphatic malformations (LM)	**Genes**
Milroy disease	FLT4/VEGFR3
Primary hereditary lymphoedema	VEGFC
Primary hereditary lymphoedema	GJC2/Connexin 47
Lymphedema-distichiasis	FOXC2
Hypotrichosis-lymphoedema-telangiectasia	SOX18
Primary lymphoedema with myelodysplasia	GATA2
Hennekam lymphangiectasia-lymphoedema syndrome	CBE1
Microcephaly ± chorioretinopathy, lymphoedema, or mental retardation syndrome	KIF11
Lymphoedema-choanal atresia	PTPN14
Venous malformations (VM)	**Genes**
Common VM	TIE2 somatic
Familial VM cutaneo-mucosal	TIE2
Glomuvenous malformation – VM with glomus cells	Glomulin
Cerebral cavernous malformation – CCM1	KRIT1
Cerebral cavernous malformation – CCM2	Malcavernin
Cerebral cavernous malformation – CCM3	PDCD10
Vascular malformations associated with other anomalies	**Genes**
Klippel–Trenaunay syndrome	PIK3CA
Parkes Weber syndrome	RASA1
Sturge–Weber syndrome	GNAQ
Macrocephaly-CM – M-CM or MCAP	PIK3CA
Microcephaly-CM – MICCAP	STAMBP
CLOVES syndrome	PIK3CA
Proteus syndrome	AKT1
Bannayan–Riley–Ruvalcaba syndrome	PTEN
PTEN hamartoma of soft tissue – 'angiomatosis' of soft tissue	PTEN

Source: Wassef M, et al. *Pediatrics* 2015;136:203–14. http://pediatrics.aappublications.org/content/pediatrics/early/2015/06/03/peds.2014-3673.full.pdf

- Use B-mode to measure the breadth and depth and whether it extends into underlying muscle and other tissues. Relate the lesion to adjacent normal arteries and veins and to surface landmarks. Determine tissue characteristics.
- Use spectral and colour Doppler to determine whether flow is present and, if so, slow indicating a venous malformation, or fast with a haemangioma. Determine if flow is continuous or low resistance pulsatile. Measure mean or peak systolic velocities. These usually allow classification.

Capillary and venous malformations

- B-mode ultrasound for VM shows compressible multi-spacial hypo- or anechoic vascular spaces in the subcutaneous or intra-muscular tissues, while thrombosed veins appear as a solid echogenic mass with phleboliths.[2] Spectral Doppler demonstrates monophasic venous flow or flow only on augmentation.
- MR venography with imaging using gadolinium is essential before interventions for VM unless ultrasound has shown that the lesion is small and well demarcated. They confirm the extent and type of VM, delineate feeding and draining vessels and distinguish between different soft tissues and vascular structures. It is necessary to confirm that there is no high flow or arterial component, for this would greatly alter treatment, although this is often best assessed with Doppler ultrasound. However, infants and children need anaesthesia for MR, so the test should be selective and carefully planned. The area to be studied can be considerable, particularly for KTS limbs.
- Angiography is seldom needed to establish a diagnosis for most VMs, but may be required for intervention. Ascending or descending phlebography provide anatomical information, and percutaneous direct puncture angiography may be needed for treatment by embolization or sclerotherapy.
- Venography determines haemodynamic characteristics of VMs and allows their classification into four types:

- Type I – isolated VM without appreciable venous drainage.
- Type II – normal-sized venous drainage.
- Type III – enlarged venous drainage.
- Type IV – ectatic dysplastic draining veins.
- This helps to plan treatment as it is found that sclerotherapy can be safely performed in patients with Type I and Type II VMs, whereas there is an increased risk of efflux of sclerosant from a VM during sclerotherapy causing potentially lethal distal embolism with Type III and Type IV VMs.

Lymphatic malformations

- B-mode ultrasound for an LM shows a variable non-compressible multi-cystic mass with or without fluid and debris. Doppler ultrasound for a LM shows no flow except in septa.
- MRI for an LM shows no enhancement except within septa, but is required for anatomical assessment of the lesion.

Arterio-venous malformations

- Initial evaluation should combine several relatively non-invasive investigations including ultrasound, MRI and CT angiography, then angiography in selected patients.[1]
- Ultrasound determines flow characteristics. B-mode for a fast-flow AVM shows clusters of vessels with no intervening well-defined mass. Spectral and colour Doppler show mixed arterial and venous signals.
- Dynamic contrast enhanced MRI using gadolinium demonstrates the extent of the lesion, flow characteristics, soft tissue involvement and the relationship to normal anatomy (Figure 26.15). Quantitative MR angiography can measure relative blood flow and is a non-invasive technique to follow the response to treatment. However, MRI does not precisely demonstrate the nidus or arteriovenous connections. This would be better shown by CT angiography but this is rarely performed due to radiation hazards in children.
- Whole-body blood pool scintigraphy using radioisotope-tagged erythrocytes is very useful in selected patients to assess the vascularity of AVM.

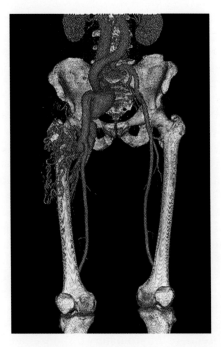

Figure 26.15 MRI of an arterio-venous malformation of the right thigh.

- Angiography is required to define a lesion to plan the best treatment, and is usually performed at the time of treatment in children so as to minimize radiation exposure. The study may be by selective arteriography, percutaneous direct puncture arteriography or percutaneous direct puncture venography.

> ### *26.1 Workup of a baby with a birth mark*
> - Was it present at birth?
> - Has it grown in proportion to child or showed rapid growth then involution?
> - Does B-mode ultrasound show a soft tissue mass with no or slow flow indicating a malformation?
> - Does Doppler ultrasound show a low-resistance arterial waveform for an AVM, venous waveform for a VM or semi-compressible cyst with no wave form for an LM?
> - Does B-mode thickness of the wall or compression suggest a VM?
> - Does B-mode echogenicity of the cavity indicate a thrombosed or treated VM or treated LM?

Associated platelet and coagulation disorders

These are shown in Table 26.2.

Treatment

General principles

- It is best to manage a dormant malformation expectantly.[2,3] However, early aggressive treatment may be required for cosmetic

Table 26.2 Vascular tumours and malformations associated with platelet and coagulation disorders

Anomalies	Haematological disorders
Kaposiform haemangioendothelioma. Tufted angioma.	Kasabach–Merritt phenomenon – profound sustained thrombocytopoenia, profound hypofibrinogenaemia, consumptive coagulopathy, elevated D-dimer.
Rapidly involuting congenital haemangioma.	Transient mild to moderate thrombocytopenia, ± consumptive coagulopathy, elevated D-dimer.
Venous malformations. Lymphatic–venous malformations.	Chronic localized intravascular coagulopathy, elevated D-dimer, ± hypofibrinogenaemia, ± moderate thrombocytopoenia.
Multifocal lymphangioendotheliomatosis with thrombocytopenia. Cutaneovisceral angiomatosis with thrombocytopoenia.	Sustained fluctuating moderate to profound thrombocytopenia, gastrointestinal tract bleeding or pulmonary haemorrhage.
Kaposiform lymphangiomatosis	Mild to moderate thrombocytopoenia, ± hypofibrinogenaemia, D-dimer elevation.

reasons or to prevent limb- or life-threatening complications. It is essential to ensure that the benefits from intervention exceed morbidity from treatment, since ill-planned interventions can make subsequent treatments more difficult. VMs are treated less aggressively than AVMs. Children usually wait until they are more than two years old. The drug sirolimus is now being used to treat LM and VM in many centres. A multidisciplinary team of dermatologists, paediatricians, radiologists, plastic surgeons and vascular surgeons, is necessary for complicated malformations.

- Indications for intervention include:
  - Cosmetically severe deformity.
  - Severe functional impairment.
  - Lesions located at a life-threatening region, such as adjacent to the airway,
  - Lesions at a region threatening vital functions, such as vision
  - Lesions in a region with potentially high risk of complications, such as haemarthrosis.
  - Disabling pain.
  - Haemorrhage or lymph leakage.
  - Secondary arterial ischaemia.
  - Secondary complications from chronic venous hypertension.
  - Infection, thrombosis, bone destruction or growth changes.
  - High-output heart failure.
- Treatment may involve a combination of compression, embolization, sclerotherapy and surgical resection, and requires a multidisciplinary team. If intervention is required, then it should be deferred if possible until a child is older enough to minimize anaesthetic risk and to allow easier surgical dissection of complex lesions. Non-vascular surgery for associated deformity should be deferred until the primary lesion is controlled.
- Long-term follow-up after ablation of these malformations is essential given the high risk of recurrence. Clinical and ultrasound surveillance are recommended, for example at six weeks and six months then at yearly intervals.

- Making the wrong diagnosis can lead to giving the wrong treatment, such as unnecessary sclerotherapy for a haemagioma instead of watching and waiting, or giving unnecessary propranolol for a VM.

Embolisation

- Embolisation can be performed with particles, coils or liquid adhesive materials via a venous or arterial approach or by direct injection. Contour particles such as Ivalon® tend not to be useful for treating malformations. Coils occlude larger vessels but are unable to penetrate into the nidus and can actually stimulate growth, and are best used placed in outflow veins to reduce vascularity prior to other treatment. Liquid agents are best able to penetrate into the nidus. N-butyl cyanoacrylate in oil produces immediate mechanical obstruction and a subsequent inflammatory response causing long-term occlusion, although this may not be sufficient to cure the lesion and is frequently no more than palliative. Onyx® is a less adhesive agent which is a copolymer of ethylene and vinyl alcohol dissolved in dimethyl sulphoxide. It is extremely effective in reaching into small vessels in the nidus, allowing better control, but again it is not necessarily curative, although in combination with other treatments causes lesion shrinkage and hardening to permit surgical excision.

Sclerotherapy

- Various sclerosants have been used and multiple sessions are often required. Absolute ethanol is the most potent sclerosant but carries a risk of adjacent nerve and skin damage and can precipitate pulmonary hypertension, either due to pulmonary artery spasm or extensive micro-thromboembolism, with a danger of cardiac arrest. Treatment requires monitoring and the maximum safe volume of ethanol is less than 1 mL/Kg. Radio-opaque ethylcellulose–ethanol gel is a newly developed sclerosant with a higher viscosity. Ethylcellulose traps ethanol to form a framework in the malformation which allows prolonged contact between ethanol and the vascular endothelium, reducing the quantity of absolute ethanol needed. Ethylcellulose spontaneously dissolves within about three months unless an excessive amount is used. Sodium tetradecyl sulphate or polidocanol either as liquid or foamed are less effective than ethanol but have few side effects (see Chapter 5). OK-432 (Picibanil) is an exotoxin derived from a low-virulence strain of *Streptococcus pyogenes*, and is a selective lymphatic sclerosant that can be easily and safely injected into macrocystic LM.

Surgical excision

- Surgical resection is simple in principle, although it may need to be radical, but surgical reconstruction is usually complex, depending on the site of operation. Excision should include all involved tissues, the extent based on preoperative imaging, normal bleeding patterns at the margins and frozen sections of the resection margin. Anatomical technique depends on the site of the lesion and is particularly important for surgery on the face and hands. Emergency surgery may be limited to decompression to relieve acute symptoms until a later more definitive treatment can be planned. Extensive excision may necessitate skin grafting or tissue transfer for adequate wound closure. Massive lesions causing intolerable complications occasionally necessitate major amputations. Intra-lesional laser ablation is increasingly being used to destroy the nidus.

Capillary malformations

- These are usually treated for cosmetic reasons. The initial approach is with laser photocoagulation. Most small fibrovascular lesions can easily be excised. More extensive CM would require excision with full- or split-thickness skin grafts. Facial lesions might also require facio-maxillary reconstruction.
- Capillary malformations confined to the upper dermal plexus respond well to 595 nm PDL. In adult CM with thickening and widening of vessels, more deeply penetrating

lasers and light treatments are required, such as long pulsed 1064 nm lasers, Alexandrite laser or certain IPL systems.

Venous malformations

- Initial treatment of VMs may be with elastic compression to reduce swelling and pain. A period of anticoagulation with low molecular weight heparin is warranted to attempt to control pain if thrombosis occurs, and to anticipate the risk of thrombosis during diagnostic or therapeutic intervention.
- Sclerotherapy under general anaesthesia with ultrasound guidance is the primary treatment for refractory lesions. Ethanol should be used sparingly for treating low-flow VMs due to the risk of complications, and foam sclerotherapy with detergents using sodium tetradecyl sulphate or polidocanol is now favoured (see Chapter 5).
- Superficial lesions with obvious blue raised lumps do well with long-pulsed 1064 nm lasers, which may be preferred to sclerotherapy in this setting.
- Surgery may be offered, or a planned combination of surgery and sclerotherapy. Sclerotherapy performed prior to surgery can make dissection more difficult and increase the risk of nerve injury, so, involvement of the surgeon from the beginning is important if there is a plan for combined treatment.

Lymphatic malformations

- Treatment is directed towards preventing infection and bleeding, correcting cosmetic deformity and improving function. Macrocystic lesions can be effectively treated with sclerotherapy. Carbon dioxide, argon, and yttrium–aluminum–garnet (YAG) laser therapy can also be used to treat mucosal lesions. Surgical resection is the principal treatment and staged operations may be used for complex lesions.
- Compared to other malformations, LM are usually not life- or limb-threatening and treatment should be limited to relatively safe methods such as OK-432 or doxycycline, even though they have a higher risk of lesion

recurrence. More aggressive treatment with sclerotherapy and surgical excision are reserved for lesions located near vital organs and those causing complications such as lymph leakage, bleeding, recurrent infections, severe deformities or functional disability. Other malformations take priority for treating combined lesions. If extratruncular and truncular LM occur together, the extratruncular lesion should be treated first. In particular, primary lymphoedema is treated by conservative measures.

- The sclerosant Picibanil (OK432) is a specific agent used to fibrose macrocystic LM. However, this is ineffective for a combined LM and VM lesion where more powerful sclerotherapy with ethanol is required. Sclerotherapy is usually best avoided for microcystic LM as treatment is less effective and complications more likely. Multiple sessions may be required, and treatment thickens the lesions making subsequent surgical excision easier even if they recur. Surgical excision is effective as long as there is a defined aesthetic or functional aim. Complete excision of an LM is rarely possible, but good long term improvements in appearance and function can be achieved.
- Most LM have both macrocystic and microcystic components or are combined with VM, and this limits the use of sclerotherapy. This means that most are best treated by surgical excision, if necessary, with or without preoperative OK-432 to thicken the lesion to make it easier to excise. Incomplete excision sparing vital anatomic structures may be an acceptable alternative to radical resection to avoid morbidity.

Arteriovenous malformations

- Patients should be advised to avoid factors that might trigger progression, particularly at times of puberty, menarche, pregnancy or surgery. This includes not using oral contraception and avoiding unnecessary surgery. It is necessary to direct treatment to aggressive control of the nidus either by occlusion or excision. It is vital to avoid improper treatment strategies which are likely to compromise future treatment options, such as incomplete resection or ligation or proximal embolization of feeding arteries. Recurrence is likely even after appropriate treatment as it is very difficult to remove all cells in the nidus, so that long-term surveillance is required.

- Quiescent AVM should be managed expectantly, if possible. However, development of complications suggests that intervention might have been appropriate at an earlier time. Medical treatment plays little part in management, except for measures such as compression to improve swelling and relieve discomfort as palliation if comorbidity means that the risk of intervention is too high.
- If intervention is required, embolization is considered as the initial treatment, either for definitive control or by aiming to convert high to lower flow. Preliminary embolization to reduce vascularity increases likely success from subsequent sclerotherapy or reduces bleeding with subsequent surgical resection. These treatment measures may be sequential or combined.
- Sclerotherapy with ethanol is still the most effective treatment, but requires careful monitoring in an experienced environment because of the considerable risk of local and systemic complications.
- The angiographic appearance helps to predict the outcome of endovascular treatment. The rate for complete occlusion or obliteration is highest for Types I and II and lowest for Type III. Generally, Types I and II are best treated by a trans-arterial or trans-venous approach, whereas Type III should be treated by the arterial route or by direct puncture of the nidus.
- Deep intracranial and complex craniofacial AVMs present a unique challenge, since surgical excision may be impossible. Embolization is the usual treatment. Radiotherapy has also been claimed to be successful, but compromises any other treatment method and should only be considered when other treatment options have been fully excluded.

Klippel–Trenaunay syndrome and other combined malformations

- Surgery for varicose disease with the Klippel–Trenaunay syndrome is notoriously difficult, so that many rarely recommend surgery for cosmetic reasons alone and reserve intervention for patients who develop complications from venous hypertension.[12] The veins are large, and perioperative bleeding can be a problem, though usually controlled by appropriate use of tourniquets. It is essential to confirm that the deep venous system is adequate to cope with loss of superficial veins. Recurrence rates are far higher than for usual venous surgery and patients must be warned of this in advance. Endovenous thermal ablation or foam sclerotherapy can be used.
- Surgery may be required to correct limb overgrowth and orthopaedic deformity to improve appearance and function, but only after vascular disease has been corrected as best as possible.
- Anticoagulation in KTS and extensive VMs has an analgesic effect and protect from the significant risk of pulmonary embolism.

History

- Birthmarks were believed to be secondary to the mother's past experiences and were called the 'mother's mark', a belief that persists in many cultures around the world. The colloquial term for a birthmark is a 'wish' in Italian, Spanish and Arabic, referring to unsatisfied wishes of the mother during pregnancy, or 'mother spots' in Dutch, German and Danish.
- In Iranian folklore, a birthmark appears when the pregnant mother touches a part of her body during a solar eclipse. A birthmark is considered a 'kiss of St Mary the virgin' in Ethiopian Orthodox Christianity folklore.
- Other beliefs hold that a birthmark is an omen that determines a person's traits or future depending on its site and shape, or that it results from an event in a person's past life.

References

1. Wassef M, Blei F, Adams D, Alomari A, Baselga E, Berenstein A, Burrows P et al. Vascular anomalies classification: Recommendations from the International Society for the Study of Vascular Anomalies. *Pediatrics* 2015;136:203–14. http://pediatrics.aappublications.org/content/pediatrics/early/2015/06/03/peds.2014-3673.full.pdf

2. Lee BB, Baumgartner I, Berlien P, Bianchini G, Burrows P, Gloviczki P, Huang Y et al. Diagnosis and treatment of venous malformations. Consensus document of the International Union of Phlebology. *Int Angiol* 2015;34:97–149. https://www.ncbi.nlm.nih.gov/pubmed/24566499

3. Lee BB, Baumgartner I, Berlien HP, Bianchini G, Burrows P, Do YS, Ivancev K et al. Consensus document of the International Union of Angiology (IUA)-2013. Current concept on the management of arterio-venous malformations. *Int Angiol* 2013;32(1):9–36. http://www.angiologie.insel.ch/fileadmin/angiologie/angiologie_user/Pdf/Guidelines_IUA.pdf

4. Lee BB, Antignani PL, Baraldini V, Baumgartner I, Berlien P, Blei F, Carrafiello GP et al. ISVI-IUA consensus document diagnostic guidelines of vascular anomalies: Vascular malformations and hemangiomas. *Int Angiol* 2015;34:333–74. https://www.ncbi.nlm.nih.gov/pubmed/25284469

5. Ma EH, Robertson SJ, Chow CW, Bekhor PS. Infantile hemangioma with minimal or arrested growth: Further observations on clinical and histopathologic findings of this unique but underrecognized entity. *Pediat Dermatol* 2017;34:64–71. https://www.ncbi.nlm.nih.gov/pubmed/?term=Ma+EH%2C+Robertson+SJ%2C+Chow+CW%2C+Bekhor+PS.+Infantile+hemangioma+with+minimal+or+arrested+growth%3A+further+observations+on+clinical+and+histopathologic+findings+of+this+unique+but+underrecognized+entity

6. DermNet New Zealand. http://www.dermnetnz.org/topics/

7. Boscolo E, Bischoff J. Vasculogenesis in infantile hemangioma. *Angiogenesis* 2009;12:197–207. https://www.ncbi.nlm.nih.gov/pubmed/19430954

8. Harbi S, Wang R, Gregory M, Hanson N, Kobylarz K, Ryan K, Deng Y, Lopez P, Chiriboga L, Mignatti P. Infantile hemangioma originates from a dysregulated but not fully transformed multipotent stem cell. *Sci Rep* 2016;6:Article 35811. http://www.nature.com/articles/srep35811

9. Kleinman ME, Greives MR, Churgin SS, Blechman KM, Chang EJ, Ceradini DJ, Tepper OM, Gurtner GC. Hypoxia-induced mediators of stem/progenitor cell

trafficking are increased in children with hemangioma. *Arterioscler Thromb Vasc Biol* 2007;27;2664–70. https://www.ncbi.nlm.nih.gov/pubmed/?term=Mark+E.+Kleinman%2C+Matthew+R.+Greives%2C+Samara+S.+Churgin%2C+Keith+M.+Blechman%2C+Eric+I.+Chang%2C+Daniel+J.+Ceradini%2C+Oren+M.+Tepper%2C+Geoffrey+C.+Gurtner

10. Boon LM, Ballieux F, Vikkula M. Pathogenesis of vascular anomalies. *Clin Plastic Surg* 2011;38:7–19. https://www.ncbi.nlm.nih.gov/pmc/articles/PMC3031181/

11. Myers KA, Clough A. *Practical Vascular Ultrasound. An Illustrated Guide.* 2014. Boca Raton, FL:CRC Press. https://www.crcpress.com/Practical-Vascular-Ultrasound-An-Illustrated-Guide/Myers-Clough/p/book/9781444181180

12. Noel AA, Gloviczki P, Cherry KJ Jr, Rooke TW, Stanson AW, Driscoll DJ. Surgical treatment of venous malformations in Klippel-Trénaunay syndrome. *J Vasc Surg* 2000;32:840–7. https://www.ncbi.nlm.nih.gov/pubmed/11054214

Techniques can be used to assess how well a diagnosis is made and how effective treatment has been.

Methods to evaluate outcome

- Studies to determine how effective management has been involve selecting methods to measure diagnostic accuracy and technical and clinical success from treatment, and then using them to analyse outcomes by case reports, observational studies or clinical trials.[2]
- Outcomes measured can be assessed by the physician or by the patient. Evaluation is frequently subjective which makes it difficult to standardize the methods.
- Physician evaluation of outcome:
  - Ultrasound surveillance for technical success
  - Haemodynamic studies
  - Venous severity scores
- Patient evaluation of outcome:
  - Quality of life
  - Analogue pain chart

This chapter incorporates recommendations from the European Society for Vascular Surgery.[1]

- Side-effects
- Return to work and other activities

Ultrasound surveillance

- The vein diameter and length treated can be measured and used as covariates for multivariate analysis of outcome.[3]
- Surveillance is performed before and at intervals after treatment, usually until the treated vein disappears and then at less frequent intervals to detect new disease in other veins. Common intervals planned are at six weeks, six months, one year, two years then two- to three-yearly.
- Early post-operative scans look for deep vein thrombosis or sclerosis (see Chapter 13), but routine scanning for this reason alone is not cost-effective. Each post-treatment ultrasound scan notes whether the vein is occluded, absent or patent, and whether there is reflux in any patent segments. Defining success or failure is difficult with no universal consensus. Success is defined as absence or continuing occlusion with no flow and no visible reflux in the treated vein. Failure is defined as patency in a segment of treated vein, some would contend over an arbitrary 5 cm length, or reflux from the top end into a major tributary. If the vein is occluded above or below then it may not be possible to elicit reflux by a calf squeeze or Valsalva manoeuvre.

Venous severity score (VSS)

- The Clinical, Etiology, Anatomy, Pathology (CEAP) classification does not estimate the severity of disease and is not designed to measure changes in patients' condition.[1,4] VSS was designed to supplement CEAP for follow-up after treatment by grading the variables used in CEAP. It is based on physician assessment of patient responses to subjective questions, and each limb is scored separately.
- Telangiectases and reticular veins are not included and remain without a score except for corona phlebectatica. Focal pigmentation confined to the skin over a varicose vein is not considered to signify the same severity as more diffuse pigmentation and is given a score of 0. Skin colour changes occurring at the site of a previous venous procedure such as endovenous ablation, phlebectomy or sclerotherapy are not included in assessment of skin pigmentation.
- Treatment by compression is a measure of compliance with conservative measures and leads to diminished symptoms or signs and a lower VCSS score. However, compression therapy has no effect on VCSS if its use does not change during treatment.
- VSS has three components.

Venous disability score

- An extension of CEAP to evaluate the level of ability to work with or without support.

Venous segmental disease score

- This is based on anatomical and pathophysiological components of CEAP.

Venous clinical severity score (VCSS)

- This is a dynamic form of CEAP evaluation designed to include hallmarks of the most severe complications, and is the most clinically relevant and widely used method. VCSS has a three-point per item scoring system for ten common stigmata of chronic venous disease and the use of compression stockings to produce a 30-point score (Table 27.1).

Table 27.1 VCSS scores

Attribute	Absent (0)	Mild (1)	Moderate (2)	Severe (3)
Pain or other discomfort	None	Occasional	Daily, interfering with but not preventing regular daily activities	Daily, limiting most regular daily activities
Varicose veins	None	Few, scattered Includes corona phlebectatica	Confined to calf or thigh	Involve calf and thigh
Venous oedema	None	Limited to foot or ankle	Extends above ankle but below knee	Extends to knee or above
Skin pigmentation	None or focal	Limited to perimalleolar area	Diffuse over the lower third of calf	Wider distribution above lower third of calf
Inflammation	None	Limited to perimalleolar area	Diffuse over the lower third of calf	Wider distribution above lower third of calf
Induration	None	Limited to perimalleolar area	Involving lower third of calf	Involving more than lower third of calf
Number of active ulcers	None	One	Two	>2
Active ulcer duration	None	<3 months	>3 months but <1 year	>1 year
Active ulcers size	None	Diameter <2 cm	Diameter 2–6 cm	Diameter >6 cm
Compression therapy	Not used	Intermittent use of stockings	Uses stockings most days	Full compliance with stockings

Villalta–Prandoni scale

- The Villalta–Prandoni scale is specific to the post-thrombotic syndrome and consists of five patient-rated symptoms and six clinician-rated physical signs, with each of the 11 factors scored as mild (1), moderate (2) or severe (3) to give a total possible score of 33.[1] (Table 27.2). A drawback to be noted, is that it does not take into account venous claudication or venous ulcer severity.
- The post-thrombotic syndrome is rated as:
  - Severe – score >14 or the presence of venous ulceration
  - Moderate – score 10–14
  - Mild – score 5–9
  - Absent – score <5.

Table 27.2 Villalta–Prandoni scale

Symptoms	Signs
Pain	Oedema
Cramping	Induration
Heaviness	Hyperpigmentation
Pruritus	Venous ectasia
Paraesthesia	Redness
	Calf tenderness

Quality of life

- Quality of life (QOL) scores provide information regarding the patient-perceived burden of illness.[1,4] Generic assessments include Short Form 36 (SF-36), Short Form 12 (SF-12]) and EuroQol 5 Dimension (EQ-5D). Disease-specific assessments are more popular, and include the Aberdeen Varicose Veins Questionnaire (AVVQ), Specific Quality Of life Response – Venous (SQOR-V), Chronic Venous Disease Questionnaire 2 (CIVIQ-2), the VEnous INsufficiency Epidemiologic and Economic Study (VEINES) and the Charing Cross Venous Ulcer Questionnaire.
- Disease-specific CIVIQ2 poses questions for physical, psychological, social and pain aspects of chronic venous disease. VEINES focuses more on symptoms rather than the psychological and social aspects. The Aberdeen Varicose Vein Questionnaire addresses physical symptoms, social issues and cosmetic manifestations. The CIVIQ-2 and Aberdeen Questionnaire are the two most widely used. As yet there is no validated QOL scoring for cosmetic outcomes alone.
- The items assessed for CIVIQ2 are in answer to 'In the past four weeks, to what extent did your leg problems interfere with/cause you to ...' (Table 27.3):

Table 27.3 CIVIQ2 questions

Physical Items	Psychological Items	Social Items	Pain Items
Climbing stairs	Feel on edge	Going out in the evening	Pain in the ankles or legs
Crouching/kneeling	Become tired easily	Practicing a sport	Interference with work or daily activities
Walking briskly	Feel like a burden to people	Travelling by car/bus/plane	Interference with sleeping
Doing housework	Need to take precautions		Interference with standing for a long time
	Be embarrassed to show one's legs		
	Be easily irritable		
	Feel handicapped		
	Have difficulty getting going in the morning		
	Not feeling like going out		

Cost-effectiveness

- New technologies should be shown to be at least as cost-effective as existing techniques. Outcome is measured by direct costs of materials and staff for the procedure, time lost from work or other activities for patients and their carers, and the likelihood of recurring costs for repeat treatment resulting from failure of the first procedure.
- The National Institute for Health and Clinical Excellence (NICE) studied cost-effectiveness for treatment strategies.[5] It observed that conservative care has traditionally been considered a low-cost intervention for symptomatic patients and has been routinely offered before interventional treatment, but that interventional treatment is more clinically effective and cost-effective than conservative care in the long-term.
- Endovenous techniques provide better comfort in the early post-treatment period and shorter delays in returning to work, and it is hoped that increased use of the procedures will drive down procedural costs in the future.
- Ultrasound-guided sclerotherapy is the least expensive option for initial treatment, but has a considerably higher chance of failure, requiring repeat treatment. Accordingly, studies show that endovenous thermal ablation is at least as cost-effective as ultrasound-guided sclerotherapy, as well as more traditional surgery.[6,7]

Observational studies

- There are several types of observational studies.
  - Cross-sectional studies report the prevalence of a disease in a population at any time.
  - Case–control studies assess the natural history of disease compared to normal subjects.
  - Cohort studies follow individuals for a time to see how disease evolves and how well it responds to treatment.
- It is better to collect prospective data rather than to perform a retrospective analysis.

- A cohort study to observe the outcome of patient management requires a computer database to list patient details and covariates that could influence outcome. Patients are observed over a defined period during which various outcomes develop, particularly success or failure. Data may simply be recorded as being present or absent, or it may be given a numeric value. All relevant information should be recorded without being overzealous to include irrelevant 'orphan data'. Selected patients are studied with clear definition of who is to be included and reasons for exclusion.
- Statistical techniques can then be used to test the hypothesis that treatment is effective, rather than the null hypothesis that there is no benefit, although an observational study cannot prove an association. Statistics are further used to measure how effective the treatment is. The larger the group studied, then the more robust the statistical analysis.
- Meta-analysis refers to statistical methods for contrasting and combining results from multiple studies to identify patterns of results and sources of disagreement about results or other relationships. A weighted average can help to achieve a higher statistical power.

Descriptive statistics

- Parametric data is a group of measured observations that has a homogeneous distribution about an average or mean. Non-parametric data has skewed data, best represented by its median value.
  - The variance measures how far a set of numbers are spread out from their mean.
  - The standard deviation is the square root of the variance and is more frequently used to define the degree of variation.
  - The standard error also represents this degree of variation adjusted for the number of observations.
  - The confidence interval measures the range of values; for example, a measure of all values that fall within 95% of the range either side of the mean.

The variance (V) is

$$V = \frac{[\Sigma(x_1 - x_n)^2]}{n - 1}$$

The standard deviation (SD) is $\sqrt{variance}$

$$= \sqrt{\frac{[\Sigma(x_1 - x_n)^2]}{n - 1}}$$

The standard error (SE) is

$$SE = \frac{SD}{\sqrt{n}}$$

The 95% confidence intervals (CI) shows the reliability that the estimation procedure lies within 95% of the range

$$95\%CI = (x_n - 1.96SE)\,to\,(x_n + 1.96SE)$$

Inferential statistics

- Different methods are then used to analyse data according to whether it is parametric or non-parametric and whether there are two or more groups studied. This may be to compare the groups to determine whether or not they are different, or to use regression analysis to determine whether or not they are related to each other. Calculations are made by statistical software packages, but the details are beyond the scope of this text and should be reviewed in standard texts. Appropriate techniques are listed in Table 27.4.

p-values and confidence intervals

- The null hypothesis is that there is no difference between two sets of data. The p-value is the probability that the null hypothesis is or is not correct. A *significant* p-value <0.05 simply means that there is considerable evidence that the null hypothesis is not correct, but that it is likely that such a difference will occur once in every 20 times by chance alone, in which case the null hypothesis is correct.
- Demonstrating a significant difference by measuring a p-value does not mean that the difference is clinically important. A way to show this is to compare confidence intervals for two groups, and this can be used for either parametric or nonparametric data. The null hypothesis cannot be rejected if the confidence levels overlap and may be rejected if they do not.

Errors

- A Type I error (α) is present if statistical testing shows a difference between groups when in reality no difference exists. A type II error (β) is present when a clinically important difference exists between groups but the difference is not shown to be statistically significant. Calculations can be made to determine the likelihood of either error.

Life table analysis

- Life table analysis should be used to measure long-term follow-up for success or failure rates.[8] The duration is measured from the date of treatment to a date selected to finish the study.

Table 27.4 Statistical techniques

Parametric data	Method
Comparison	
Means of two groups	Student t-test
Confidence intervals two groups	Chi-square analysis
Means of three or more groups	Analysis of variance
Relationships	
Two groups	Linear regression analysis
Three or more groups	Analysis of covariance Multiple regression analysis
Non-parametric data	**Method**
Comparison	
Means of two groups	Wilcoxon rank sum test Mann–Whitney U-test
Means of three or more groups	Friedman's analysis Kruskal–Wallis analysis
Relationships	
Two groups	Non-linear regression Kendall's rank correlation Spearman's coefficient

Patients enter and leave a study on different dates but the duration for each procedure is adjusted to start at an entry-point which is the date of intervention and to continue to an end-point which is when the procedure fails, the patient has been followed to the finishing date or has been withdrawn or *censored* because of loss to follow-up or death. It is inevitable to have an increasing number of censored observations with each interval, but calculations assume that censored procedures would have continued to behave the same as those remaining in the study and that on average they would likely to have been withdrawn midway through the observation interval.

- This allows cumulative success or failure rates to be calculated, which more accurately represents outcome for all patients rather than the rates in the smaller numbers of patients remaining in the study at each interval.

Publications that quote interval rather than cumulative success rates should be ignored.

- An example is to use serial ultrasound scans to determine technical success following intervention for varicose disease. *Primary failure* is the development of a patent or refluxing segment after initial treatment. *Secondary failure* is subsequent failure to occlude the vein if further treatment is unsuccessful or if a decision is made not to proceed with further treatment.
- Either actuarial or product-limit (Kaplan–Meier) life table analysis is used to calculate success or failure rates. For example, the time to failure after treatment for varicose disease is the difference between the date of treatment and date that recurrent patency or reflux is demonstrated at follow-up ultrasound. All patients present for the first post-procedure scan a few days after treatment and if failure is noted at this scan, then this is used as the failure date for analysis even though it is probable that the procedure had failed from the time it was performed. If a patient noted to have recurrent saphenous reflux had missed a previous scheduled visit, then failure should be dated back to the time of that missed visit.

- Actuarial life-table analysis calculates the change in cumulative success rates for each selected interval. If N is the number entering each interval, w is the number of censored observations in the interval and r is the number that risk failure during the interval, then assuming that censored observations are withdrawn halfway through the interval

$$r = N - \frac{w}{2}$$

If f is the number that failed during the interval, q is the proportion that fail and p is the proportion that remain successful through the interval, then

$$q = \frac{f}{r} = \frac{f}{N - \frac{w}{2}} \quad \text{and} \quad p = (1 - q)$$

The cumulative success rate (P) is obtained by successively multiplying the values for p calculated for each interval.

- The standard error for each interval is

$$SE = P\sqrt{[(1 - P)/N]}$$

and it is generally considered that the size of the sample becomes too small for confident analysis beyond the interval when the SE exceeds 10%.
- The product-limit or Kaplan–Meier technique calculates a change in the graph for each event but provides the same cumulative success rates as the actuarial technique

$$q = [1 - (n - r)(n - r + 1)] \cdot X$$

where $X = 1$ if the event is a failure and $X = 0$ if the event is a censored observation.
- The significance of difference between two life table curves is calculated by the log-rank test, which is based on a progressive chi-square test for each interval.
- Multivariate Cox regression proportional hazard analysis is used to correlate success or failure with various covariates considered independently. For venous disease, these relate to the patients, limbs and treated veins, and may include age, sex, side, clinical

CEAP category, treating doctor, vein treated, primary disease without previous treatment or recurrence after previous treatment, time to the date of procedure from the date for commencement of each doctor's experience, length of vein treated, representative diameter of the vein and treatment technique.

Observer agreement

- The ability of an observer to reproduce results on different occasions represents the intra-observer agreement or variability, and the ability of two observers to agree is the inter-observer agreement or variability. These can be measured using the Bland–Altman technique.
- If a and b represent each pair of observations to be compared and n is the number of observations then
  - the mean for each pair is $X = (a + b)/2$
  - the difference between a pair of observations is $Y = (a - b)$
  - the mean for the difference for all observations is $Z = \Sigma(a + b)/n$
  - the coefficient of variability (2SD) is $2\Sigma[(a - b)^2/(n - 1)]$
- Intra- and inter-observer variability is assessed by plotting the means X against the differences Y. The baseline Z ideally should be zero, but there is usually a systematic difference which sets a baseline that is slightly more or less than zero. An example of the resultant Bland–Altman figure for observer variability with the mean and limits from the coefficient of variability is shown in Figure 27.1.

Contingency tables

- Two-by-two contingency tables are used to compare a new unknown test with an established standard of reference commonly, referred to as the 'gold standard', to determine how well they agree (Figure 27.2). A decision threshold for the new test is selected to indicate whether disease is present or absent. However, there is always an overlap in values for the new test compared to the standard of reference. The new test will apparently show many true positive (TP) and true negative

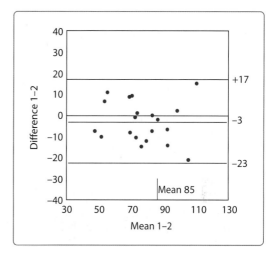

Figure 27.1 Variability for measurements of reflux time (ms) for all observations from venous ultrasound scans performed by two different sonographers. There was a mean difference of −3 ms and limits for agreement for all measurements of −23 to + 17 ms.

(TN) results as well as a few false positives (FP) or 'false alarms' and false negatives (FN) or 'misses'.

		Gold standard	
		Positive	Negative
New test	Positive	TP	FP
	Negative	FN	TN

- The accuracy of a new test is the proportion of all correct results to all tests performed. The sensitivity is the likelihood that a test result will be positive if the subject actually has the disease, and the specificity is the likelihood that a test result will be negative when the subject is truly free from disease. A positive predictive value is the likelihood that a subject with a positive test actually has the disease, and the negative predictive value is the likelihood that a subject with a negative test does not have the disease. The formulae can be used to determine the approximate numbers of observations required for a chosen level of precision, and to compare different techniques. Calculations are shown in Table 27.5.

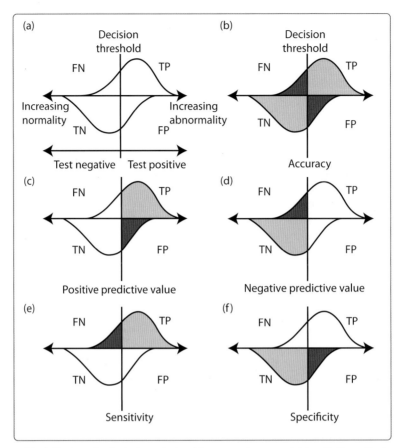

Figure 27.2 A graphical display of calculations derived from contingency tables. Ratios refer to cross-hatching/ entire hatching. There is an overlap between values so that there are true positive (TP) and true negative (TN) as well as false positive (FP) and false negative (FN) tests. The figures depict (a) the overlap between results in patients with disease and no disease, and calculations of (b) accuracy, (c) positive predictive value, (d) negative predictive value, (e) sensitivity and (f) specificity.

Table 27.5 Contingency table calculations

Prevalence	(TP + FN)/(TP + TN + FP + FN)
Accuracy	(TP + TN)/(TP + TN + FP + FN)
Sensitivity	(TP)/(TP + FN)
Specificity	(TN)/((TN + FP)
Positive predictive value	(TP)/(TP + FP)
Negative predictive value	(TN)/(TN + FN)
Likelihood of a positive test	Sensitivity/(1-Specificity)
Likelihood of a negative test	(1-Sensitivity)/Specificity
Odds ratio	(TP×TN)/(FP×FN)
Hazard ratio	TP(TP + FP)/FN(TN + FN)

- For example, 150 patients had both a new diagnostic test and the gold standard diagnostic test, 70 of the new and gold standard were positive, 55 had negative results on both tests, 10 had negative results on the new test but were positive on the gold standard and 15 had positive results on the new test but were negative on the gold standard. The table below is

		Gold standard	
		Positive	**Negative**
New test	Positive	70	15
	Negative	10	55

Accuracy = 125/150 = 83%
Sensitivity = 70/80 = 88%
Specificity = 55/70 = 79%
Positive predictive value = 70/85 = 82%
Negative predictive value = 55/65 = 85%

Receiver operating characteristics (ROC) curves

- It is best to settle on one value for the threshold chosen to calculate sensitivity and specificity. This can be arbitrary or can be calculated using ROC curves. A range of threshold values is chosen and sensitivity and specificity are calculated for each value then plotted against each other (Figure 27.3). The point chosen on the curve to allow decisions to be made is the *operating position*.
- The best compromise for the operating position may be the point on the turn of the curve where the sum of sensitivity and specificity is greatest. The upper right section corresponds to the high sensitivity and low specificity range that indicates a lenient threshold for diagnosis, and the lower left section corresponds to the low sensitivity and high specificity range for a strict threshold.
- Calculations are independent of prevalence, but it is as well to move towards the strict left

part of the curve if prevalence is low so as to not risk over-diagnosing disease, and to move the right section if prevalence is high so as not to miss too many opportunities to make the diagnosis. The larger the area under the curve, the better the investigation, and if the results produce no more than a diagonal straight line, then the investigation is useless.

The Kappa statistic

- The kappa statistic (κ) is used to measure true agreement between two observers after adjustment for chance. Confidence in their ability is high if they usually agree but on the other hand they would agree about half the time if they simply guessed the outcome. Indeed, they would agree most of the time if they both decided it was easiest to guess that the finding was normal if disease prevalence is low or abnormal if disease prevalence is high. The findings are shown in a table for a positive or negative result (yes or no) for each observer for N findings:

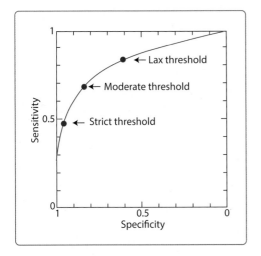

		Observer 1	
		Yes	No
Observer 2	Yes	a	b
	No	c	d

The observed proportion of agreement (P_o) is

$$P_o = \frac{a+d}{N}$$

The proportion of agreement expected by chance (P_c) is

$$P_c = \frac{\left[\dfrac{(a+b)(a+c)}{N} + \dfrac{(c+d)(b+d)}{N}\right]}{N}$$

The likelihood of agreement after adjustment for chance is

$$\kappa = \frac{P_o - P_c}{1 - P_c}$$

Figure 27.3 Receiver operating characteristics (ROC) curves showing their use to (a) select operating points and (b) compare tests.

- The maximum value for κ is $+1$ for perfect agreement, the minimum value is -1 for perfect disagreement, and a value of approximately 0 means that there is no agreement other than expected by chance. It is agreed that $\kappa < 0.4$ represents poor agreement and $\kappa > 0.75$ represents excellent agreement.
- For example, two phlebologists wish to determine how astute they are at detecting saphenous reflux from clinical examination. They record whether reflux is present or absent in a number of patients:

		Phlebologist 1			
		Present	Absent	Sum	Sum/n(P)
Phlebologist 2	Present	19(a)	6(b)	25	0.57(P1)
	Absent	3(c)	16(d)	19	0.43(P3)
	Sum	22	22	44	1
	Sum/n	0.50(P2)	0.50(P4)		

$$P_o = \frac{19 + 16}{44} = 0.795$$

$$P_c = (0.57 \times 0.50) + (0.43 \times 0.50)$$
$$= 0.285 + 0.215 = 0.5$$

$$\kappa = \frac{0.795 - 0.5}{1 - 0.5} = 0.59$$

indicating that agreement is quite good.

Randomized clinical trials

Design

- A clinical trial involves measuring outcome after allocating a particular treatment compared to another more standard treatment or placebo. Subjects are allocated to each arm in a way that allows the trial to be *randomized*. Ideally, they should not know which study treatment they receive so as to be *blinded*, although this is difficult

for many forms of intervention for venous disease. Ideally, treatment is performed by trial members unaware of the results and measurement are made by observers unaware of the chosen treatment, so that the trial is *double-blinded*. A randomized trial can provide statistical evidence that a new technique for treatment is more effective or no more or less effective than past established treatment or no treatment. All patients allocated to either arm should be included in the final analysis, even if they do not complete treatment on the basis of *intention to treat*.

- Usually, a trial design does not allow management to be modified after it begins or results to be examined until the study is complete. However, it may be elected in advance to allow changes to be made based on data accumulated during the trial, and this requires provision for the trial to be *broken* from being *blinded*. This can be taken a step further with provision to modify management and patient selection progressively as results become available to speed up the outcome referred to as an *adaptive trial*.
- There are phases for trials of a drug prior to it being approved by a regulatory authority for use in the general population after animal studies have been completed. Phase 0 involves giving the drug to a small number of volunteers to record the interactions between drug and patient. Phase 1 involves screening a small group to determine safety, safe dosage ranges and side-effects.

Phase 2 establishes efficacy of the drug against a placebo. Phase 3 involves testing a large group for efficacy and safety. Phase 4 involves gaining further data after the drug is released.

Informed consent

- Patients are required to sign an *informed consent* which should detail the reason for the trial and its nature, its likely duration and requirements expected of the patient and potential risks and side-effects. The patient can elect to withdraw at any stage.

Ethics committee approval

- There is a need to obtain approval from an ethics committee that evaluates risks and benefits from a trial, although this does not guarantee its safety.

Conflict of interest

- Financial support from vested interests that could potentially lead to conflict of interest must be declared. Editors of major journals have strengthened restrictions to counter control over clinical trials exerted by sponsors, particularly the use of contracts that allow them to review studies prior to publication or even withhold publication.

Inclusion and exclusion criteria

- It is desirable to randomize all consecutive patients able to be treated by the selected technique to make the study representative. A poor recruitment rate can make it impossible to apply results to the general community. However, patients are excluded and not randomized if they do not fulfil entry criteria. If a trial is to continue for several years, it is usual to exclude patients who are old or who have severe general medical diseases that make it unlikely that they will survive for the required time.

- Other patients are withdrawn after being randomized if they do not continue to meet the requirements of the study. Some were never really eligible in the first place, others did not comply with the treatment regimes and a few may be withdrawn because their course and outcome were not adequately recorded.
- Exclusion criteria include those at high risk from the procedure such as endovascular intervention for varicose disease during pregnancy or lactation, or those at high risk of complications such as deep vein thrombosis.

Outcome measures

- Outcome measures are defined as being primary or secondary in importance, and include technical success, relief of symptoms and quality of life.

Power of the study

- The trial must contain a sufficient number of patients to provide adequate *power* with the least chance of error, though with appreciation of ever-increasing cost with larger numbers.
- A *type I error* is present if statistical testing shows a difference between groups when in reality no difference exists. The chance of a type I error is designated by 2α, which represents the cut-off point for two tails of the standard normal distribution. For $p = 0.05$ this means that $2\alpha = 0.05$ with a 5% chance of a type I error. A *type II error* is present when a clinically important difference exists between groups but the difference is not large enough to be statistically significant. The chance of a type II error is designated by β which represents the cut-off point for the lower tail of the standard normal distribution, and the power of a study is $1-\beta$. Accessible values for 2α and β should be defined for any study from tables for standard normal curves. From this, the number of observations required can be calculated.

Level of proof

- The criteria used by a European consensus group is as follows:[1]

Levels of evidence

A	Data derived from multiple randomized clinical trials or meta-analyses.
B	Data derived from a single randomized clinical trial or large non-randomized studies.
C	Consensus of opinions of experts and/or small studies, retrospective studies or registries.

Classes of recommendation

I	Evidence and/or general agreement that a given treatment or procedure is beneficial, useful, effective.
II	Conflicting evidence and/or a divergence of opinion about the usefulness/efficacy of the given treatment or procedure.
IIa	Weight of evidence/opinion is in favour of usefulness/efficacy.
IIb	Usefulness/efficacy is less well established from evidence/opinion.
III	Evidence or general agreement that the given treatment or procedure is not useful/effective and in some cases can be harmful.

References

1. Wittens C, Davies AH, Bækgaard N, Broholm R, Cavezzi A, Chastanet S, de Wolf M et al. Management of chronic venous disease. Clinical practice guidelines of the European Society for Vascular Surgery. *Eur J Vasc Endovasc Surg* 2015;49:678–737. https://www.research-gate.net/publication/280483468_Editor's_Choice_-_Management_of_Chronic_Venous_Disease_Clinical_Practice_Guidelines_of_the_European_Society_for_Vascular_Surgery_ESVS

2. Krousel-Wood MA, Chambers RB, Muntner P. Clinicians' guide to statistics for medical practice and research. *Ochsner J Part 1* 2006;6:68–83. Part 2. 2007;7:3–7. http://www.ncbi.nlm.nih.gov/pmc/articles/PMC3121570/; http://www.ncbi.nlm.nih.gov/pmc/articles/PMC3096336/

3. Myers KA, Clough A. *Practical Vascular Ultrasound. An Illustrated Guide.* 2014. Boca Raton, FL: CRC Press. https://www.crcpress.com/Practical-Vascular-Ultrasound-An-Illustrated-Guide/Myers-Clough/p/book/9781444181180

4. Vasquez MA, Munschauer CE. Venous Clinical Severity Score and quality-of-life assessment tools: Application to vein practice. *Phlebology* 2008;23:259–75. http://www.venousinstitute.com/app/webroot/img/File/PHLEB-08-018.PDF

5. Marsden GI, Perry M, Kelley K, Davies AH; Guideline Development Group. Diagnosis and management of varicose veins in the legs: Summary of NICE guidance. *BMJ* 2013;347: f4279. http://www.ncbi.nlm.nih.gov/pubmed/?term=Marsden+G%2C+Perry+M%2C+Kelley+K%2C+et+al.+Diagnosis+and+management

6. Brittenden J, Cotton SC, Elders A, Tassie E, Scotland G, Ramsay CR, Norrie J et al. Clinical effectiveness and cost-effectiveness of foam sclerotherapy, endovenous laser ablation and surgery for varicose veins: Results from the Comparison of LAser, Surgery and foam Sclerotherapy (CLASS) randomised controlled trial. *Hlth Technol Assess* 2015;19:27. http://www.ncbi.nlm.nih.gov/pubmed/25858333

7. Marsden G, Perry M, Bradbury A, Hickey N, Kelley K, Trender H, Wonderling D, Davies AH. A cost-effectiveness analysis of surgery, endothermal ablation, ultrasound-guided foam sclerotherapy and compression stockings for symptomatic varicose veins. *Eur J Vasc Endovasc Surg* 2015;50:794–801. http://www.ncbi.nlm.nih.gov/pubmed/26433594

8. Lee ET. *Statistical Methods for Survival Data Analysis.* 1980. Belmont: Lifetime Learning Publications. http://www.popline.org/node/459899

Index